DANGEROUS LIAISONS: A SOCIAL HISTORY OF VENEREAL DISEASE IN TWENTIETH-CENTURY SCOTLAND

THE WELLCOME INSTITUTE SERIES IN THE HISTORY OF MEDICINE

Forthcoming Titles

Lesion and Metaphor:
Chronic Pain in British, French and
German Medical Writings, 1800–1914
Andrew Hodgkiss

Malthus, Medicine, & Morality:
'Malthusianism' after 1798
Brian Dolan (ed.)

Academic enquiries regarding the series should be addressed
to the editors C. J. Lawrence, V. Nutton and Roy Porter at
the Wellcome Institute for the History of Medicine,
183 Euston Road, London NW1 2BE, UK

DANGEROUS LIAISONS:
A SOCIAL HISTORY OF
VENEREAL DISEASE IN TWENTIETH-
CENTURY SCOTLAND

Roger Davidson

Amsterdam – Atlanta, GA 2000

First published in 2000
by Editions Rodopi B. V., Amsterdam – Atlanta, GA 2000.

Roger Davidson © 2000

Design and Typesetting by Alex Mayor, the Wellcome Trust.
Printed and bound in The Netherlands by Editions Rodopi B. V.,
Amsterdam – Atlanta, GA 2000.

British Library Cataloguing in Publication Data
A catalogue record for this book is available from the British
Library
ISBN 90-420-0618-8 (Paper)
ISBN 90-420-0628-5 (Bound)

Dangerous Liaisons:
A Social History of Venereal Disease
in Twentieth-Century Scotland –
Amsterdam – Atlanta, GA:
Rodopi. – ill.
(Clio Medica 57 / ISSN 0045-7183;
The Wellcome Institute Series in the History of Medicine)

Front cover:
Poster issued by Scottish Health Education Unit, 1970.

© Editions Rodopi B. V., Amsterdam – Atlanta, GA 2000
Printed in The Netherlands

All titles in the Clio Medica series (from 1999 onwards) are available to
download from the CatchWord website: http://www.catchword.co.uk

For Mo

Contents

Abbreviations

AMSH	Association for Moral and Social Hygiene
ARI	Aberdeen Royal Infirmary
BJVD	*British Journal of Venereal Diseases*
BMA	British Medical Association
BMJ	*British Medical Journal*
BSHC	British Social Hygiene Council
CAMO	Chief Administrative Medical Officer
CANO	Chief Area Nursing Officer
CEHD	City of Edinburgh Health Department
CMA	Contemporary Medical Archives Centre
DCA	Dundee City Archives
DHS	Department of Health for Scotland
ECA	Edinburgh City Archives
EHSSD	Edinburgh Health and Social Services Department
EMJ	*Edinburgh Medical Journal*
EPHD	Edinburgh Public Health Department
EUL	Edinburgh University Library
EWCA	Edinburgh Women Citizens' Association
GCA	Glasgow City Archives
GGHBA	Greater Glasgow Health Board Archive
GMJ	*Glasgow Medical Journal*
HC	House of Commons
HEBS	Health Education Board for Scotland
HL	House of Lords
LHSA	Lothian Health Services Archives
MAC	Medical Advisory Committee
MOH	Medical Officer of Health
MSSVDSB	Medical Society for the Study of Venereal Diseases Scottish Branch
NAS	National Archives of Scotland
NCCVD	National Council for Combating Venereal Diseases

i

N-ERHB	North-Eastern Regional Hospital Board
NHSA	Northern Health Services Archives
NLS	National Library of Scotland
NSU	Non-Specific Urethritis
NUSEC	National Union of Societies for Equal Citizenship
NVA	National Vigilance Association
PHC	Public Health Committee
PP	*Parliamentary Papers*
PRO	Public Record Office
RCPLRD	Royal Commission on the Poor Laws and the Relief of Distress
RCVD	Royal Commission on Venereal Diseases
RIE	Royal Infirmary of Edinburgh
SAMO	Senior Administrative Medical Officer
SBH	Scottish Board of Health
SCBSHC	Scottish Committee, British Social Hygiene Council
SCHE	Scottish Council for Health Education
SED	Scottish Education Department
SHEG	Scottish Health Education Group
SHEU	Scottish Health Education Unit
SHHD	Scottish Home and Health Department
SHMO	Senior Hospital Medical Officer

List of Plates

Plate 2.1: Advert for Lock Hospital and Magdalene Asylum [*Handbook of Glasgow Charitable and Beneficent Institutions (1907)*]

Plate 3.1: Plan of Black Street VD Clinic in Glasgow [*Glasgow MOH Annual Report (1927)*]

Plate 3.2: Black Street VD Clinic in 1929 [courtesy of Greater Glasgow Health Board Archives]

Plate 3.3: Joseph Patterson, outside Ward 45, Royal Infirmary of Edinburgh, 1920s [courtesy of Lothian Health Services Archives]

Plate 3.4: Robert Lees operating in Ward 45, Royal Infirmary of Edinburgh, *c.*1935 [courtesy of Dr Lorna Lees]

Plate 3.5: The New Dermatology and Venereal Diseases Pavilion, Royal Infirmary of Edinburgh, 1936 [*Edinburgh Medical Journal* (1936)]

Plate 4.1: Interior of Black Street Clinic in 1929, showing irrigation cubicles [courtesy of Greater Glasgow Health Board Archives]

Plate 6.1: Local authority VD propaganda, 1922 [*Haddington Courier and East Lothian Advertiser*, 3 March 1922]

Plate 6.2: Transcript of cinema announcement, Dundee 1917 [courtesy of Dundee City Archives]

Plate 6.3: Three of the cinemotors used by the British Social Hygiene Council in rural areas in interwar Scotland [*Scotsman*, 2 April 1935]

Plate 6.4: British Social Hygiene Council Appeal, 1935 [*Scotsman*, 2 April 1935]

Acknowledgements

Many people have helped me in the preparation of this book. I greatly appreciate the financial support of the Wellcome Trust, whose research grants and a Research Leave Fellowship for the 1996–97 academic year were critical to the completion of the project. Funding from the University of Edinburgh's Social Sciences Travel and Research and Research Initiatives Committees is also gratefully acknowledged.

I have also received invaluable support from many archivists. In particular, I would wish to thank Stephen Connelly (Perth and Kinross District Archive), Ian Flett (Dundee City Archives and Record Centre), Emily Naish (BMA Archive), Alison Scott (Edinburgh City Archives), Alistair Tough (Greater Glasgow Health Board Archive) and Arnot Wilson (formerly Edinburgh City Archives). Two archivists, Fiona Watson (Northern Health Services Archives) and Alison Lindsay (National Archives of Scotland), have been a constant source of inspiration and new lines of enquiry, and have added enormously to the range and productivity of my research. I would like to thank the Keeper of the Records of Scotland and the Keeper of the Public Record Office for permission to quote from central government archives. I am also greatly indebted to the Scottish Office and to the Department of Health for permission to consult closed files relating to VD/STD policy-making. The help of their Departmental Record Officers, Ken Glasgow and Mike Marsh, in facilitating such access, has been especially valued.

I have benefited enormously from the shared expertise of many historians and social scientists. Margaret Bennett, Andrew Blaikie, Viviene Cree, Anne Crowther, Leah Leneman, Ian Levitt, Sandy McCall Smith, Linda Mahood, Rosalind Mitchison, Graeme Morton and Alison Nuttall have all provided much-needed enlightenment on the history of Scottish culture, law, medicine, social work and folklore. As a relative newcomer to the social history of medicine, I have especially appreciated the encouragement and advice of Virginia Berridge, Debbie Brunton, and Steve Sturdy. Helen Coyle, Gayle Davis, Susan Lemar, and Elaine Thomson have all generously shared with me their sources and ideas relating to the social history of VD, while as both social historians and departmental heads, Mike Anderson and Bob Morris have always ensured a very supportive and challenging intellectual environment at the University of Edinburgh.

I wish also to thank Ann McCrum who has laboured long and devotedly to provide me with bibliographical and prosopographical material for this study. The assistance of Janet Pearse in formatting the manuscript, of John Banasik in advising on quantitative techniques, and of Ian Goddard in producing the plates is equally appreciated.

In addition, I am indebted to many contact tracers and venereologists for allowing me to interview them on their past experiences in the field of VD/STD work, for commenting on earlier drafts of the book, or for their permission to consult private correspondence. In particular, I wish to thank Dr M. Taylor Brown, Dr A. J. Downie, Dr J. Finnie, Dr J. M. Harvey, Mrs M. MacLellan, Dr G. Masterton, Dr S. I. A. Mathieson, Dr R. S. Morton, and Dr C. B. S. Schofield. Thanks are also due to Dr Lorna Lees, Mrs L. J. Lees, and Dr Alastair Batchelor for permission to use photographs and other papers in their private possession. As well as correcting technical inaccuracies in my text, Dr Sandy McMillan contributed greatly to the quantitative aspects of the study by facilitating access to surviving VD registers at the Royal Infirmary of Edinburgh for the purposes of anonymous random sampling.

I should like to thank the editors of the Journal of the History of Sexuality, Medical History, the Social History of Medicine, and the Scottish Historical Review for permission to use material which previously appeared in article form.

Two colleagues have played a major role in sustaining my research and richly deserve a special mention. As both a medical historian and Lothian Health Services Archivist, Mike Barfoot has furnished me with a constant stream of ideas and archival material, along with constructive criticism of my work. Lesley Hall has been similarly selfless in sharing with me her expertise as a social historian of medicine and sexuality and in ensuring that I always had ready access to the rich variety of social hygiene and medical archives at the Wellcome Institute.

Above all, I have to thank my wife, Mo. Not only has she endured my intrusion of 'soft chancres' and 'syphilitic sores' into meal-time conversations, she has also, with her warmth, humour and affection, made the preparation of this book a genuine labour of love.

1

Introduction: The Context

The Historiography of VD

Society's response to venereal disease [VD][1] has been shown to be a central strand in that 'whole web of discourses' that has constructed and regulated sexuality in modern society. During the late nineteenth and early twentieth centuries, VD became in many countries a metaphor for physical and moral decay, for the forces of pollution and contamination that appeared to threaten the institutions of social order and racial progress. Alarm over the issue of VD therefore offered an opportunity to express concern about the moral direction of society and changing standards of conduct. Given the supposedly wilful nature of its diffusion and its threat to 'social hygiene', it also provided a powerful justification for the social construction and proscription of dangerous sexualities.

The significance of VD in shaping and reflecting perceptions of sexuality, and in defining the response of the State to patterns of sexual behaviour in the twentieth century has, in recent years, been the focus of extensive research.[2] In particular, feminist and Foucaultian concepts of social control, initially used to analyse the social politics of nineteenth-century prostitution,[3] have been redeployed to interpret both the formal and informal strategies of the central and local state in the twentieth century aimed at identifying and penalizing those women who deviated from appropriate norms of sexual behaviour. Within this framework of analysis, the medical and legal discourses surrounding VD have come to be seen as integral to the processes of moral regulation in modern society, and VD measures to be interpreted not primarily as health legislation, but as legislation concerned with social order and control in a sexually repressive society.

Moreover, an understandable preoccupation of feminist historians with the sexual discrimination underpinning VD measures has been supplemented by increased awareness of other interlocking dimensions of stigmatization and control, including class, generation, and race, and by increasing evidence of the social complexity of the cultural and institutional factors shaping VD

1

policy in different countries. Social historians now recognize that, within the process of moral regulation, 'women's interests were fractured by age, class, and race as well as gender' and that medical policy and provisions were shaped not only by the proscriptions of a patriarchal legal system.[4]

They were, it is argued, equally determined by class considerations and an ideology that sought to impose bourgeois concepts of social and sexual hygiene as a means of remoralizing the poor. In the final analysis, it was primarily working-class female sexuality that was scrutinized (or more accurately stereotyped) by public health and police authorities. Accordingly, the social response to VD has been increasingly located by social historians within a general framework of regulatory, reformative and medical procedures designed to counter the perceived moral dangers confronting the 'working girl' within a rapidly changing urban economy.[5] In addition, class values and assumptions are seen to cut across considerations of gender in defining strategies of negotiation and resistance adopted by women's movements in their efforts to modify VD provisions.

Such studies have also come to highlight the role of social hygiene panics and provisions in regulating the sexual behaviour of the young. In a range of countries, during and after both World Wars, and again during the 'permissive' sixties, public health debate surrounding VD was informed by acute concern at the apparent breakdown of familial and community controls upon the social and sexual behaviour of adolescents. VD has therefore been depicted as a metaphor for the threat posed to rational, responsible sexuality posed by shifts in the income and consumption patterns of youth and their addiction to new forms of disinhibited entertainment.

The social history of VD has also been advanced as a means of illustrating the links between medicine, sexuality and imperialism, and how European conceptions of medical and moral danger were transferred overseas.[6] Within this historiography, discourses surrounding the medical control of VD have emerged as central to the regulation of socio-sexual relations between races. Moreover, imperial constructions of sexuality and disease are seen to have fed back into the social politics of VD at home with concepts such as 'racial degeneration' and 'sexual atavism' conflating fears of native and female sexuality.[7] Conversely, within this literature, 'social hygiene' has also been located in certain countries as an important part of the rhetoric of emerging national or ethnic identity, with implications for 'moral' devolution from 'metropolitan' vice and 'old world degeneracy'.[8]

The development of VD and sexually transmitted disease [STD] policy and administration in twentieth-century Britain has attracted increasing attention from medical and social historians. Various strands of public health policy, along with their broader socio-medical implications, have been documented. Some studies have focused upon the emergence in interwar Britain of a State-funded, voluntary system of provisions for the diagnosis and treatment of VD, with public clinics and associated laboratory facilities.[9] Others have examined the lasting debate within government circles over the relative merits of moral education and medical prophylaxis as preventive strategies, charting the influence and interplay of contesting professional groups within the social hygiene movement, and highlighting the powerful moral agenda which has shaped institutional responses to VD at both central and local government levels.[10]

Further studies have focused upon the process by which VD has been deployed by legal and medical authorities to identify and proscribe dangerous (predominantly female) sexualities, perceived as a threat to racial health and national efficiency, and upon patterns of resistance from within feminist organizations.[11] Attention has also been paid to the 'association of war, vice and venery as associated disruptions of natural order', the significance of VD in defining the interface between military and civilian health and sexuality, and the impact of war on the surveillance and regulation of sexual behaviour.[12] Finally, several studies have analysed the impulses and constraints determining the course and outcome of campaigns for compulsory VD controls, including compulsory notification and treatment, or explored their implications for current issues of public health and civil liberties surrounding the threat of AIDS.[13]

This book seeks to integrate and advance many of these strands of enquiry within a wide-ranging study of VD in twentieth-century Scotland. It examines how civic, medical and political authorities responded to the perceived threat of VD and how far that perception was shaped by social anxieties surrounding sexual behaviour and social change, in addition to the pressure of medical events and ideology. It seeks to locate community and governmental responses to sexually related diseases within contemporary epidemiological debate and to explore the socio-medical contours and politics of suffering, treatment and prevention.

The study is based on the archives not only of the central health departments of State and local health authorities, but also of the major pressure groups involved, including women's organizations, the Churches, social hygiene and moral welfare agencies and medical societies, along with oral evidence from venereologists and other staff employed within the VD service. Documentary evidence has been supplemented by surviving photographic and film archive.

It is important to recognise a Scottish dimension to the social history of VD. Much of existing British research has centred on the socio-medical politics of VD at a national level, in Westminster and Whitehall, and there is a lack of regional and local studies of the interrelationship between VD, sexual morality and public health, and of the interface between health authorities and dispensaries and those in society who were venereally infected. Moreover, as will become evident, the ideology and practice of the VD service in twentieth-century Scotland continued to be shaped by distinctive traditions of law, local government, and medical practice, as well as arguably a distinctive civic and sexual culture.

An introductory overview of the early history of VD in Scotland highlights the role of such traditions. Thereafter, Chapter 2 surveys the health provisions for the treatment of VD prevailing in Scotland around 1900 and explores the relationship between public health, public morality and the social politics of VD in the pre-war years. It documents the Scottish contribution to contemporary debate culminating in the proceedings of the Royal Commission on Venereal Diseases and the authorization in 1916 of a comprehensive, public system of medical diagnosis and treatment for VD.

Chapters 3–7 deal in turn with the development, resourcing, ideology and achievements of VD provisions in interwar Scotland. Chapter 3 examines the gradual establishment of VD schemes under the 1916 Scottish VD Regulations, along with more detailed case studies of the major urban schemes in Aberdeen, Dundee, Edinburgh and Glasgow, and of provisions specifically designed for merchant seamen and prisoners.

Chapter 4 evaluates the treatment regimes for syphilis and gonorrhoea in the hospitals and clinics, treatment provided privately by general medical practitioners, unqualified treatment, and self-disinfection. The social characteristics of VD patients attending interwar VD clinics are analysed, as is the status of venereology as an emerging specialty within Scottish medicine.

Chapter 5 focuses on the social ideology informing the administrative and medical philosophy of the VD service in interwar Scotland. In particular, it explores how a fundamentally conservative moral agenda shaped the categories and content of treatment, the focus of epidemiology and public health debate, and the broader

4

socio-sexual engineering of the dispensaries and Public Health Committees. This agenda was most clearly articulated in the 'propaganda' work of Scottish health authorities and social hygiene agencies, and its organization and content are duly analysed in *Chapter 6* with the aid of surviving posters, pamphlets and film material.

In *Chapter 7*, an attempt is made to assess the impact of public health provisions upon the incidence and repercussions of VD in interwar Scotland. Limitations in the scope of treatment and the success of 'propaganda' measures are identified. In particular, it examines contemporary concerns over the extent of default and venereal recidivism which questioned the adequacy of purely voluntary strategies. This forms the preamble to an analysis in *Chapter 8* of the major impulses and constraints shaping the course and outcome of the campaign for compulsory VD controls in interwar Scotland.

Chapter 9 addresses the impact of the Second World War on civilian VD policy and provisions. It narrates the continuing struggle of Scottish public health authorities to obtain powers of compulsory notification and treatment, and focuses especially on the debates surrounding Defence Regulation 33B and the more discriminatory aspects of its operation.

Chapters 10–12 trace the social history of VD in Scotland under the National Health Service from 1948 to 1980, developing many of the themes raised in Chapters 3–9 through to the onset of AIDS. In *Chapter 10*, the incidence and social distribution of VD in post-war Scotland is discussed along with the epidemiological debate shaping professional and public responses to the issue of sexual permissiveness and disease. The resource and disease control strategies of the Regional Hospital and Area Health Boards form the subject of *Chapters 11* and *12*. *Chapter 11* reviews the struggle of Scottish venereologists to secure adequate funding and recognition as a specialty under the National Health Service. *Chapter 12* documents the continuing, sporadic attempts of local authorities to use public order and child welfare legislation to contain female 'sexual delinquency' in the interests of public health. Thereafter, it explores the main developments in treatment regimes and the content and limitations of health education initiatives in the post-war period. Finally, the chapter outlines the development of contact tracing for VD/STDs in late twentieth-century Scotland and the institutional and legal constraints affecting tracing procedures.

This volume focuses in particular on the social history of the two main 'classic' venereal diseases: syphilis and gonorrhoea. Syphilis is a sexually transmitted disease produced by *Treponema pallidum*, a corkscrew shaped bacterium known as a *spirochaete*. Within twentieth-century medical literature, the course of the disease has conventionally been divided into three stages. The primary stage is normally characterized by the development of a chancre, usually on the genitals, which may frequently go undetected in women. Although the chancre heals after a few weeks, the infection has by that time become systemic. The secondary stage, during which the sufferer remains infectious, develops some six to eight weeks after the primary lesion first appears. It is most commonly characterized by the outbreak of a widespread skin rash which persists for weeks or months if left untreated. Eventually, primary and secondary lesions disappear and the disease enters a latent period.

In a proportion of untreated patients, a third stage of syphilis may develop from two to twenty years after the disappearance of the secondary lesions. Late or tertiary syphilis may manifest itself in a number of ways: the development of a soft gummy tumour in the skin, mucous membrane or bone, life-threatening damage to the heart and blood vessels, or acute deterioration of the central nervous system. Neurosyphilis manifests itself primarily in tabes dorsalis (locomotor ataxia) involving progressive degeneration of the spinal cord and the loss of bodily functions, or in general paresis (general paralysis of the insane) resulting in insanity. In addition, syphilis can be transmitted from an infected woman to her unborn baby. A significant proportion of infected unborn babies die in the womb. Of the babies born alive with congenital syphilis, many will die early in life if no treatment is given. Of the remainder, a good proportion will develop the signs of tertiary syphilis between the ages of seven and fifteen with, in many cases, a range of characteristic deformities in the eyes, ears and teeth combined with mental disabilities.

Gonorrhoea is caused by the *Neisseria gonorrhoeae* or *gonococcus* and is almost invariably transmitted by means of sexual intercourse. The first symptoms of infection appear within days of exposure and if untreated, the sufferer will long remain infectious. In men, the condition is rapidly evident in acute inflammation of the urethra, increasing discomfort on passing urine, and a purulent discharge from the penis. Eventually, the condition may spread and severely impair the whole genito-urinary and reproductive systems. In women, the initial infection is usually located in the cervix. Although there is frequently a discharge from the vagina, women often suffer little or no pain despite their remaining infectious for prolonged periods. In many women, the early stages of gonorrhoea are asymptomatic. If the disease remains untreated, it can spread into the uterine cavity and fallopian tubes, causing sterility. Some bacteria may also be carried in the blood stream to other parts of the body, especially the joints, causing chronic arthritis. The infection may also be transmitted during delivery to the eyes of new-born babies (ophthalmia neonatorum), frequently leading to blindness if it is not treated immediately.

Three disclaimers are necessary. First, while the impact of war and of the military on VD policy and administration is an important theme in this study, it mainly deals with the incidence and attempted control of VD within the civilian population. Secondly, this book primarily focuses on the earlier, infective stages of VD that were to dominate public health debate and the moral agenda that shaped it. The social history of VD within the Scottish asylums as a psychiatric disorder is not therefore explored but awaits the outcome of ongoing research.[14] Finally, this study does not attempt to provide a social history of AIDS in Scotland. As Virginia Berridge's exhaustive investigation of *AIDS in the UK* bears witness, this would both require and merit a separate book.[15] Nonetheless, a concluding chapter does briefly examine the fate of the 'classical' venereal diseases in Scotland since 1980, and explores the implications of this study, not only for the social historiography of VD, but also as a pre-history of AIDS.

'This Loathsome and Horrible Distemper': An Historical Perspective

VD was deeply rooted within Scottish cultural, legal, literary and medical traditions. As early as 1497, repressive controls had been introduced by Aberdeen Town Council and the Privy Council of Scotland to contain the spread of 'glengore' or 'grandgore', as syphilis was commonly named in Scotland, supposedly introduced by the foreign mercenaries of Perkin Warbeck. The Aberdeen edict especially targeted sexually active women, demanding that all 'light [loose] women dicist from thair vices and syn of venerie' and work for 'thair support on pain of being branded' or being banished from the town.[16] The Edinburgh Statute of the same year, known as the Glengore Act and drawn up by James IV himself, ordered the immediate transportation of all infected individuals and their medical attendants to the Islands of Inchkeith in the Firth of Forth, and the branding of those who sought to evade the edict.[17]

However, these measures to contain the disease appear to have been ineffective and evidence suggests that, within a few years, syphilis spread into most of the sizeable towns in Scotland.[18] Certainly, its rapid diffusion both at court and within the community was celebrated by contemporary Scottish poets. Thus, William Dunbar, in his *General Satyre of Scotland* (1507), recorded that:

> Sic losing sarkis, so mony Glengoir markis,
> Within this land was nevir hard nor sene.[19]

Scotland appears to have experienced a series of epidemics of syphilis during the sixteenth century which triggered an array of coercive measures on the part of civic authorities. In 1507, a second edict in Aberdeen attempted to quarantine syphilitics by confining them to their homes and banning them from entering the vicinity of butchers, bakers, and launderers,[20] and similar measures were subsequently proclaimed in many urban centres. Contemporary observers frequently ignored the 'venereal' aspects of the disease and often focused on the secondary symptoms rather than the 'primary affection of the sexual organs'.[21] It was widely regarded as a highly contagious and infectious disease communicated by shared clothing and utensils and bathing arrangements, by kissing, 'and by the slightest contact of the sick with the healthy, or even by inhaling the same air'.[22]

However, by the mid-sixteenth century, there was growing stress on the sexual transmission of the disease and regulations increasingly targeted women perceived to be promiscuous. Thus, under an Edinburgh Act of 1560, in the interests of public health, prostitutes were subject to penalties ranging from public rebuke and carting to branding or torture and death. The segregation of syphilitics was confined to women only, as the Act directed that 'all "whores", whether infected or not, were to be banished from the town and suburbs'.[23] By the end of the century, the fear of VD was prompting kirk sessions to introduce draconic measures against women who failed to conform to Church laws of morality and particularly brutal executions were proscribed where syphilis and witchcraft were associated in the indictment.[24]

Meanwhile, regulations frequently stigmatized medical attendants along with their syphilitic patients. As a result, the more respectable members of the medical profession 'refused to attend patients attacked by the disease, and the sufferers were left to the mercies of barbers, quacks, and old women'.[25] There is circumstantial evidence that mercury and its derivatives were prescribed in sixteenth-century Scotland, and medical practitioners, such as Peter Lowe, Glasgow's town surgeon, were publicizing their experience of treating syphilis, or 'the Spanish sickness' as he called it.[26] However, the main response of Scottish civic authorities remained one of coercion and isolation. Thus, the central recommendation of Glasgow Kirk Session in the 1590s, having consulted medical experts, was that a special house should be designated as a quarantine hospital for women 'affected with the Glengore'.[27]

Fresh and possibly more virulent epidemics of syphilis spread across Scotland in the seventeenth and eighteenth centuries. The 'sibbens', as it was popularly called in the Highlands, allegedly introduced by Cromwell's army during the Civil War, was regarded as a new disease, distinct from the Glengore. Over the next century, this 'loathsome and horrible distemper' spread south into the Lowlands and south-west of Scotland, creating widespread panic.[28] Writing from Dumfries in 1769, Ebenezer Gilchrist observed that: 'Great are the perplexity and distress, the suspicion and terror caused by it wherever it comes; and hitherto nothing has been able to prevent the spreading of it'.[29] Along with other commentators, he emphasized the hereditary nature of the disease and echoed Pennant's foreboding that it seemed to have 'accomplished the divine menace, in visiting the sins of the father upon the children to the third and fourth generation'.[30]

While sexual incontinence remained one important strand of explanation, the spread of epidemics was increasingly attributed to the customs of the poor and their lack of general hygiene, and particularly to the lifestyle of migrant workers.[31] According to Gilchrist, it was propagated:

> by using the same spoons and knives, and wiping with the same cloth the infected have used, without cleaning or washing them; drinking out of the same glass or cup; smoking with the same pipe; sleeping with the infected, or in the same bedclothes they have lain in; and handling their sores; by sucking or giving suck; saluting or kissing; and fondling children, or feeding them in an uncleanly way.[32]

The response of public authorities and medical commentators was to advocate rigorous vetting of servants and wet-nurses and their use of separate facilities and utensils.[33] A range of quarantine procedures operated for those suspected of carrying the infection. In the northern islands, huts were built in the fields and sufferers rigorously isolated. In the south, an isolated cottage often had its guard of soldiers, and the dramatic symptoms of the disease made outcasts of those infected. According to one Scottish surgeon: 'Whole families must perish, the infected being detested as lepers whom nobody would receive or go near'.[34] This strategy of isolation and quarantine was coordinated by the Convention of Scottish Royal Burghs with its pro-active commitment to the regulation and containment of venereal and other 'pestilential infections'.[35]

Advances in the diagnosis and treatment of VD in Scotland remained limited. Venereal wards *were* opened in the mid-eighteenth century at the Royal Infirmary of Edinburgh, and by the final decades of the century VD was by far the most common ailment seen at the Infirmary.[36] Edinburgh practitioners, such as the surgeon Benjamin Bell, made significant advances in the nosology of VD, arguing that gonorrhoea and lues venerea were distinct diseases.[37] Moreover, both medical and legal evidence would suggest that many Scottish practitioners increasingly specialized in the treatment of venereal diseases and that treatment was becoming somewhat more 'regularized'.[38] Nevertheless, most voluntary hospitals regarded VD cases as undeserving of philanthropy and unfit for admission, or allowed access only to 'innocent' sufferers.[39] Thus, at the Town's Hospital of Glasgow, the original City Poorhouse, the Directors determined in 1750 that: 'These who are Recommended to be taken into the house. That they bring along with them and produce a Certificate from a phisician or surgeon of their being free of all Venerial Distemper'.[40] As a result, the majority of those infected either remained untreated or had recourse to quack remedies. Prevailing therapies included purging, blood-letting and a variety of 'mercurial physic', much of which was highly toxic, if not fatal, together with sinister notions of cure by means of transmitting the disease to others, especially virgins.[41] Even at Edinburgh Royal Infirmary, VD patients were heavily stigmatized, and virtually incarcerated in the lock ward so as to confine their perceived moral and physical corruption.[42]

Although there are many similarities between the social response to VD in early modern and modern Scotland, three strands of continuity are particularly significant.

First, there is the compulsionist stance of Scottish administration towards VD and the pronounced tradition of civic authoritarianism and interventionism in issues relating to public health. The overriding concern of early edicts relating to VD was to contain rather than to cure infection, with a consequential erosion of civil liberties. This trend was consolidated in the nineteenth century. Scottish medical and legal ideology had been heavily influenced by the European enlightenment, and by the early decades of the century, the German tradition of 'medical police' involving wide-ranging powers of surveillance and intervention in personal and civic life in the cause of health, had begun, albeit in a more moderate form, to shape Scottish administration. Medical Officers of Health were primarily appointed to aid the police and the magistracy, and this ideological and institutional conflation of health and public order was to prove decisive in shaping the response of local authorities to VD in nineteenth- and twentieth-century Scotland.[43]

Secondly, the history of VD in Scotland prior to 1800 reveals a vigorous tradition of church and community disciplining of sexual behaviour, strongly reinforcing secular law. While patterns of church discipline administered by the kirk sessions, and most vividly enshrined in the stool of penitence, were largely undermined by the mid-nineteenth century, the churches continued to play a critical role in defining the moral climate of Scottish civil society. In particular, church views and institutions remained central in shaping the response of the local state to VD, especially its continuing integration of public order, public morality and public health in regulating forms of social intercourse that threatened the hygiene of the family and community.[44]

Finally, the history of the surveillance and control of VD in Scotland prior to 1800 enables us to see how the antecedents of nineteenth-century discourses surrounding female prostitution and VD were rooted in heavily gendered and discriminatory practices of social medicine which date back centuries.[45] From the outset, many regulations to contain the spread of VD had been targeted at women and their sexual behaviour, despite continuing uncertainty as to how precisely it was transmitted. Social fear of female 'promiscuity' engendered a powerful moral epidemiology that was to inform the social response to VD, arguably until the present day. Moreover, as issues of sexual immorality and sexual disease became increasingly medicalized, legal and medical agencies worked in collaboration to institutionalize and reform the promiscuous and the venereally infected woman and to isolate her from respectable society.[46] As Linda Mahood has so vividly documented, these processes were further developed within the local 'city states' of nineteenth-century Scotland in which newly established lock hospitals for venereally infected females formed part of a general strategy of legal repression and moral regulation operated by the police and by the Magdalene and other reformatory asylums in an effort to contain prostitution.[47] As a result, VD became increasingly engrossed within the social politics surrounding prostitution, and medical provisions and debate shaped primarily by contemporary fears over female immorality and vice;[48] a feature that was to persist well into the twentieth century.

Notes

1 In twentieth-century Britain, the term 'venereal disease' has been commonly used to describe those diseases arising from infection transmitted during sexual intercourse. In public health regulations, VD has been narrowly defined as syphilis, gonorrhoea, and soft chancre. However, from the early 1930s, for most non-legal purposes, the term was also regarded as covering other forms of non-specific venereal infection such as septic balanitis. From the 1970s, the term 'sexually transmitted diseases' was increasingly substituted for 'VD' in recognition of the wide range of other infections spread by means of sexual contact, and as a means of reducing the social stigma associated with the disease category.

2 See especially, R. Davenport-Hines, *Sex, Death and Punishment: Attitudes to Sex and Sexuality in Britain since the Renaissance* (London: William Collins, 1990); F. Mort, *Dangerous Sexualities: Medico-Moral Politics in England since 1830* (London: Routledge and Kegan Paul, 1987); L. Bland, '"Cleansing the Portals of Life": The Venereal Disease Campaign in the early Twentieth Century', in M. Langan and B. Schwarz (eds), *Crises in the British State, 1880–1930* (London: Hutchinson, 1985), ch. 9; A. Brandt, *No Magic Bullet, A Social History of Venereal Disease in the United States since 1880* (Oxford: Oxford University Press, 1985); A. Mooij, *Out of Otherness: Characters and Narrators in the Dutch Venereal Disease Debates, 1850–1990* (Amsterdam/Atlanta: Rodopi Press, 1998); M. Murnane and K. Daniels, 'Prostitutes as "Purveyors of Disease": Venereal Disease Legislation in Tasmania 1868–1945', *Hecate*, 5 (1979), 5–21; P. J. Fleming, 'Fighting the "Red Plague": Observations on the Response to Venereal Disease in New Zealand 1910–45', *New Zealand Journal of History*, 22 (1988), 56–64; A. Corbin, *Women for Hire: Prostitution and Sexuality in France after 1850* (London/Cambridge, Mass.: Harvard University Press, 1990), pt 3.

3 See especially, J. Walkowitz, *Prostitution and Victorian Society: Women, Class, and the State* (Cambridge: Cambridge University Press, 1980).

4 For a detailed discussion of the concept of moral regulation, see especially, J. Sangster, 'Incarcerating "Bad Girls": The Regulation of Sexuality through the Female Refuges Act in Ontario 1920–45', *Journal of the History of Sexuality*, 7 (1996), 241–6.

5 See, e.g., C. Strange, *Toronto's Girl Problem, The Perils and Pleasures of the City: 1880–1930* (Toronto: University of Toronto Press,

1995); R. M. Alexander, *The 'Girl Problem': Female Sexual Delinquency in New York, 1900–30* (Ithaca: Cornell University Press, 1995).

6   See especially, M. Vaughan, *Curing Their Ills: Colonial Power and African Illness* (London: Polity Press, 1991), ch. 6; P. Levine, 'Venereal Disease, Prostitution, and the Politics of Empire: The Case of British India', *Journal of the History of Sexuality,* 4 (1994), 579–602; L. Mandelson, *Sickness and the State: Health and Illness in Colonial Malaya: 1870–1940* (Cambridge: Cambridge University Press, 1996), ch. 6; A. L. Stoler, 'Making Empire Respectable: The Politics of Race and Sexual Morality in Twentieth-Century Colonial Cultures', *American Ethnologist,* 16 (1989), 634–60; J. M. Kehoe, 'Medicine, Sexuality and Imperialism: British Medical Discourses surrounding Venereal Disease in New Zealand and Japan', Victoria University, New Zealand, Ph.D. thesis, (1992).

7   Such approaches have drawn heavily on the insights of S. L. Gilman, *Difference and Pathology: Stereotypes of Sexuality, Race and Madness* (Ithaca: Cornell University Press, 1985). See also, A. McKlintock, *Imperial Leather: Race, Gender and Sexuality in the Colonial Conquest* (New York: Routledge, 1995).

8   See, e.g., Fleming, *op. cit.* (note 2), 60; D. R. Tibbits, 'The Medical, Social and Political Response to Venereal Diseases in Victoria 1860–1980', Monash University, Ph.D. thesis, (1994), 161.

9   See, e.g., D. Evans, 'Tackling the "Hideous Scourge": The Creation of the Venereal Disease Treatment Centres in Early Twentieth-Century Britain', *Social History of Medicine,* 5 (1992), 413–33.

10 See, e.g., B. A. Towers, 'Health Education Policy 1916–26: Venereal Disease and the Prophylaxis Dilemma', *Medical History,* 24 (1980), 70–87; S. M. Tomkins, 'Palmitate or Permanganate: The Venereal Prophylaxis Debate in Britain, 1916–1926', *Medical History,* 37 (1993), 382–98; Davenport-Hines, *op. cit.* (note 2), ch. 7.

11 See, e.g., Bland, *op. cit.* (note 2); L. Bland, '"Guardians of the Race" or "Vampires upon the Nation's Health"?: Female Sexuality and its Regulation in Early Twentieth-Century Britain', in E. Whitelegg *et al.,* (eds), *The Changing Experience of Women* (Oxford: Martin Robertson, 1982), 375–88; L. Bland and F. Mort, 'Look out for the "Good Time" Girl: Dangerous Sexualities as a Threat to National Health', in *Formations of Nation and People* (London: Routledge and Kegan Paul, 1984), 131–51.

12 See, e.g., L. Bland, 'In the Name of Protection: The Policing of Women in the First World War', in J. Brophy and C. Smart (eds), *Women-In-Law: Explorations in Law, Family and Sexuality* (London:

Routledge and Kegan Paul, 1985), 23–49; E. H. Beardley, 'Allied against Sin: American and British responses to Venereal Disease in World War I', *Medical History*, 20 (1976), 189–202; S. Buckley, 'The Failure to Resolve the Problem of Venereal Disease among the Troops in Britain during World War I', in B. Bond and I. Roy (eds), *War and Society: a Yearbook of Military History*, Vol. 2 (London: Croom Helm, 1977), 65–85; L. Hall, '"War always brings it on": War, STDs, the Military, and the Civil Population in Britain 1850–1950', in R. Cooter, M. Harrison, and S. Sturdy (eds), *Medicine and the Management of Modern Warfare* (Amsterdam/Atlanta: Rodopi Press, 2000), 205–23.

13 See, e.g., R. Davidson, '"A Scourge to be Firmly Gripped": The Campaign for VD Controls in Interwar Scotland', *Social History of Medicine*, 6 (1993), 213–35; D. Porter and R. Porter, 'The Enforcement of Health: The British Debate', in E. Fee and D. M. Fox (eds), *AIDS: The Burdens of History* (Berkeley/London: University of California Press, 1988).

14 Gayle Davis is currently undertaking an ESRC doctoral thesis on 'Social Disease and Psychiatry in Edinburgh and Glasgow *c.*1870–1930'.

15 V. Berridge, *AIDS in the UK: The Making of Policy, 1981–1994* (Oxford: Oxford University Press, 1996).

16 A. Duncan, *Memorials of the Faculty of Physicians and Surgeons of Glasgow* (Glasgow: Maclehose, 1896), 14; J. Y. Simpson, 'Notices of the Appearance of Syphilis in Scotland in the last years of the Fifteenth Century', *Edinburgh Medical Journal [EMJ]*, 6 (1861), 683; R. S. Morton, 'Some Aspects of the Early History of Syphilis in Scotland', *British Journal of Venereal Diseases [BJVD]*, 38 (1962), 176.

17 Simpson, *op. cit.* (note 16), 684; Duncan, *op. cit.* (note 16).

18 Simpson, *ibid.*; T. Ferguson, *The Dawn of Scottish Social Welfare* (London: Thomas Nelson, 1948), 109; J. Y. Simpson, *Antiquarian Notices of Syphilis in Scotland in the 15th and 16th Centuries* (Edinburgh: Edmonston and Douglas, 1862), 10–11.

19 Cited in Morton, *op. cit.* (note 16), 177.

20 *Ibid.*

21 Simpson, *op. cit.* (note 18), 25.

22 D. Newman, 'The History and Prevention of Venereal Disease', *Glasgow Medical Journal [GMJ]*, 81 (1914), 94.

23 K. M. Boyd, *Scottish Church Attitudes to Sex, Marriage and the Family 1850–1914* (Edinburgh: John Donald, 1980), 176.

24 Simpson, *op. cit.* (note 18), 12; Morton, *op. cit.* (note 16), 177.

25 Newman, *op. cit.* (note 22), 93.

26 Morton, *op. cit.* (note 16), 177; Duncan, *op. cit.* (note 16), 15.

27 Morton, *ibid.*, 176; Ferguson, *op. cit.* (note 18), 107–8.

28 T. Pennant, *A Tour in Scotland, 1772,* Vol. 2 (Fourth Edition, London: Benj. White, 1776), 44; E. Gilchrist, *An Account of a Very Infectious Distemper Prevailing in Many Places* (Edinburgh: John Balfour, 1770); G. Risse, *Hospital Life in Enlightenment Scotland* (Cambridge: Cambridge University Press, 1986), 128. In the south of Scotland, it was frequently called 'the Yaws'.

29 Gilchrist, *op. cit.* (note 28), 4.

30 *Ibid.*, 26; Pennant, *op. cit.* (note 28), 44. On contemporary fears of hereditary infection elsewhere in Britain and in France, see B. J. Dunlap, 'The Problem of Syphilitic Children in Eighteenth-Century France and England' in L. E. Merians (ed.), *The Secret Malady: Venereal Disease in Eighteenth-Century Britain and France* (Lexington: University Press of Kentucky, 1996), 114–27.

31 G. M. Cullen, 'Concerning Sibbens and the Scottish Yaws', *Caledonian Medical Journal,* 8 (1909–11), 348–9.

32 Gilchrist, *op. cit.* (note 28), 13.

33 Cullen, *op. cit.* (note 31), 349. In the Highlands, servants were stripped naked and carefully examined for sibbens before being engaged. See Ferguson, *op. cit.* (note 18), 110.

34 Risse, *op. cit.* (note 28), 128.

35 J. D. Marwick (ed.), *Records of the Convention of Royal Burghs 1711–38* (Edinburgh: Scottish Burgh Records Society, 1885), 267–70, 299–301. The practice of isolating patients with 'sibbens' or banishing them to their district of birth was maintained in small parishes well into the nineteenth century. See Cullen, *op. cit.* (note 31), 342.

36 Risse, *op. cit.* (note 28), 105–6, 128. This was, in part, a consequence of a contract that the Infirmary had concluded with the military authorities to treat men in the army and navy.

37 For details, see *ibid.*, 127–8.

38 See W. F. Bynum, 'Treating the Wages of Sin: Venereal Disease and Specialism in Eighteenth-Century Britain', in W. F. Bynum and R. Porter (eds), *Medical Fringe and Medical Orthodoxy, 1750–1850* (London: Croom Helm, 1987), 5–28; L. Leneman, 'Venereal Disease in Eighteenth-Century Scotland: Evidence From the Divorce Courts', *Proceedings of the Royal College of Physicians of Edinburgh,* 27 (1997), 242–5.

39 Risse, *op. cit.* (note 28), 105.

40 Mitchell Library, Glasgow, Acc. 641982. Minutes of Directors Meetings, 1732–64, 142. I am indebted to Dr Fiona A. Macdonald

for this reference.

41   Gilchrist, *op. cit.* (note 28), 19–25; Risse, *op. cit.* (note 28), 126; Cullen, *op. cit.* (note 31), 349–50; *The Third Statistical Account of Scotland: The County of Banff,* edited H. Hamilton (Glasgow: Collins, 1961), 174.

42   Risse, *op. cit.* (note 28), 105–6.

43   B. White, 'Training Medical Policemen: Forensic Medicine and Public Health in Nineteenth-Century Scotland', in M. Clark and C. Crawford (eds), *Legal Medicine in History* (Cambridge: Cambridge University Press, 1994), 145–63; K. Carson and H. Idzikowska, 'The Social Production of Scottish Policing 1795–1900', in D. Hay and F. Snyder (eds), *Policing and Prosecution in Britain 1750–1850* (Oxford: Oxford University Press, 1989), 267–97. The authoritarian nature of Scottish civil government also reflected a legal system based heavily upon Canon or Roman Law, as distinct from English Common Law. On the contrasting traditions of health administration in Scotland and England, see K. Underhill, 'Science, Professionalism and the Development of Medical Education in England: An Historical Sociology', University of Edinburgh, Ph.D. thesis (1987), 275–83.

44   See especially, A. Blaikie, *Illegitimacy, Sex and Society: Northeast Scotland, 1750–1900* (Oxford: Oxford University Press, 1993), ch. 7; A. Blaikie, '"The Map of Vice in Scotland": Victorian Vocabularies of Causation', in J. Forrai (ed.), *Civilization, Sexuality and Social Life* (Budapest: Semmel University of Medicine Institute, 1996), 117–32; Boyd, *op. cit.* (note 23), 4–12.

45   L. Mahood, *The Magdalenes: Prostitution in the Nineteenth Century* (London: Routledge, 1990), 17.

46   *Ibid.,* 27–8.

47   *Ibid., passim.*

48   See, e.g., W. Tait [House Surgeon to Edinburgh Lock Hospital], *Magdalenism: An Inquiry into the Extent, Causes, and Consequences of Prostitution in Edinburgh* (Edinburgh: P. Richard, 1840); W. Logan, *The Great Social Evil: Its Causes, Extent, Results, and Remedies* (London: Hodder and Stoughton, 1871). For a general discussion of this process, see M. Spongberg, *Feminizing Venereal Disease: The Body of the Prostitute in Nineteenth-Century Medical Discourse* (Basingstoke: Macmillan Press, 1997).

2

Public Health, Public Morality and VD in Early-Twentieth-Century Scotland

'Every Possible Indignity':
The Pattern of VD Provisions in Edwardian Scotland

The first decade of the twentieth century witnessed dramatic advances in venereology. The discovery in 1905 of the causal organism of syphilis, *Spirochaeta pallida*, was succeeded by the development of a reliable serological test for syphilis, the Wassermann Test, in 1906, and the introduction of an effective chemotherapeutic agent, Salvarsan '606', the first of the antitreponemal organic arsenical compounds, in 1910. Significant advances were also taking place in the aetiology of neuro-syphilis and congenital syphilis and in the medical awareness of the more serious sequelae of gonorrhoea, especially sterility. Yet, provisions for the diagnosis and treatment of VD in Edwardian Scotland were widely regarded as woefully inadequate. As Dr Leslie Mackenzie, Medical Member of the Local Government Board for Scotland, observed in 1907, it was customary to place 'every difficulty in the way of treatment and every possible indignity on the patient'.[1]

Practitioner Treatment

Members of the middle and upper classes suffering from VD were treated almost exclusively by private practitioners or by consultants in the first instance, and did not normally go to institutions for cure.[2] Evidence is sparse on the content and calibre of private professional practice relating to VD. However, it would appear that, due to the lack of medical training, many practitioners failed to appreciate the seriousness of these diseases and their threat to public health.[3] They were often ignorant of new forms of diagnosis and treatment, and failed to convey to patients the health risks to themselves and their families of incomplete treatment and premature sexual indulgence.[4] General practitioners were averse to examining patients with acute VD, let alone treating them. As David Watson, Dispensary Surgeon to Glasgow Royal Infirmary, noted: 'The prospect of drops of pus falling on the carpet, or pus-contaminated hands fingering the furniture or door-handle, makes the unfortunate patient too often an

17

unwelcome intruder, and the fight between the doctor's conscience and his feelings one in which the right may not always win'.[5] According to the skin physician at Glasgow Victoria Infirmary, 'the majority of doctors gave the matter [of VD] the cold shoulder, their attitude being one of indifference, if not disgust'.[6] Moreover, evidence suggests that practitioners often shared the view of many civic leaders in Edwardian Scotland that gonorrhoea and syphilis were 'appropriate and necessary punishments for acts of disobedience to the moral code'.[7]

The Voluntary General Hospitals

While traditionally there had been a more liberal admissions policy for VD patients in Scottish voluntary hospitals than elsewhere in Britain,[8] the stigma attached to the disease as a just punishment 'for the sins of the flesh and the transgression of Christian morality' remained a potent force in limiting provisions. Perversely, while surgical cases arising out of advanced syphilis and gonorrhoeal infection occupied a significant number of beds, those suffering from the early, most infective and most treatable stages of VD were rarely admitted.[9] 'Only when the ravages of syphilis in the central nervous and the cardio-vascular systems and those of gonorrhoea in the genito-urinary and articular systems had made their victims interesting cases were they admitted to the teaching hospitals.'[10] According to J. Kerr Love, surgeon to Glasgow Royal Infirmary, in many general hospitals, physicians and surgeons were not interested in early cases of VD. In his experience, they did not want 'dirty cases' of any kind in their wards. Not only did they lack adequate medical expertise and facilities, they often shared the moral reservations of their Directors and subscribers about the allocation of resources to VD patients, especially where infection was perceived to be primarily a function of prostitution.[11] Indeed, some general hospitals in Scotland 'would not admit female venereal cases without a character reference or other proof of "respectability"'.[12]

'Lock wards', dedicated to VD cases, did exist in the Royal Infirmaries of Aberdeen, Edinburgh and Glasgow, with, in total, some 33 beds allocated for male patients and 20 beds for female patients. However, evidence would suggest that facilities for diagnosis and treatment were often seriously inadequate and that inmates were heavily regimented and stigmatized.[13] A 'strong body of medical opinion' considered that the care of venereal patients at the new Royal Infirmary of Edinburgh, established in 1879, was inferior to the more specialized treatment previously received at the former Lock Hospital. Female patients were confined in daytime to basement rooms called

18

the 'Duck Pond', so called because they were forced into a humiliating routine each night of waddling along the corridors single file in heel-less slippers to their sleeping quarters.[14] Male patients were normally attended to by inexperienced students and their ward-masters frequently dismissed 'for bad conduct and general irregularity'.[15] Out-patient facilities for primary cases of acquired VD at the general hospitals were equally deficient and characterized by an indiscriminate prescription of 'pills, potions or mercury solutions' with little regard for the need to educate patients as to the seriousness of their disease and the likely repercussions on family and public health of default from treatment. According to Dr Carl Browning, Director of the Laboratory of Clinical Pathology at Glasgow Western Infirmary, out-patient therapy for VD was extremely ineffective and probably failed 'to affect cure in more than a small proportion of cases'.[16]

Poorhouse Provisions

In many Scottish poorhouses, special wards were provided for infective VD cases. In addition, many patients, especially women, in the later, non-infectious stages of VD, lingered on in the general wards of the parish hospitals. Leslie Mackenzie estimated that during the period 1902–6, on average, 587 VD patients were admitted each year into the poorhouse system.[17]

Such provisions were widely regarded by contemporary observers as inadequate. Parochial managers, with their concern for strict economy and commitment to the principle of 'less eligibility', were highly discriminatory in their admissions policies.[18] In some parishes, able-bodied paupers suffering from primary syphilis were refused treatment in the poorhouse, regardless of the consequences for public health.[19] Fears and assumptions surrounding the sexual habits and contaminating influence of female patients, most of whom were presumed to be prostitutes, also led to differential admissions practices. Thus, in Glasgow, while male patients were housed in Barnhill Poorhouse, apart from maternity cases, the parish council made no special provision for acute cases of VD in women, who were referred to the Lock Hospital.[20]

The quality of treatment and life within poorhouse 'foul wards' varied greatly, but, as in England, conditions were in general 'grossly inadequate'. In practice, 'the concern of parish authorities to curtail severely the physical comfort and moral sympathy for their "test" cases necessarily rebounded on the paupers and particularly on their sick patients' and on none more so than those in the lock wards. These were typically allocated the worst accommodation, in cramped, often damp, insanitary buildings. Patients shared the stringent regime of discipline and restraint of other indoor paupers. Their clothing and tasks were often designed to attract additional stigma.[21] Adequate indoor ventilation and open-air space for exercising, vital for a range of mercurial therapies, was often lacking. Moreover, as in other areas of medicine, poor law hospitals lagged behind in the employment of new diagnostic and treatment procedures for VD, and especially the new laboratory and therapeutic advances such as Wassermann testing and the use of Salvarsan.[22] The deterrent effect of poorhouse conditions coupled with inadequate medical provisions led to a large proportion of patients either defaulting from treatment or being prematurely discharged back into the community, with inevitable consequences for the spread of venereal infection.[23]

Lock Hospitals

By 1900, Glasgow retained the only surviving lock hospital in Scotland specifically dedicated to the treatment of female VD patients *(see Plate 2.1)*. Since its foundation in 1805, it had admitted over 32,000 patients and had become, with over eighty permanent beds, the largest specialist hospital in Scotland. Although a charitable institution with a number of subscribers, the Hospital 'was mostly given over to pauper or police cases' and was regularly supported by annual grants from the City, Barony, and Govan parochial authorities.[24] In the late nineteenth century, the majority of patients were young women involved in prostitution, but inmates also included shop girls, mill girls, domestic servants and field labourers, along with the wives of soldiers and tradesmen.[25] On average, 321 patients were admitted each year during the period 1900–1910, with some 50–55 patients resident at any one time.[26] As Mahood has demonstrated, along with the police courts and Magdalene Asylums, the Glasgow Lock Hospital was part of an overall strategy of containing the 'dangerous sexuality' of alleged prostitutes within the City.[27] Their medical isolation in the Lock Hospital was conceived as the first stage in a process of moral regulation. Indeed, until after 1910, the Lock Hospital Directors were 'unwilling to recognise any policy of [outdoor] dispensary treatment' precisely because it lacked the same potential for moral controls.[28] Although officially denied, women entering the Lock Hospital had to submit to a compulsory medical examination. Thereafter, 'although the hospital had no legal power to detain patients against their will', its management resembled a reformatory or prison.[29]

Glasgow Lock Hospital was chronically under-resourced.

Traditional philanthropic resistance to assisting those infected through their own wilful, 'vicious indulgence' was reinforced by a lingering fear that assistance to the venereally diseased might prove an encouragement to 'vice and immorality'.[30] As a result of

APPENDIX. 135

LOCK HOSPITAL

(1805),

41 ROTTENROW STREET.

Object.—The cure of unfortunate females. **Management.**—By Directors chosen annually, and consisting of 1 from the Clergy, 1 from the Town Council, 1 from the Merchants' House, 1 from the Trades' House, 2 from the Faculty of Physicians and Surgeons, and 8 from the general body of Subscribers. **Admission.**—Open daily. Patients treated—Annual number about 360. Ordinary income, £1,120. Ordinary expenditure, £1,296. Centenary appeal for additional funds and Subscribers has just been made.

Secretary and Treasurer.

R. C. GREIG, C.A., 104 West George Street.

Chairman.

JOHN YOUNG, Esq., 142 Queen Street.

Glasgow Magdalene Institution

(Incorporated by Royal Charter).

President—Preceptor JAS. H. DICKSON, D.L.

Hon. Treasurer—ALEXANDER SLOAN, Esq., C.A.

Secretary and Treasurer—JAMES G. ROSS, 268 Cathedral Street.

And a General Board of 42 Directors.

Objects.—The repression of Vice, and the Reformation of penitent women. The rescue and protection of young females who may be in imminent danger of being led astray.

Appeal.—Owing to the great increase in the number of women benefited by the Institution., the Directors appeal for £300 additional Subscriptions, £700, in addition to Donations and Legacies, being required annually.

Subscriptions and Donations will be received by the Charity Organisation Society, 212 Bath Street; or the Treasurer, J. G. Ross, 268 Cathedral Street.

Plate 2.1
Advert for Lock Hospital and Magdalene Asylum
(*Handbook of Glasgow Charitable and Beneficent Institutions* (1907))

insufficient funding, only half the available beds were used, and there was a serious lack of segregated accommodation for the young girls under sixteen (frequently the victims of sexual assault or abuse) who formed a significant proportion of inmates and required more lengthy and careful treatment.[31] Treatment regimes in the Hospital continued to rely on mercurial therapies well after 1900 and were slow to adapt to new developments in venereology.[32] As Checkland concludes, insofar as patients recuperated: 'It is possible that the women in the Lock Hospitals, isolated as they were from society, may have recovered by means of rest and plain feeding as much as by treatment'.[33]

Quack Treatments

Evidence would suggest that a significant proportion of patients seeking institutional treatment for VD in Edwardian Scotland only did so after consulting a chemist or herbalist, or trying some advertised cure. The use of self-administered, 'alternative' potions and washes for sexual problems and infections was widespread, especially within working-class communities. An official inquiry reported in 1910 that 'in many of the great towns the treatment of venereal diseases [was] in the hands of unqualified persons' and this view was subsequently endorsed by Scottish evidence before the Royal Commission on Venereal Diseases.[34]

In part, widespread recourse to quacks and patent medicines was due to the enduring moral stigma attached to VD and the inevitable desire to conceal infection from family and community. A 'conception of venereal diseases as the just retribution of sin' which continued to shape public and philanthropic opinion towards institutional provisions for venereal patients, served merely to reinforce this tendency.[35] Even under the National Health Insurance Act of 1911, 'misconduct clauses' retained the traditional exclusion from friendly society benefits of those afflicted with VD.[36] In part, recourse to 'quack' treatment was also due to the widespread lack of interest and training of many medical practitioners in venereal cases. Thus, David Watson, Surgeon to the Glasgow Lock Hospital, blamed the apathy of the medical profession for the fact that quacks controlled 'the larger proportion of gonorrhoea practice'.[37]

In addition, avoidance of professional treatment stemmed from an understandable aversion to the prevailing therapies for syphilis and gonorrhoea which were often painful, protracted and dangerous. Medical practices in Edwardian Scotland had not advanced significantly from those in the lock wards of the 1880s.[38] Although salivation had become discredited as a cure for syphilis, mercurial treatment, by pills, by inunction using strong ointments, by fumigation with vapour of calomel, or by intramuscular injection, remained the most common therapy for primary and secondary syphilis. Such treatment, commonly prescribed over a period of eighteen months or more, produced a range of symptoms of heavy metal poisoning. Moreover, even if a patient with primary syphilis subjected himself to the rigours of mercurial treatment, there was still a high probability of clinical relapse and/or the development of secondary syphilis.[39] For patients with gonorrhoea, the pills and salves dispensed by chemists and the 'rapid, painless, curative treatment' promised in quack advertisements must also have appeared an appealing alternative to the often brutal, invasive regime of the hospital wards. Thus, cases of acute gonorrhoea were treated in Glasgow Royal Infirmary either with a urethral injection of an antiseptic solution of silver salts every 3–4 hours or by gravity-fed irrigation of the urethral tract from a reservoir of potassium permanganate suspended up to five feet above the patient. Leeches were not infrequently applied to the scrota of patients with gonococcal epididymitis, while patients suffering from chronic gonococcal urethritis were subjected to an equally painful and hazardous course of dilatation with heated, steel sounds or bougies.[40]

As a result of the inadequacies of medical provisions and the fear and stigma surrounding hospital therapies, it is likely that the bulk of active and infectious VD in Edwardian Scotland remained undiagnosed and untreated. Patients commonly submitted to institutional treatment only after a protracted period of infectivity and the development of intractable and debilitating secondary and chronic symptoms, incurring a heavy price in sickness and mortality and presenting to contemporary observers a major threat to racial health and national efficiency.[41] It was to countering this threat that Scottish public health and public order reformers were to turn their attention after 1900.

The Social Politics of VD 1900–1918

As in many other countries during the early years of the twentieth century, the social politics surrounding VD in Scotland came to enshrine broader concerns over changing standards of social and sexual conduct, and the desire to regulate and stigmatize 'deviant' behaviours. Issues of public health, public order and public morality were increasingly conflated in contemporary debate over VD in Scotland. Not infrequently, proposals were advanced by a broad alliance of health authorities, social purity campaigners, magistracy and the police and were informed as much by moral anxieties as by the medical dimensions of the problem. Moreover, the relative autonomy of the Scottish cities gave such proposals real significance in shaping Scottish social policy. Early twentieth-century commentators compared Edinburgh and Glasgow to the city-states of classical antiquity,[42] and along with Aberdeen and Dundee and the larger Scottish burghs, they jealously defended their traditional independence from departmental 'rule and regulations'.[43] As with the Board of Supervision in the nineteenth century, the Local Government Board for Scotland and its twentieth-century successors had much more limited powers of intervention in local issues than their English counterparts, and it was often local initiatives North of the Border that set the agenda of medico-moral debate.

Four main strands of reform dominated the response of Scottish urban government to VD in the period 1900–1914: the reduction of infant mortality and congenital diseases; the suppression of 'immoral traffic'; the regulation of 'farmed-out' housing' and the policing of entertainment venues likely to excite sexual promiscuity amongst the young – pre-eminently the ice-cream parlours.

Infant Health and Mortality

Between 1900 and World War 1, infant welfare and mortality in Britain 'became defined by contemporaries as one of the major social problems of the time'.[44] Concerns over the physical deterioration of the race and the impact of 'urban degeneration' upon national efficiency served to position the issue high on the agenda of public health debate in Scotland. Initially, attention focused on the improvement of milk supplies and infant hygiene, but after 1906, Scottish health authorities broadened their remit to confront additional aspects of maternal and child mortality and morbidity, including the impact of VD.

Health officials were heavily influenced by the proceedings of the national conferences on infantile mortality held annually in London from 1906, in which Dr A. K. Chalmers, Medical Officer of Health for Glasgow, was a leading activist.[45] In particular, Scottish representatives were vocal in their support of proposals for more prompt and systematic birth registration, for the extension of the 1902 Midwives Act to Scotland, and for the introduction of infant welfare centres.[46] Procedures under the Notification of Births Act 1907 were adopted by Scotland's leading health authorities in 1908.

This enabled health visitors to operate more promptly and to identify more clearly the factors endangering infant life. In particular, it fuelled the growing campaign for the compulsory notification and regulated treatment of ophthalmia neonatorum (gonococcal infection of the eye in the newborn child) conducted by a broad alliance of ophthalmic surgeons, obstetricians, Medical Officers of Health and directors of blind asylums.[47] Powers to include ophthalmia neonatorum under the Infectious Diseases (Notification) Act of 1889 were subsequently adopted by local health authorities in Glasgow (1911), Edinburgh (1912), Dundee (1912) and Aberdeen (1913), with the active encouragement of the Local Government Board for Scotland.

Meanwhile, evidence from infant consultations at child welfare centres was revealing the devastating impact of VD upon child health. In Glasgow, some 17.1 per cent of children brought to infant consultations in 1911–12, whose state of nutrition was classified as bad, were diagnosed as suffering from the effects of VD; 6.3 per cent from ophthalmia neonatorum and 10.8 per cent from congenital syphilis.[48] Along with the reports of health visitors, such revelations prompted a drastic review of VD provisions. In Glasgow, as part of the more general campaign for improved child and maternity welfare, Chalmers pressed for free public laboratory and hospital facilities for the early diagnosis and treatment of VD in women and children.[49] The provision of Wassermann testing for all cases of notified ophthalmia neonatorum served further to demonstrate the extent of congenital syphilis in the poorer areas of Glasgow, and in turn led to a call for more comprehensive provisions for adults.[50] By 1913, a diagnostic laboratory service for suspected VD cases had been introduced for general practitioners and extended to all poorhouse infirmaries and hospitals, and as in Edinburgh, dispensaries and lock wards were making increasing use of Salvarsan preparations to supplement mercury therapies.[51] Significantly, Chalmers proposed that, in exchange for free diagnostic testing, general practitioners should provide information on the age, sex, clinical symptoms and address of each patient as a means of generating a data base upon which further measures of treatment and control might be based.[52] Progress in other cities was slower and more *ad hoc*, but by degrees, Scottish local health authorities had begun to redefine their responsibilities and the relationship of the local State to the venereally infected, and anticipated some of the recommendations of the Royal Commission on Venereal Diseases.

Immoral Traffic

A central issue overshadowing contemporary debate concerning the incidence, epidemiology and prevention of VD was 'the social evil' of prostitution or so-called 'immoral traffic'. Here again, in the formulation of general legislation and local byelaws, medical and moral agendas were closely interwoven. On the one hand, the suppression of vice was seen as essential for 'draining the reservoir' of venereal infection. On the other, the discourse surrounding sexual diseases was frequently used to validate wider social fears and proscriptions of moral deviance and degeneration, and the issue and imagery of VD served as powerful propaganda for the social purity movement in its quest to mobilize the criminal law to regulate public morality.

As in England, private, voluntary initiatives continued to play a major role in the Scottish regulation of sexuality, and purity groups remained central to the enactment and enforcement of criminal law legislation – organizing, investigating and petitioning the State to act. The Scottish Office played an essentially reactive rather than pro-active role in moves to criminalize immoral behaviour and was often a relatively passive partner in the dialogue with purists and feminists. Nonetheless, within Scottish local government, public health officials, magistrates and senior police officers worked closely with the Scottish churches and vigilance associations to form a powerful alliance for moral reform.[53]

One strand of policy-making focused on the need to detain prostitutes and other venereal 'recidivists' for the protection of public and racial health and the preservation of public order. The Contagious Diseases Acts, allowing for the coercive detention and medical examination of any woman suspected of being a prostitute in certain sea-ports and garrison towns, had never applied in Scotland. However, within the major Scottish cities, similar 'technologies of power' had developed in an attempt to reduce the level of prostitution. Under local Burgh Police Acts, the police, in association with the lock wards/hospitals and reformatory asylums, had operated a policy of legal repression and medico-moral regulation for suspected prostitutes.[54]

After 1900, Scottish magistrates and public health committees sought additional powers to detain prostitutes and other 'habitual offenders of the dissipated and dissolute class' in farm colonies, Magdalene Institutions, poorhouses and lock hospitals for an appropriate period of medical treatment and moral rehabilitation.[55] Growing awareness of the degree of default from VD treatment by allegedly promiscuous 'young girls', and the high incidence of re-infection in patients from rate-funded hospitals, served to fuel public support for such controls.[56] A range of Scottish Poor Law Medical Officers subsequently pressed for similar powers in their evidence before the Royal Commission on the Poor Laws and endorsed its recommendation that 'an order for detention should be obtainable whenever sufficient proof is adduced that an individual suffering from venereal disease is a danger to the community'.[57]

In addition, asylum doctors such as Thomas Clouston and George Robertson, Physician Superintendents to the Royal Edinburgh Asylum, concerned at the role of VD in the process of 'urban degeneration', and especially at emerging evidence of its links with infertility and general paralysis of the insane [GPI], argued for additional powers of medical detention for prostitutes known to be communicating the disease, as part of a broader programme of segregation of 'the socially unfit'.[58] Admissions and deaths attributed to GPI in Scottish asylums had escalated since the 1880s.[59] While this rise partly reflected changes in methods of tabulation and partly the establishment of the Scottish Asylums' Pathological Scheme under W. Ford Robertson, it formed the basis of much contemporary criticism of the 'vicious and degenerative impact' of urban values and 'dissipation'. In particular, an apparent disproportionate rise in female GPI in some asylum admissions had reinforced an emerging association within the medical discourse surrounding VD between female sexual promiscuity and 'moral imbecility'.[60] Within this disease model, prostitutes had come to be perceived not just as vectors of disease but a principal source of physical and moral degeneracy.[61] In addition, the promiscuity or 'amateur' prostitution of feeble-minded 'problem girls' was increasingly identified as a central threat to racial health.

The Local Government Board for Scotland remained evasive on the issue of general powers of detention for prostitutes, reluctant to become involved in the contentious politics of sexual and moral behaviour, and sensitive to the fears of some sections of the Scottish vigilance and feminist movements that the more discriminatory aspects of the Contagious Diseases Acts might be resurrected. However, it *was* prepared to endorse proposals under the Mental Deficiency and Lunacy (Scotland) Act of 1913 for the institutionalization of girls who had contracted VD and who were deemed a risk to public health by virtue of their feeble-mindedness or 'moral imbecility'.[62]

A second strand of the campaign against 'immoral traffic', led by the Scottish Churches and social purity groups, centred on securing

27

more effective protection under the Criminal Law for women and girls against sexual exploitation by brothel-keepers and pimps. After a vigorous campaign in the Roman Catholic press, Glasgow magistrates had successfully promoted the Immoral Traffic (Scotland) Act in 1902, significantly increasing the penalties for men living on 'immoral earnings'.[63] In 1906, an Edinburgh Corporation Act extended the penalties for brothel-keeping to every owner, factor, or agent who knowingly let property for the purposes of prostitution.[64] Meanwhile, reflecting the xenophobia surrounding much of the contemporary panic over so-called 'white slavery', Glasgow magistrates sought to deploy existing powers under the 1892 Burgh Police (Scotland) Act in order to secure the deportation of foreign pimps, especially Italians, alleged to be corrupting and abducting Glaswegian girls, often after accosting them in local ice-cream parlours.[65]

Thereafter, a major campaign was launched in the period 1909–12 by vigilance and purity groups to increase further the penalties for procuring and brothel-keeping.[66] Across Scotland, city magistrates came under increasing pressure from church leaders, from the National Vigilance Association [NVA] and the newly established Scottish Council on Public Morals, from women's organizations such as the Women's Temperance Association, and from Poor Law and lock hospital administrators, to undertake a fresh offensive against 'immoral traffic'.[67] Evidence of the history of sexual abuse and exploitation of girls seeking medical treatment for VD, and of their sacrifice to a continuing belief 'among the lower classes that connection with a virgin [would] cure a venereal disease', was widely cited in the press and at a series of public conferences on 'public morals' in support of fresh legislation.[68] By 1910, an Immoral Traffic (Scotland) Amendment Bill had been drafted facilitating the arrest and conviction of pimps and the suppression of brothels and significantly increasing the penalties for procurers. After sustained lobbying of the Lord Advocate and the Scottish Office, the bill was incorporated within the Criminal Law Amendment (White Slave Traffic) Bill of 1912 already being promoted in England.[69] An unintended outcome of this conflation was that flogging was reintroduced to Scots Law in the case of second or subsequent male convictions under the Act.[70]

While a minority of Scottish MPs had libertarian qualms about such penalties, Scottish professional and public opinion generally welcomed them as a just reward for the entrepreneurs of such 'a Devilish trade'.[71] Thus, Dr D. Yellowlees, former Physician Superintendent to Glasgow Royal Asylum, a Director of the Glasgow

Lock Hospital and Chairman of the NVA for Scotland, applauded the introduction of the lash for immoral trafficking. In his view: 'There were some people who could be reached only through their hides. He was quite sure that nothing would be such a deterrent to those miserable scoundrels as a sense of flogging.'[72] There was also a widespread belief, informed by eugenics, that traffickers should be severely sanctioned for facilitating the spread of racial degeneration by 'seek[ing] out innocent girls, the potential mothers of a healthy race, and turn[ing] them against their will into a curse to their generation and to posterity'.[73] Convictions under the Act were closely monitored by the press and purity organizations, and on the eve of the First World War, additional local powers to reduce evasion of its provisions by male pimps were still being sought.[74]

Farmed-Out Houses

In addition, throughout the period 1900–14, Edinburgh and Glasgow Corporations sought, with the support of a variety of religious, medical, philanthropic, judicial and purity groups, to contain the threat of prostitution to public health and morality by the regulation of farmed-out houses. These were houses leased from the owners by so-called 'house-farmers' and sub-let or rented for multiple occupancy for limited periods as furnished apartments.[75] Such houses suffered from acute overcrowding. In the press, and in the deliberations of the police and public health departments, they were identified as a major source of prostitution and VD. According to the Superintendent of Police for the Western District of Glasgow, they were 'hotbeds of vice and immorality and a menace to the welfare of the community'. It was calculated that in Glasgow, some 20 per cent of the inhabitants of farmed-out houses were prostitutes, and that a large proportion of those prosecuted for involvement in 'immoral traffic' resided in these apartments. Evidence obtained under the 1908 Children Act suggested that they were widely used for the purposes of child prostitution and 'the defilement of young girls', and that most of the young women referred to the Lock Hospital by the Parish Councils came directly from farmed-out housing, as did the bulk of male VD admissions to the lock wards of the poorhouses. In the view of the authorities, they constituted a reservoir of vice and disease, 'a great festering mass of humanity, rotten and degraded and obscene, all mixed up together without any control'. In addition, they were perceived as a major source of the 'rapid and alarming increase of general paralysis of the poorer classes'.[76]

As with other local authority initiatives relating to immorality and VD in early twentieth-century Scotland, Glasgow took the lead in attempting to secure greater moral and sanitary controls over farmed-out houses. In 1901, responding to an exposé by the Inspector of Glasgow Parish Council of the 'social evils' arising from the system, the City magistrates successfully promoted a Glasgow Corporation (Police) Provisional Order Bill, sanctioning byelaws to require that persons of different sexes above the age of ten (other than husband and wife) should not occupy the same sleeping apartment.[77] However, the measure remained largely a dead-letter. During 1907–9, under pressure from the presbyteries of the Established and United Free Churches of Scotland, Glasgow and Edinburgh Corporations sought to introduce a Public Health Amendment Bill further regulating the use of farmed-out houses, by excluding from residence young girls under the age of eighteen and persons convicted of prostitution and procuring, with increased penalties for those 'farming' or inhabiting such premises for immoral purposes. However, the Local Government Board for Scotland was reluctant to accept within a local public health measure what in effect represented significant changes in the Criminal Law.[78]

In response to growing moral panic over the incidence and 'racial poisoning' of VD, Aberdeen, Edinburgh and Glasgow continued to press the issue over the period 1909–12 as part of the general 'crusade against immorality' being orchestrated by the press and the Vigilance Associations.[79] Thereafter, frustrated in their efforts to address the issue through public health legislation, each city attempted to smuggle additional powers over farmed-out houses into the miscellaneous provisions of their private Corporation Acts. In 1913, Edinburgh succeeded in obtaining additional powers of access and registration but was forced in Parliamentary Committee to confine its regulations to 'sanitary purposes'. Undeterred, Glasgow's Corporation Bill of 1914 again endeavoured to eliminate prostitution from farmed-out housing. As before, however, while sympathetic to both the health and moral objectives of the promoters, the Scottish Law Officers were not prepared to permit local acts to redefine the role of the State in the highly contentious area of sexual behaviour, and the clauses had to be dropped from the bill.[80]

Ice-Cream Parlours

Meanwhile, in response to widespread public concern at the apparent breakdown in family and community controls over the sexual mores of the younger generation, Scottish social purity groups sought to regulate other alleged sources of 'moral depravity' and disease among the young. A prime example was their ceaseless efforts to regulate the Italian ice-cream shops which formed a major focus for youth culture and entertainment in the cities. Initially, sabbatarian pressures had been primarily responsible for the imposition of byelaws regulating the opening hours of the parlours, but after 1906, a broader moral (and to a significant extent anti-alien) attack on their layout and conduct was launched by community leaders and by the newly established vigilance societies. Along with picture houses and other 'dangerous resorts', the parlours, with their ill-lit, intimate booths and late opening hours, were alleged to be a sinister source of 'venery' and 'moral depravity'. The NVA reported 'gross acts of familiarity between young persons' in the shops. Poor Law and welfare officials identified them as a source of prostitution and VD, and they were commonly cited in evidence submitted to the police by juvenile girls receiving treatment in the lock wards. It was alleged that 'the tone and atmosphere' of such premises 'lowered the moral nature' of young girls and made them 'ready victims' for the procurers and 'white slave traffickers' who also frequented them.[81]

As a result, the Burgh Police (Scotland) Amendment Act was passed in 1911 increasing local authority powers over ice-cream shops with a view 'to their orderly conduct and control'. Subsequent byelaws, as in Glasgow, imposed a set of moral planning controls. The parlours had to have sufficient lighting to enable all customers 'to be distinctly seen by anyone at the front or back of the premises'. To frustrate their use for prostitution, no entry was permitted from the refreshment room to any private dwelling house or living room and no female (unless employed on the premises) was allowed to loiter in the shop. Above all, the refreshment area had to be 'entirely open from back to front and from side to side' and not partitioned into 'compartments' or 'sitting rooms' where illicit intercourse was allegedly rampant.[82] Similar regulations, ensuring access to places of public refreshment for the purposes of moral surveillance, were passed in other urban centres such as Dundee.[83]

Wartime Controls

With the onset of the First World War, such initiatives by moral welfare and purity groups were subsumed within a broader process of moral regulation. The central and local State sought to criminalize and to police female promiscuity, especially that of the newly identified 'amateur' [prostitute], allegedly indulging in gratuitous but unsafe sex, which, it was claimed, threatened to undermine the manhood and efficiency of the nation. As elsewhere in the United

31

Kingdom, numerous allegations emerged in Scotland that young women were infesting military camps, 'preying' upon soldiers, and spreading VD.[84] Three main strategies were adopted to try and counter this perceived threat to the sexual hygiene and military efficiency of troops: the amendment of the Criminal Law, the imposition of controls under the Defence of the Realm Act, and the introduction of women patrols.[85]

Opinion in Scotland over the Criminal Law Amendment Bills of 1917 and 1918 was divided. Public Health Committees generally approved of their repressive clauses against prostitutes and medical clauses penalizing the transmission of VD.[86] However, Scottish Office officials voiced serious reservations. They considered that, given the stigma of contracting VD, few people would accuse others of transmitting the disease. More seriously, it was felt that such coercive measures might deter sufferers from seeking treatment at the new clinics, and that prostitutes would avoid official treatment centres for fear of prosecution.[87] Moreover, as in England, while wanting to restrain and remoralize 'amateurs' and other 'problem girls', many Scottish women's organizations were concerned at the likely discriminatory aspects of punitive purity legislation.[88]

Their fears had already been realized in the arbitrary use by military and police authorities of the Defence of the Realm Act (DORA) to regulate the movement and social intercourse of women.[89] In various towns, curfews and drinking restrictions were placed on women, and police surveillance of servicemen's wives authorized. Due to heavy pressure from feminists, central government ruled such controls illegal but fresh regulations under DORA soon emerged in order to protect the military from VD. In 1916, DORA 13A sanctioned the expulsion of prostitutes from military areas but this failed to address the problem of so-called 'amateurs'. Thus, in March 1918, under mounting pressure from Allied commanders to protect their troops from contamination, the British government introduced a more comprehensive Regulation 40D making it an offence for any woman suffering from VD in a communicable form to have or to solicit sexual intercourse with any member of His Majesty's Forces.

In practice, the law operated in very similar ways to the Contagious Diseases Acts. In order to establish their innocence, women were forced to undergo a medical examination. Conviction rested only on having intercourse while diseased, and did not require proof of actual transmission. Nor was ignorance of infection held to be a legitimate defence, as three cases sentenced before Edinburgh

Sheriff Court in August 1918 clearly indicated. There was a marked absence of safeguards against wrongful accusation, victimization and infringement of civil liberties. As with the Criminal Law Amendment Bills, DORA 40D met with vigorous opposition from libertarian and feminist groups in Scotland. Moreover, given the few cases successfully proceeded against, Scottish Law Officers considered that the cost in social and political disaffection occasioned by the measure far outweighed its benefits to public health, and did not recommend that it be permanently incorporated in the Criminal Law. Faced by mounting opposition in Parliament and the media, orchestrated by the Association for Moral and Social Hygiene, and concerned not to alienate further the mass of newly enfranchised women, the Government revoked the regulation in November 1918.[90]

Meanwhile, voluntary women patrols had been operating in Scotland since the early months of 1915 under the auspices of the Scottish Union of Women Workers, and with official backing from the Scottish Office and from police and military authorities. They had undertaken some positive protective work involving the provision of recreation, training and welfare facilities for girls. However, from the outset, their primary role was one of moral surveillance and control, 'to work in the neighbourhood of camps and other places where troops [were] being trained, with the object of meeting as far as possible the difficulties caused by the presence of women and girls of loose behaviour'. In association with the vigilance and rescue organizations and the police, the patrols sought to contain the sexual urges of girls disinhibited by the 'excitement of war' and their ability to 'contaminate' the forces. The 'silent presence' of patrols on 'moonlight evenings' was designed to break up dangerous liaisons in parks and alleys. Suspected prostitutes were reported to the authorities as were female sexual 'delinquents' who were often institutionalized in 'training homes'. In particular, 'amateurs' suspected of being vectors of VD were identified to the police and troop commanders, and soldiers consorting with them warned of the potential risks.[91]

'Revealing the Skeleton in our National Cupboard':
The Royal Commission on Venereal Diseases:
The Scottish Dimension

However, it was the deliberations of the Royal Commission on Venereal Diseases which came to dominate VD debate and policy after 1913. Recent research has extensively explored the social politics surrounding the origins, proceedings, and recommendations of the Commission.[92] However, it has been mainly analysed from a London perspective, with particular focus on the essentially metropolitan controversy over prophylaxis, and with little regard to evidence submitted from the regions.

The Scottish evidence was curiously limited in its representation. In contrast to its English, Welsh and Irish counterparts, the Local Government Board for Scotland declined to give evidence. Moreover, all the clinical and public health department witnesses from Scotland were based in Glasgow, perhaps reflecting its distinctively pro-active stance towards VD since 1900.[93]

Scottish medical opinion was divided over the issue of the compulsory notification and treatment of VD. Some venereologists, such as Dr Carl Browning, Director of the Laboratory of Clinical Pathology in Glasgow, and Dr J. Kerr-Love, aural surgeon at Glasgow Royal Infirmary, advanced interventionist views. Browning advocated the compulsory notification and treatment of VD in the interests of community health and racial efficiency, with the imposition of Wassermann testing on all hospital patients, and the use of the Infectious Diseases Act to harass and segregate those who defaulted from treatment. Kerr-Love proposed that congenital syphilis be notifiable and that all infected mothers be subject to compulsory treatment.[94]

However, other witnesses advocated a voluntarist strategy towards the problem of VD. Although he personally favoured some form of notification and the criminalization of the wilful transmission of VD, according to Dr John Barlow, President of the Royal Faculty of Physicians and Surgeons of Glasgow, many practitioners were generally opposed to legal controls on the grounds that they would undermine the concept of medical privilege and the confidence of patients in qualified medical practice. Patients would be deterred from seeking early, effective treatment and be more likely to rely on the advice and 'remedies' of quacks.[95] The most influential evidence in favour of voluntarism came from Dr A. K. Chalmers, Medical Officer of Health for Glasgow and President of the Society of Medical Officers of Health. In his view, because of the stigma attached to VD, compulsory notification, even of a confidential type, would prove seriously counter-productive in discouraging patients in the acute, infectious stages of the diseases from obtaining medical advice, and would frustrate recent advances in the local provision of public diagnostic and treatment facilities in some Scottish cities.[96]

Scottish witnesses to the Royal Commission were nonetheless at one in calling for the State-subsidized provision of free and accessible, local authority provisions for the diagnosis and treatment of VD. Where possible, it was hoped to minimize the stigma of attending clinics by locating them within general hospitals and by allowing patients to seek treatment outwith their residential areas. In addition, Scottish evidence stressed the need for venereal diseases to be included in medical training so that general practitioners were more conversant with recent advances in venereology. An educational campaign was also canvassed as a means of reducing the stigma attached to VD, of promoting earlier recourse to treatment, and of eliminating the ignorance which quacks so readily exploited. However, treatment was perceived as the primary means of prevention, with sex instruction and hygiene propaganda an essential but secondary approach.[97]

The subsequent recommendations of the Royal Commission closely conformed to the tenor of the Scottish evidence. While advocating compulsory treatment for infected Poor Law patients and prisoners, and conceding the *prima facie* need to restrain wilful sexual recidivists in the interests of public health, the Commission subscribed to a broadly voluntarist strategy. It advised against compulsory notification, fearing that it would act as a deterrent to early treatment. The major medical recommendations were for the provision by local authorities of free diagnostic and treatment services in negotiation with the general hospitals, the free supply of Salvarsan or its substitutes to general practitioners, and 75 per cent exchequer funding. A ban on the advertisement of remedies for VD was proposed and it was recommended that instruction 'in regard to moral conduct as bearing upon sexual relations' should be provided under the auspices of the National Council for Combating Venereal Diseases [NCCVD].[98]

Initial reaction in Scotland to the Report of the Royal Commission in 1916 was generally favourable. The *Edinburgh Review* welcomed it 'as an event of national importance deserving the attention of all well-wishers of humanity, even in the stress and strain of a world-war'.[99] The Scottish medical press broadly endorsed its proposals and considered it the 'bounden duty of the profession' to 'impress upon the government the necessity of giving immediate effect' to its recommendations, especially in view of the likely impact of the war upon the incidence of VD.[100] Leading Medical Officers of Health, such as A. K. Chalmers, who was a Council member of the NCCVD, were keen to develop the new local authority provisions outlined in the Royal Commission Report. Social purity and feminist groups favoured the treatment scheme, but criticized the recommended limited powers of compulsory detention for Poor Law patients and prisoners as a potential source of sexual discrimination. They were also frustrated at the failure of the Commission to investigate the more systemic socio-economic forces underlying prostitution and VD.[101] Along with the purity lobby, the United Free Church Assembly noted with satisfaction that the Report had concluded that 'no advantage would accrue from a return to the system of the Contagious Diseases Acts'. Its revelations of the incidence of VD and of its impact upon the health and fertility of the nation were viewed by elders as 'one of the great historical disillusioning documents of these times', 'a destructive bomb' which 'had torn down the curtain' which had continued to hang 'over a most disagreeable subject', revealing 'the skeleton in our national cupboard'.[102]

The startling conclusion of the Royal Commission that the 'number of persons ... infected with syphilis, acquired or congenital, [could not] fall below ten per cent of the whole population in the large cities, and the percentage affected by gonorrhoea must greatly exceed this proportion' fuelled contemporary crisis perceptions of VD and its implications for the health, efficiency, and social morality of the nation.[103] As the *Edinburgh Review* observed, with the possible exception of TB and cancer, VD had been revealed as a 'scourge' which was 'chief among the Captains of Death and Disease'.[104] Faced with a growing demand for action, the government used emergency powers under the Public Health Acts to introduce a wide-ranging set of regulations and administrative guidelines for the diagnosis, treatment, and prevention of VD.[105]

The Public Health (Venereal Diseases) Regulations (Scotland) which were to form the legal basis of the Scottish VD Services until the National Health Service (Scotland) Act of 1947, were circulated along with an explanatory memorandum on 31 October 1916.[106] Every local authority was required to prepare and submit for approval a 'scheme' for the diagnosis, treatment and prevention of the 'three great venereal diseases' (syphilis, gonorrhoea, and soft chancre). To ensure more effective diagnosis of VD, medical practitioners were to be provided, 'without difficulty or delay', free access to the existing bacteriological and pathological laboratories of the medical schools, hospitals and local health authorities, and in particular to the technical expertise required for the Wassermann Test for syphilis. Provision had to be made by local authorities for the free and voluntary treatment of VD cases from 'all classes of the community' in hospitals or other institutions or in their homes. It was anticipated that the bulk of cases would be referred by medical practitioners to the hospitals and clinics, but where home treatment was more appropriate, 'skilled assistance by men trained in the technicalities of the modern methods of diagnosis and treatment of the venereal infections' was to be made available to the practitioner 'free of cost to him or his patient'. In addition, practitioners demonstrating proof of competence in the administration of new forms of chemotherapy were to be freely supplied with Salvarsan or its substitutes. In order to attract as many cases as possible, the regulations stressed the vital need for strict confidentiality in dealing with information relating to VD patients, and there were no provisions for any form of notification.

As with the recommendations of the Royal Commission on Venereal Diseases, the Regulations were markedly reticent on the issue of preventive measures other than medical treatment and moral instruction. Mention of alternative strategies involving condoms, prophylactic self-disinfection packets, or the introduction of public ablution centres was significantly absent. Local authorities were merely empowered to provide for 'instructional lectures' and 'the diffusion of information' relating to VD, with priority to be given to its 'far-reaching and disastrous effects on the social efficiency of the family'. To ensure adequate resourcing and expertise, local health authorities were urged to combine in joint schemes and were to receive a Treasury grant-in-aid of 75 per cent of approved expenditure incurred in implementing the Regulations.

Notes

1 *Royal Commission on the Poor Laws and Relief of Distress, [RCPLRD], Oral and Written Evidence from Scottish Witnesses, Parliamentary Papers [PP] 1910 (Cd. 4978) XLVI*, 185.

2 *Local Government Board, Report on Venereal Diseases by Dr R. W. Johnstone, PP 1913 (Cd. 7029) XXXII*, 24.

3 W. H. Brown, 'A Plea for the Early Recognition of Syphilis', *Glasgow Medical Journal [GMJ]*, 94 (1920), 203–5. Thus, many practitioners were taught not to treat a suspected syphilitic sore until after the appearance of 'a secondary eruption'.

4 *Final Report of the Royal Commission on Venereal Diseases [RCVD], PP 1916 (Cd. 8189) XVI*, 41–2; L. W. Harrison, *Medical Practitioners and the Management of Venereal Disease in the Civil Community* (London: National Council for Combating Venereal Diseases [NCCVD], 1919), 4–5.

5 D. Watson, *Gonorrhoea and its Complications in the Male and Female*

(London: Henry Kimpton, 1914), 101.

6   Brown, *op. cit.* (note 3), 203.

7   M. Archibald, 'The Position of the General Practitioner in Anti-Venereal Disease Schemes', *Proceedings of the Imperial Social Hygiene Congress* (London: NCCVD, 1924), 186. See also D. Newman [Surgeon to the Glasgow Royal Infirmary], 'The History and Prevention of Venereal Disease', *GMJ*, 81 (1914), 167–8.

8   J. Woodward, *To Do the Sick no Harm. A Study of the British Voluntary Hospital System to 1875* (London: Routledge and Kegan Paul, 1974), 48–51; G. B. Risse, *Hospital Life in Enlightenment Scotland* (Cambridge: Cambridge University Press, 1986), 125–6.

9   *RCVD, PP 1914 (Cd. 7475) XLIX*, evidence of Dr A. K. Chalmers, Medical Officer of Health for Glasgow, qq. 10474–5; Newman, *op. cit.* (note 7), 168. As Dr Carl Browning, Director of the Laboratory of Clinical Pathology in Glasgow, observed: 'The hospital does not take the patient just at the time when a hospital might be most useful to him' (*RCVD, PP 1914 (Cd. 7475) XLIX*, 231).

10 L. W. Harrison, 'Those were the days! or Random notes on then and now in VD', *Bulletin of the Institute of Technicians in Venereology*, n.d. ? 1950s, Wellcome Institute Library Reprint Collection.

11 See especially, *RCVD, Minutes of Evidence, op. cit.* (note 9), 136–43; O. Checkland, *Philanthropy in Victorian Scotland: Social Welfare and the Voluntary Principle* (Edinburgh: John Donald, 1980), 325. Evidence in criminal proceedings involving the communication of VD to young girls as a result of sexual assault frequently revealed medical ignorance and apathy on the part of hospital staff towards such cases. See, for example, National Archives of Scotland [NAS], AD 15, High Court Precognitions.

12 L. Mahood, *The Magdalenes: Prostitution in the Nineteenth Century* (London: Routledge, 1990).

13 R. Lees, 'The "Lock Wards" of Edinburgh Royal Infirmary', *BJVD*, 37 (1961), 187–9; A. Logan Turner, *Story of a Great Hospital: The Royal Infirmary of Edinburgh* (Edinburgh: Oliver and Boyd, 1937), 273; F. W. Lowndes, *Lock Hospitals and Lock Wards in General Hospitals* (London: J. and A. Churchill, 1882), 20–2.

14 Checkland, *op. cit.* (note 11), 195; Logan Turner, *op. cit.* (note 13), 273–4.

15 C. W. Cathcart, 'Four and a Half Years' Work in the Lock Wards of the Edinburgh Royal Infirmary', in G. A. Gibson *et al.* (eds), *Edinburgh Hospital Reports, Vol. 5* (Edinburgh: Y. J. Pentland, 1898), 337–8; Lees, *op. cit.* (note 13), 188–9.

16 C. H. Browning, 'Investigations of Syphilis as Affecting the Health

of the Community', *British Medical Journal [BMJ]*, 10 Jan. 1914,
81. For a critique of treatment provisions for VD in general hospitals
in England and Wales, see *Local Government Board, Report on
Venereal Diseases, op. cit.* (note 2), 19–21.

17 *RCPLRD, op. cit.* (note 1), q. 56732. These included 43 cases
diagnosed as primary syphilis, 218 as secondary syphilis, and 326 as
'other VD'.

18 See especially, R. Gaffney, 'Poor Law Hospitals 1845–1914', in O.
Checkland and M. Lamb (eds), *Health Care and Social History: The
Glasgow Case* (Aberdeen: Aberdeen University Press, 1982), ch. 3. As
late as 1914, A. K. Chalmers noted the reluctance of local health
authorities 'to expend money out of the rates for treating a class of
disease which they regard[ed] as largely due to personal misconduct'.
See, *RCVD, op. cit.* (note 9), q. 10479.

19 See, for example, *RCPLRD, op. cit.* (note 1), evidence of C. B.
Williams, Inspector of Poor, Aberdeen, qq. 64316–25.

20 *Ibid.*, Appendix XL. See also, J. Walkowitz, *Prostitution and Victorian
Society: Women, Class and the State* (Cambridge: Cambridge
University Press, 1980), 58.

21 Gaffney, *op. cit.* (note 18), 49; *Local Government Board, Report on
Venereal Diseases, op. cit.* (note 2), 21–3. It was common for female
VD patients in poorhouse wards to be made to wear yellow dresses,
hence the nickname 'canary wards'.

22 Gaffney, *op. cit.* (note 18), 49; *RCVD, op. cit.* (note 9), 232–4,
evidence of Dr C. Browning; *op. cit.* (note 4), para. 128.

23 *RCPLRD, op. cit.* (note 1), qq. 56732, 58665, p. 361.

24 Checkland, *op. cit.* (note 11), 195; *Glasgow Herald*, 22 Feb. 1906.

25 Lowndes, *op. cit.* (note 13), 10.

26 *Glasgow Herald*, 22 Feb. 1906; 25 Feb. 1908; 24 Feb. 1910.

27 Mahood, *op. cit.* (note 12), ch. 2.

28 *RCVD, Minutes of Evidence, op. cit.* (note 9), q. 17885; Glasgow
City Archives [GCA], *Annual Reports of Glasgow Lock Hospital,
1904–7, 1910*.

29 Mahood, *op. cit.* (note 12), 126. According to the rules of the
Hospital, patients discharging themselves prematurely would be
denied any further treatment.

30 Checkland, *op. cit.* (note 11), 194; Lowndes, *op. cit.* (note 13), 1.

31 *Glasgow Herald*, 25 Feb. 1908; *RCVD, Minutes of Evidence, op. cit.*
(note 11), 353. Other hospitals were not prepared to 'take depraved
girls of that age' (*Report of Departmental Committee on Reformatory
and Industrial Schools in Scotland, PP 1914–16 (Cd. 7886), Minutes
of Evidence*, q. 5732).

32 RCVD, *Minutes of Evidence, op. cit.* (note 11), q. 7042.

33 Checkland, *op. cit.* (note 11), 195–6.

34 *Report on the Practice of Medicine and Surgery by Unqualified Persons,*
   PP 1910 (Cd. 5422) XLIII, 15–16; RCVD, *Minutes of Evidence, op.*
   cit. (note 9), *PP 1914 (Cd. 7475),* 351. Proceedings in the
   celebrated prosecution of 'Professor' Abraham Eastburn under the
   1917 Venereal Diseases Act reveal such quackery to have been a very
   lucrative and well-organized business both before and after the First
   World War. See *Glasgow Herald,* 25 Feb. 1920. See also below, ch. 4.

35 *Local Government Board, Report on Venereal Diseases, op. cit.* (note 2),
   26.

36 *Report of Departmental Committee on Sickness Benefit Claims under*
   the National Insurance Act, Minutes of Evidence, PP 1914–16 (Cd.
   7690) XXXI, 252; Newman, *op. cit.* (note 7), 67.

37 Watson, *op. cit.* (note 5), vi.

38 A. G. Miller [Surgeon to the Royal Infirmary of Edinburgh], 'Four
   and a Half Years' Experience in the Lock Wards of the Edinburgh
   Royal Infirmary', *Edinburgh Medical Journal [EMJ],* 28 (1882),
   386–403.

39 A. Wheeler and W. R. Jack [Assistant Physician to Glasgow Western
   Infirmary], *Handbook of Medicine and Therapeutics* (Edinburgh: E.
   and S. Livingstone, 1908), 91–2; T. K. Monro [Physician to
   Glasgow Royal Infirmary], *Manual of Medicine* (London: Bailliere,
   Tindall and Cox, 1903), 138–9; *Local Government Board, Report on*
   Venereal Diseases, op. cit. (note 2), 17. Tertiary syphilis, when
   diagnosed, was commonly treated with a solution of iodide of
   potassium along with mercury and a range of 'iron and other tonics'.
   See, Monro, *ibid.,* 134–5.

40 Watson, *op. cit.* (note 5), chs 5, 7; Cathcart, *op. cit.* (note 15),
   343–4; Harrison, *op. cit.* (note 10), 5. In Harrison's view, 'more
   damage was being done by the treatment than by the disease'.

41 It was, in part, the advanced state of the disease in women admitted
   to lock wards and hospitals that prompted efforts by the BMA and
   Royal Medical Colleges in 1899 to obtain a government inquiry into
   the prevalence and treatment of VD. See *BMJ,* 22 April 1899, 984;
   Royal College of Physicians of Edinburgh, Council Minutes, 7
   March 1899.

42 J. H. Muir, *Glasgow in 1901* (Glasgow: William Hodge & Co.,
   1901), 46–7.

43 I. Levitt (ed.), *Government and Social Conditions in Scotland*
   1845–1919 (Edinburgh: Scottish History Society, 1988), xviii–xix,
   xxxviii; I. Levitt, *Poverty and Welfare in Scotland 1890–1948*

(Edinburgh: Edinburgh University Press, 1988), 13, 191–2.

44   C. Dyhouse, 'Working-Class Mothers and Infant Mortality in England, 1895–1914', *Journal of Social History*, 12 (1978), 248.

45   For the broader significance of these conferences in shaping health legislation, see J. L. Brand, *Doctors and the State: The British Medical Profession and Government Action in Public Health, 1870–1912* (Baltimore: Johns Hopkins, 1965), 181–2.

46   Glasgow City Archives [GCA], C1/3/35, C/1/3/40, Health Committee Minutes, 27 June 1906, 24 March 1909; *Dundee Medical Officer of Health* [MOH] *Annual Report, (1908)*, 63; Edinburgh City Archives [ECA], Minutes of Town Council, 14 Jan. 1908. A bill regulating the training and practice of midwifery in Scotland was eventually enacted in 1915.

47   *Local Government Board for Scotland, Report by Thomas F. Dewar on the Incidence of Ophthalmia Neonatorum in Scotland* (Edinburgh: HMSO, 1912), 10–31.

48   *Glasgow MOH Annual Report (1911)*, 21; *(1912)*, 21.

49   *Glasgow MOH Annual Report (1913)*, 30; *RCVD, Minutes of Evidence, PP 1916 (Cd. 8190) XVI*, qq. 17842–3.

50   *Glasgow MOH Annual Report (1913)*, 28–31. Memorandum by Dr A. K. Chalmers on 'Relation of the Public Health Authority to the Treatment of Venereal Diseases', 18 Oct. 1912. Test results indicated that 'about 8% of all classes of children from the poorer classes of Glasgow [gave] a positive reaction'.

51   'Report of Edinburgh Medico-Chirurgical Society', *Lancet*, 13 May 1911, 1279; *RCVD, PP 1916, op. cit.* (note 49), q. 17937, evidence of A. K. Chalmers.

52   *Ibid.*, 30.

53   For an excellent survey of the vigilance and social purity movement in early twentieth-century Scotland, see V. E. Cree, *From Public Streets to Private Life: The Changing Task of Social Work* (Aldershot: Avebury, 1995), ch. 2. For English developments, see L. Bland, *Banishing the Beast: English Feminism and Sexual Morality 1885–1914* (London: Penguin, 1995), 108–10.

54   Mahood, *op. cit.* (note 12), pt 3.

55   GCA, C1/3/33, Magistrates Committee Minutes, 30 Sept. 1904, 4 Sept. 1905; Dundee City Archives [DCA], Town Council Minutes, 22 Feb. 1905.

56   *Glasgow Lock Hospital Annual Report (1906)*, 4; GCA, D–HEW 1.2(20), 'Immoral Houses and Venereal Diseases', by J. R. Motion, Inspector and Clerk, Glasgow Parish Council, Jan. 1911, 29–30.

57   *RCPLRD, op. cit.* (note 1), *Minutes of Evidence*, qq. 57038,

58264–5, 61047; *Final Report, PP 1909 (Cd. 4499) XXXVII*, 276.

58   Lothian Health Services Archives [LHSA], *Annual Reports of the Royal Edinburgh Asylum (1911)*, 14; *(1912)*, 14. For the shifting relationship of VD to GPI as a disease category, see A. Beveridge, 'Madness in Victorian Edinburgh: a study of the patients admitted to the Royal Edinburgh Asylum under Thomas Clouston, 1873–1908', Part II, *History of Psychiatry*, VI (1995), 137–9.

59   This remained, however, a very imprecise disease category. For a discussion of contemporary developments in the nosology of GPI in Scotland, see G. L. Davis, 'The Cruel Madness of Love: Syphilis as a Psychiatric Disorder, Glasgow Royal Asylum 1900–30', University of Glasgow, M. Phil. thesis, (1997), ch. 1.

60   The proportion of admissions to the Royal Edinburgh Asylum attributed to GPI rose from 5.8% in 1874–90 to 10.3% in 1890–1907. Similarly, the proportion of deaths in Scottish asylums attributed to GPI rose from 26.3% in 1880–4 to 47.0% in 1900–4. LHSA, *Royal Edinburgh Asylum, Physician Superintendent's Annual Report (1905)*, 13; *(1907)*, 16–17; *(1911)*, 14–15; *Annual Report of Glasgow Royal Asylum (1904)*, 15; *48th Report of the General Board of Commissioners in Lunacy for Scotland, PP 1906 (Cd. 3021) XXXIX*, lix.

61   For a detailed discussion of this identification of prostitution with moral degeneracy, see M. Spongberg, *Feminizing Venereal Disease: The Body of the Prostitute in Nineteenth-Century Medical Discourse* (Basingstoke: Macmillan Press, 1997), ch. 9.

62   *Public General Acts, 3 and 4 Geo. 5, ch. 38, Mental Deficiency and Lunacy (Scotland) Act, 1913.*

63   GCA, E1/13/13, Minutes of Glasgow Magistrates Committee, 14 May 1902, 26 May 1902, 4 Aug. 1902; *Hansard [HC]* 109, 6 June 1902, cls 11–28; *Public General Acts, 2 Edw. 7, ch. 11, Immoral Traffic (Scotland) Act, 1902.*

64   *Local and Private Acts, 6 Edw. 7, ch. clxiii, Edinburgh Corporation Act, 1906.*

65   GCA, C1/3/35, Minutes of Glasgow Magistrates Committee, 7 and 21 June 1906. For subsequent efforts to target alien offenders, see C1/3/42, Magistrates Committee, 2 Dec. 1909, 27 Jan. 1910. For similar campaigns on the Continent, see A. Corbin, *Women for Hire: Prostitution and Sexuality in France after 1850* (Cambridge, Mass./London: Harvard University Press, 1990), ch. 6; A. Mooij, *Out of Otherness: Characters and Narrators in the Dutch Venereal Disease Debates, 1850–1990* (Amsterdam/Atlanta: Rodopi Press, 1998), ch. 1.

66   Cree, *op. cit.* (note 53), ch. 2; GCA, Misc. Prints, Vol. 40, 'Social

Evil in Glasgow', Report by Chief Constable, Police Procurator-
Fiscal and Town-Clerk Depute, 20 Nov. 1911, 17–19.

67 GCA, C1/3/45–47, Glasgow Magistrates Committee Minutes, 26
Jan. 1911, 23 Nov. 1911, 30 Nov. 1911, 5 Dec. 1911, 4 July 1912;
C1/3/47, Parliamentary Bills Committee Minutes, 11 Nov. 1912;
DCA, Town Council Minutes, 11 March 1911, 11 April 1911;
ECA, Lord Provost's Committee Minutes, 29 March 1911; *Glasgow
Herald*, 8 Feb. 1911, 4 March 1911, 16 Nov. 1911, 1 Dec. 1911, 6
Dec. 1911, 21 Dec. 1911; National Library of Scotland [NLS],
National Vigilance Association for Scotland , Eastern Division
Papers, Executive Committee Minutes; K. M. Boyd, *Scottish Church
Attitudes to Sex, Marriage and the Family 1850–1914* (Edinburgh:
John Donald, 1980), 243.

68 See, for example, *Glasgow Herald*, 19 Feb. 1912. The NVA for
Scotland was established in Glasgow in 1910 very much in response
to case evidence from Glasgow Lock Hospital indicating the large
number of girls infected with VD as a result of sexual assault or
exploitation. See, *Glasgow Herald*, 15 March 1910.

69 GCA, Misc. Prints, Vol. 38, Draft Immoral Traffic (Scotland) Bill,
1910. For the social politics surrounding the issue in England, see E.
Bristow, *Vice and Vigilance: Purity Movements in Britain since 1700*
(Dublin: Gill and Macmillan, 1977), ch. 5; F. Mort, 'Purity,
Feminism and the State: Sexuality and Moral Politics, 1880–1914',
in M. Langan and B. Schwarz (eds), *Crises in the British State
1880–1930* (London: Hutchinson, 1985), ch. 10.

70 *Public General Acts, 2 & 3 Geo. 5,* ch. 20; *Criminal Law Amendment
Act 1912,* clause 5.

71 *Hansard [HC]* 39, 10 June 1912, cls 618–20; 43, 12 Nov. 1912, cls
1845–7, 1885–98, 1908–18, 1938–42; *Glasgow Herald,* 1 March
1912; NLS, NVA for Scotland, Eastern Division Executive
Committee Minutes, Dec. 1912; Boyd, *op. cit.* (note 67), 242–3.

72 *Glasgow Herald,* 13 Feb. 1913.

73 Newman, *op. cit.* (note 7), 176.

74 See GCA, A3/1/267, Glasgow Corporation Act, Provisional Order
Proceedings, 238.

75 See J. Butt, 'Working-Class Housing in Glasgow 1851–1914', in
S. D. Chapman (ed.), *The History of Working-Class Housing* (Newton
Abbot: David and Charles, 1971), 76–9.

76 GCA, A3/1/199, Glasgow Corporation (Police) Provisional Order
Bill 1901, Precognitions for Promoters; A3/1/267, Glasgow
Corporation Order 1914, proofs of J. W. Pratt, MP, Reverend D.
Watson, G. Gillie [Sheriff Officer], P. Fyfe [Chief Sanitary

Inspector]; Proceedings of Inquiry, 170–9. SRA D–HEW 1.2(20),
'Immoral Houses and Venereal Diseases', Minutes of Joint
Conference, 3 Feb. 1911; Boyd, *op. cit.* (note 67), 162–3, 347–8.

77   GCA, A3/1/199, Glasgow Corporation (Police) Provisional Order
Bill, 1901, papers; *Local and Private Acts,* 1 Edw. 7, ch. clxiii.

78   GCA, C1/3/39, Minutes of Special Committee on Farmed-Out
Houses, 14 Oct. 1908; C1/3/40, Parliamentary Bills Committee, 23
Nov. 1908; A3/1/267, Glasgow Corporation Bill, 1914 Proceedings,
172–3; ECA, Town Council Minutes, 5 and 26 Oct. 1909.

79   GCA, Corporation Minutes, 2 Sept. 1910; *Glasgow Herald,* 23 Dec.
1911, 19 Feb. 1912; GCA, D–HEW 1.2(20), 'Immoral Houses and
Venereal Diseases', Minutes of Joint Conference, 3 Feb. 1911; *First
Annual Report of the National Vigilance Association for Scotland
(1910–11),* 11; Boyd, *op. cit.* (note 67), 163.

80   *Local and Private Acts, 3 & 4 Geo. 5, ch. lxxiv, Edinburgh Corporation
Act, 1913*; GCA, A3/1/267, Glasgow Corporation Order 1914, Brief
for Counsel, 41; Papers and Inquiry Proceedings; *Local and Private
Acts, 4 & 5 Geo. 5, ch. clxxviii, Glasgow Corporation Act, 1914.* The
United Free Church Assembly's Church Life and Work Committee
subsequently remarked that it was 'amazing, in face of such a
clamant case for reform, that the Department of State should
maintain a policy of masterly inactivity'. See Boyd, *op. cit.* (note 67),
163. For the continuing association of immorality, VD and housing
regulations in inter-war Scotland, see *Local and Private Acts, 24 Geo.
5, ch. v, Edinburgh Corporation Order Confirmation Act, 1933*;
Glasgow MOH Annual Reports (1921), 109–10; *(1922),* 119–20;
Dundee MOH Annual Reports (1922), 185–6; *(1929),* 185.

81   GCA, E1/13/15–16, Magistrates Committee Minutes, 1 Feb. 1904,
7 Nov. 1904, 28 Aug. 1905; C1/3/46, Glasgow Corporation
Minutes, 11 May 1911, 10 July 1911, 10 Nov. 1911; C1/3/47,
Interlocutor by Sheriff of Lanarkshire, 18 April 1913; *Glasgow
Herald,* 14 Dec. 1911; GCA, Misc. Prints, Vol. 40, 'Social Evil in
Glasgow', *op. cit.* (note 66), 5–8. On the social politics of the
Glasgow ice-cream trade, see F. McKee, 'Ice-Cream and Immorality',
in *Proceedings of the Oxford Symposium on Food and Cookery 1991:
Public Eating* (London: Prospect Books, 1991), 199–205.

82   *Public General Acts, 1 & 2 Geo. 5, ch. 51, Burgh Police (Scotland)
Amendment Act, 1911*; GCA, C1/3/47, Magistrates Sub-Committee
Minutes, 1 April 1912.

83   See, e.g., DCA, Town Clerk's Papers, NCCVD File, copy of Byelaws
with Regard to Places of Public Refreshment, 14 Feb. 1913.

84   NAS, HH 31/16, Correspondence between Scottish Office and

Home Office, Oct. 1914. The Chief Constable of Elginshire protested that 'swarms of young girls are constantly molesting the soldiers'.

85 For the broader UK context of these initiatives, see L. Bland, 'In the name of Protection: the Policing of Women in the First World War', in J. Brophy and C. Smart (eds), *Women-In-Law: Explorations in Law, Family and Sexuality* (London: Routledge and Kegan Paul, 1985), 23–49; L. Bland, '"Cleansing the Portals of Life": The Venereal Disease Campaign in the Early Twentieth Century', in M. Langan and B. Schwarz (eds), *Crises in the British State, 1880–1930* (London: Hutchison, 1985), ch. 9.

86 NAS, HH 65/111, Memorandum on Criminal Law Amendment Bill, 28 Feb. 1917; GCA, C1/3/56, Parliamentary Bills Committee, 21 March 1917. The Bills proposed to make it a criminal offence for a person suffering from VD in a communicable form to (a) have sexual intercourse with any other person, (b) solicit or invite any other person to have sexual intercourse with him or her, (c) wilfully communicate such disease in any manner to any other person. Conviction on indictment would incur penalties of up to two years' imprisonment, with or without hard labour. See, NAS, HH 65/111–12, Draft Criminal Law Amendment Bills, 1917, 1918.

87 NAS, HH 65/111, Papers on Criminal Law Amendment Act 1917. For the response of English health administration to these proposals, see D. Evans, 'Tackling the "Hideous Scourge": The Creation of the Venereal Disease Treatment Centres in Early Twentieth-Century Britain', *Social History of Medicine*, 5 (1992), 429.

88 See, for example, NLS, NVA for Scotland, Eastern Division Executive Committee Minutes, April 1917, 7 Nov. 1918.

89 For a detailed survey of this moral policing in wartime, see C. Haste, *Rules of Desire: Sex in Britain: World War I to the Present* (London: Chatto and Windus, 1992), ch. 3.

90 Bland, 'Cleansing the Portals', *op. cit.* (note 85), 204; ECA, Edinburgh Corporation Public Health Committee Minutes, 26 Nov. 1918, representations from Women's Freedom League; Fawcett Library, AMS/311, File 2, list of cases tried under DORA 40D; NAS, HH 57/566, Home Office Circular to Chief Constables on DORA 40D, 4 April 1918; *Joint Select Committee on the Criminal Law Amendment Bill and Sexual Offences Bill, PP 1918 (142) III*, evidence of Legal Secretary to the Law Advocate, qq. 2783–4. Only one in three cases were proceeded with (*ibid.*, q. 2738).

91 NAS, HH 31/16, Papers relating to Women Patrols Committee for Scotland 1915–17. For similar patterns of surveillance in England,

see Bland, 'In the name of Protection', *op. cit.* (note 85), 33–9.

92 See, for example, R. Davenport-Hines, *Sex, Death and Punishment: Attitudes to Sex and Sexuality in Britain since the Renaissance*, ch. 6; Evans, *op. cit.* (note 87), 413–33.

93 The Royal Colleges of Physicians and Surgeons of Edinburgh were scheduled to prepare a submission along with the Faculty of Medicine but no evidence appears to have been presented. Edinburgh University Library, DA43, Faculty of Medicine Minutes, 6 Jan. 1914, 27 Jan. 1914.

94 *RCVD, Minutes of Evidence, op. cit.* (note 1), qq. 4210–7; 6960–71. For similar views of Scottish clinicians expressed in the medical press, see *BMJ*, 7 Jan. 1911, 55; 8 Aug. 1914, 283–4; *EMJ*, 10 (1913), Editorial, 385–6; Newman, *op. cit.* (note 7), 100, 171–3, 177–8. Some asylum physicians, concerned at the apparent rise in syphilis-related admissions arising from 'urban degeneration', advocated additional controls to enable the medical profession to enforce the completion of treatment regimes for early, acute cases of VD and to prevent the marriage and procreation of the unfit. See, LHSA, *Royal Edinburgh Asylum, Annual Report (1912)*, 14; A. Beveridge, 'Thomas Clouston and the Edinburgh School of Psychiatry', in G. E. Berrios and H. Freeman (eds), *150 Years of British Psychiatry* (London: Gaskell, 1991), 379; *Royal Commission on Divorce and Matrimonial Causes, PP 1912–13 (Cd. 6481) XX*, 4, evidence of Sir Thomas Clouston.

95 *RCVD, op. cit.* (note 49), qq. 19198–19207, 19330. The Faculty itself had rejected a motion for anonymous notification but supported a proposal for the 'knowing' communication of VD to be created a criminal offence. See, Minutes of Faculty of Royal College of Physicians and Surgeons of Glasgow, 6 April 1914.

96 *RCVD, op. cit.* (note 9), q. 10568; *op. cit.* (note 49), qq. 17872–3, 17884, 18021. Earlier evidence by W. Leslie Mackenzie, [Medical Member of the LGB for Scotland] to the Royal Commission on the Poor Laws and Relief of Distress, *op. cit.* (note 1), 185, would suggest that, while the Local Government Board for Scotland conceded that compulsory controls would in principle be entirely consistent with the protection of public health, they feared that, in practice, it would deter acute cases from seeking treatment and would not reduce the incidence of VD.

97 *RCVD, op. cit.* (note 9), qq. 4213–14, 4336, 7098, 7190, 7205, 10453, 10463–4, 10482–507, 10573, 10805; *Final Report, op. cit.* (note 49), qq. 17891, 18012.

98 *RCVD, op. cit.* (note 4), 50–3, 70, 84–7.

 99 *Edinburgh Review*, 223 (1916), editorial, 356.

100 *EMJ*, 16 (1916), 322; *GMJ*, 85 (1916), 414–15.

101 *Annual Report of the National Vigilance Association for Scotland (1916)*, 11.

102 *United Free Church General Assembly, Debates (1917)*, 236; Boyd, *op. cit.* (note 67), 244–5.

103 *RCVD, Final Report, op. cit.* (note 4), 23.

104 *Edinburgh Review*, 223 (1916), editorial, 363.

105 For the politics surrounding government action, see Evans, *op. cit.* (note 87), 420–1; Davenport-Hines, *op. cit.* (note 92), 222–3.

106 *Local Government Board for Scotland, Venereal Diseases: Circulars Issued by the Local Government Board for Scotland on 31st October 1916* (Edinburgh: HMSO, 1916).

3

The Establishment of a VD Service

An Overview

Responsibility for preparing local schemes under the 1916 Scottish VD Regulations rested with the Public Health Committee of each local authority. In practice, the Medical Officer of Health undertook the organization, usually in consultation with the medical staff of the local hospitals and laboratories, and with representatives of local general practitioners, normally nominated by the local branch of the British Medical Association [BMA]. A range of constraints operated to frustrate the aims of the Scottish Board of Health [SBH] in the early and formative years of the VD service. On the one hand, it was faced with a massive backlog of disease previously untreated and 'the high prevalence of the more recent infections arising both at home and overseas during wartime'.[1] As a result, the early centres were overwhelmed with cases before they could become properly established.[2] On the other hand, during wartime and the period of post-war reconstruction, there was an acute shortage of medical staff, and of the physical resources for accommodating the new clinics.[3]

Despite sustained pressure from the Infectious Diseases Section of the SBH, headed by Dr Thomas Dewar, many Scottish local authorities were reluctant to establish VD schemes. Thirty per cent of local authorities had still not made any 'effective effort to comply with the regulations' by 1921 and there was an acute lack of facilities in rural areas.[4] The reasons were various. Despite substantial Treasury subsidies, the free provision of treatment for a disease widely stigmatized as the outcome of wilful promiscuity was at odds with the moral sensibilities and economy-mindedness of many local councillors and ratepayers. Local authorities were also seriously concerned at the financial implications of reciprocal agreements under joint VD schemes where there might be a net inflow of VD patients, especially in the major urban treatment centres.[5] Another major constraint was the reluctance of certain local health authorities to 'face the facts and admit the need for special arrangements'.[6] As

Thomas Dewar lamented in 1923, by virtue of their 'age, usual vocations, and social status', public health committee councillors were usually ignorant of the local incidence of VD. As a result:

> it is very hard to convince them that either syphilis or gonorrhoea is other than rare or at most quite exceptional in their respective districts. To the County Councillors of Inverdonshire or the Town Councillors of Dunnitwell, it were useless to quote the estimates given in the Report of the Royal Commission. "Oh," they will say, "these figures are for London, that abandoned place; they cannot possibly apply to Scotland."[7]

However, as in England, the overriding constraint on local authority initiatives in Scotland was frequently resistance from the voluntary hospitals, whose co-operation was vital to the viability of any VD scheme.[8] Some hospital committees, such as the Medical Committee of the Glasgow Samaritan Hospital, objected to instituting the new treatment centres on the grounds that the admission of venereal patients would contravene their constitutions and otherwise 'contaminate' their wards.[9] Other hospital directors were concerned that hospital autonomy and the status of honorary medical staff would be threatened by the VD schemes, with their emphasis on state-subsidized, free treatment and their heavy involvement of public health officers, often by implication, claiming recognition for a new area of expertise.[10] Resistance to the municipal provision of VD treatment centres also became increasingly subsumed within the wider conflict between the general hospitals and local health authorities over the reorganization of the Scottish hospital services.[11]

Meanwhile, institutions such as Glasgow Royal Infirmary and the Northern Infirmary, Inverness, pleaded acute accommodation problems when pressed to extend their facilities for in-patient care and for out-patient clinics.[12] Early refusal by the Treasury and Ministry of Health to subsidize local authority expenditure on the treatment of 'non-communicable' cases of VD also served to create friction between the infirmaries and public health committees.[13] Moreover, even where hospital authorities proved receptive to the erection of new VD clinics and/or the conversion of existing premises, such proposals were seriously delayed by the moratorium on public expenditure for additional grant-aided public health services operating under the Government's policy of retrenchment from 1921 to 1924.[14] As a result, as Dewar later admitted, the early achievements of the VD Service in Scotland were often 'a demonstration of the triumph of zeal and clinical and psychological capacity over material disadvantages'.[15]

An important outcome of the constraints and protracted negotiations surrounding the establishment of the VD centres was that each evolved 'according to local circumstances' with 'no approach to uniformity either in general situation or in design'. By the mid-1920s, some, as at Kilmarnock and Dunfermline, were in premises converted and administered directly by the local authority. A few, as at Ayr, Kirkcaldy and Motherwell, were in poorhouses or poorhouse hospitals; while the remainder, which comprised the majority, were attached to general hospitals or infirmaries. At some centres, both sexes were treated at different hours. Others dealt with one sex only. Little children of both sexes suffering from congenital syphilis were usually treated at the women's clinics. A number of centres provided treatment for out-patients only, while a few were exclusively for in-patients. In Glasgow, there were special clinics purely for juvenile patients and for those suffering from syphilitic infections of the eye.[16]

The original intention of the SBH that treatment centres should normally be integrated with the general hospitals had to be abandoned given their frequent unwillingness or inability to provide facilities. It had been feared that separate centres openly dedicated to the treatment of syphilis and gonorrhoea would be the focus of social stigma and notoriety, if not actual blackmail, and deter patients from seeking medical attention. However, the evident popularity of the Broomielaw Centre in Glasgow, set up to serve the seafaring population but rapidly frequented by the wider community, served to dispel such fears. As a result, although the SBH continued to stress the financial, clinical and research benefits of VD clinics being incorporated within hospital facilities for related medical and surgical diseases,[17] by the mid-1920s, an increasing number of so-called *'ad hoc'* clinics were being established, most notably in Constitution Road, Dundee, and in Black Street, Glasgow.[18]

Despite such compromises, by 1927, Scotland had been provided with a wide-ranging system of VD medical services. There were still some notable gaps, such as at Inverness, Clydebank, Falkirk, the textile towns of the Borders, and some of the north-eastern fishing ports, but some forty-nine treatment centres had been established. These included clinics in Glasgow (16), Edinburgh (6), Aberdeen (2), Dundee (4), Lanarkshire (5), Leith (1), Ayrshire (3), Fife (3), Stirling (1), Arbroath (1), Dumfries (1), Invergordon(1), Paisley (1), Greenock (1), Perth (1), Banff (1), and Lerwick (1).[19] In the more sparsely populated areas of the Highlands and Islands, the SBH hoped to rely on local practitioners, especially trained in the more modern methods of VD diagnosis and treatment.[20]

Certain VD centres, such as those in Glasgow, were provided by one local authority. However, their work was not restricted, as with the TB and child welfare clinics, to the population of the immediate area. For example, Glasgow centres investigated and treated cases coming from the whole of the south-west of Scotland. More usually, to ensure adequate resources, expertise and cost-efficiency, local authorities were grouped for the purposes of the VD regulations into collaborative VD schemes. Thus, forty-eight local authorities in north-east Scotland were grouped together with treatment centres at Aberdeen and Banff. The Fife and Kinross Joint Scheme with centres at Kirkcaldy and Dunfermline combined thirty-four local authorities, while another Joint Committee co-ordinated VD administration for the City of Edinburgh, the Lothians, and Peeblesshire. In order to create a fully integrated network of treatment opportunities and to preserve the confidentiality of patients, the SBH had gradually persuaded most schemes to dispense with inter-area accounting for patients seeking treatment outwith their local authorities.[21]

Each major VD scheme was provided with approved laboratory facilities for the examination of smears, purulent secretions and blood specimens, but due to its technical complexities, the Wassermann Test was confined to a small number of selected laboratories. In order to expedite diagnosis and treatment of primary syphilis, the larger treatment centres also often undertook simpler laboratory work as part of their routine examination of patients.[22]

Consequently, both Treasury and local authority funded expenditure on VD diagnosis, propaganda, and treatment rose from a mere £875 in 1917–18 to £78,000 by 1927–8. A dramatic increase in the use of the service during its first decade was reflected in a number of indicators. Despite a chronic shortage of accommodation, attendances rose by 112 per cent over the period 1920–8 *(see Figure 3:1)*, while in-patient days for VD patients treated under the 1916 Regulations rose over the same period by 69 per cent. Meanwhile, the number of specimens examined and Wassermann Tests undertaken more than doubled, as did the number of doses of Arzenobenzol compounds administered to patients.[23]

As the treatment centres continued to expand in the mid-1920s, they provided increasingly specialized facilities. In the major cities, many clinics were established in maternity and child welfare centres as a means of reducing the incidence of congenital infections.[24]

Likewise, centres such as the Broomielaw in Glasgow and Leith VD Centre were established to target seamen who were widely regarded as prime vectors of VD. The growing realization of the extent of default from treatment and of the 'sociological' problems inherent in securing the compliance of patients with often protracted and painful therapies also led to the appointment of staff for follow-up work and to rudimentary efforts at contact tracing.[25]

The operation of the various clinics varied enormously, according to the facilities and staff resource available and to the commitment and medical ideology of the senior medical officers. At a typical centre, separate sessions were held for males and females. Those for males were held once or twice a week, or on a daily basis in the large city centres. On arrival, the new patient was given an identification number by which thereafter he/she was known to ensure confidentiality, and personal details including age, address and frequently occupation and method of referral were entered onto a record sheet. Increasingly, note was also taken of the relationship of the patient to other cases (for example, whether a relative or a consort), and of whether the patient had previously defaulted on treatment. After medical examination, details of the preliminary diagnosis and recommended treatment were also recorded and the

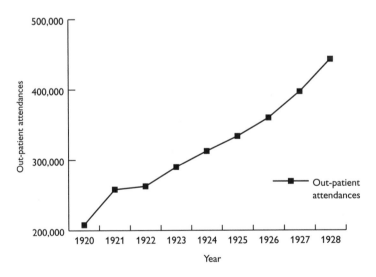

Figure 3.1
Out-Patient Attendances at Scottish VD Centres 1920–28
(*Source:* SBH Annual Reports)

prescribed treatment/tests duly performed.[26] In the larger centres, several doctors might be simultaneously engaged on examination, urethroscopy, intravenous injection, the performance of lumbar puncture, or minor operative treatment. Meanwhile, in another part of the clinic, under the supervision of an attendant, irrigation would be performed for cases of gonorrhoea.[27]

Given the varied history and location of the VD centres, their layout was inevitably diverse. Nonetheless, some of the principles that shaped the design of many of the new VD wards and *ad hoc* clinics established in Scotland between the wars *can* be discerned. The basic design of some of the major facilities such as Ward 45 at the Royal Infirmary of Edinburgh, Black Street Clinic in Glasgow and Dundee's Public Health Institute, was inspired by the ideas and example of Colonel L. W. Harrison, fleetingly designated as the Clinical Medical Officer in Charge of Edinburgh's VD Scheme in 1919 before becoming Special Adviser on Venereal Diseases to the Ministry of Health. A concern for medical efficiency and surveillance, and a desire to minimize social stigma and maximize patient compliance with treatment regimes, underpinned the spatial arrangement of the treatment centres. As a ground-floor plan of Glasgow's Black Street VD Clinic, *(see Plate 3.1)* built in 1926, and plans of the Public Health Institute in Dundee demonstrate,

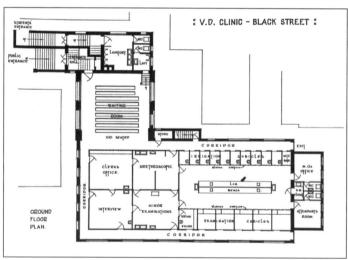

Plate 3.1

Plan of Black Street VD clinic in Glasgow
(Glasgow MOH Annual Report (1927))

54

panoptic principles were retained enabling the senior clinician to enjoy a commanding view of the patients undergoing treatment.[28] The growing emphasis of social hygienists upon recording and monitoring patterns of social contact was also reflected in the space allocated for interviewing patients and for their case records.[29]

In designing the centres, particular stress was placed upon the rapid handling of patients so as to minimize the social stigma and possible demoralization associated with lengthy waiting periods. As Dundee's VD Medical Officer observed, provisions for immediate interviewing greatly improved attendance records as new cases were less likely to be intimidated by the 'misconceived humour' of more seasoned patients.[30] Curiously, one of the central and most progressive features of the so-called 'Harrison clinics', that of individual examination and irrigation cubicles ensuring some degree of privacy but with open access to the clinician, was modelled on the layout and social psychology of the pawnbroker's. In times of student penury, Harrison had had recourse to such establishments, and his clinics borrowed their basic formula for reducing social stigma; 'a passage from which a number of small cubicles opened' but which shared in common 'a counter at which the transaction could be arranged', thus enabling the broker to keep a close eye on all the clients, but without the need for them to see one another.[31]

Glasgow

The architect of Glasgow's VD Treatment Scheme was its Medical Officer of Health, Dr A. K. Chalmers, and the Special Sub-Committee on the Treatment of Venereal Diseases, established in 1917.[32] By 1919, an assortment of treatment facilities had been established at the Royal, Western and Victoria Infirmaries, at the Hospital for Women (the Lock Hospital), Baird Street Reception House, and Bellahouston Dispensary.[33] The case-load was enormous. In addition to the large number of beds within Glasgow's hospital system already occupied by patients suffering from the more advanced symptoms of VD, there were in 1919 some 748 new in-patient cases involving 24,465 days' residence, and 4976 out-patients involving 47,127 attendances. Although case numbers began to fall after 1922–3, the introduction of new, more systematic diagnostic and therapeutic regimes, significantly lengthening the average duration of treatment, created a continuing escalation in demand upon resources.[34]

In line with guidelines from the SBH, Chalmers endeavoured to negotiate for the centres to be located within the major general hospitals, but the task proved extremely protracted. Reflecting on his efforts in 1918 at a conference convened by the National Council for

Combating Venereal Diseases, Chalmers observed that the core of the problem was that it was

> a new thing entirely for a general hospital, or its dispensary, to regard itself as responsible for providing the accommodation which a local authority may require; it takes some time to get the directorate accustomed to a position of that sort .... The Hospital Authorities have not themselves been sufficiently alive to the new burden laid on them and, whether by lack of accommodation or constitution, they are apathetic; and you have not the enthusiasm in the hospital world to provide accommodation of this sort.[35]

As a result, treatment facilities for both in-patients and out-patients at the Infirmaries remained grossly inadequate. In particular, lack of waiting facilities, shared accommodation with general wards, an acute shortage of irrigation facilities for gonorrhoea patients, and a lack of evening sessions accessible to those in employment, served to accentuate the inconvenience and stigma of out-patient treatment. In response, Chalmers opted for the local authority provision of *'ad hoc'* clinics. Thus, treatment for women and children was provided at Baird Street Reception House, while the inability of the Royal Infirmary to cope with the special needs of the seafaring population led to the opening of an *'ad hoc'* clinic at Broomielaw in 1919. The Broomielaw clinic proved exceptionally successful, in attracting not only seamen, but also patients from the surrounding community. As a result, its share of Glasgow's out-patient VD cases increased from 2 per cent in 1919 to 24 per cent in 1925, and it became a role model for the development of *ad hoc* provisions throughout Scotland.

When the Royal Infirmary subsequently withdrew from the VD Scheme after abortive negotiations by the Public Health Department and the SBH to persuade the Directors to make adequate provision for VD patients, its out-patient work was duly transferred to a newly established *'ad hoc'* 'Harrison' clinic in Black Street[36] *(see Plate 3.2)*. Consequently, the share of out-patient cases treated by the *'ad hoc'* clinics rose from 22 per cent in 1922 to 74 per cent by 1928.[37] However, a major disadvantage of these arrangements was that specialists within the clinics were increasingly distanced from infirmary physicians treating the late sequelae of VD, in contrast to the more integrated regimes in Edinburgh and London. In addition, the Infirmaries lost easy access to clinical material for student and postgraduate training in venereology.[38]

Another important development was the increased targeting of resources for the treatment of women and children, in response partly

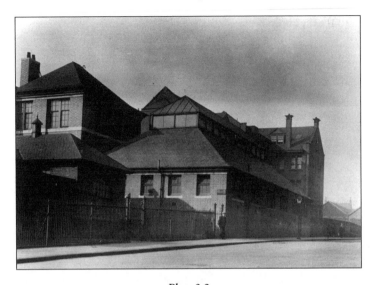

Plate 3.2
Black Street VD Clinic in 1929
(courtesy of Greater Glasgow Health Board Archives)

to sustained lobbying from women's organizations and partly to growing evidence that women were failing to seek treatment in the earlier stages of their disease, especially for gonorrhoea.[39] Provisions at the Lock Hospital were substantially upgraded. By 1928, it was furnished with 63 beds in eight wards, including a Children's Ward and a Maternity Ward. New, well-equipped out-patient facilities had also been secured and the hospital had become a recognized teaching and research centre for VD.[40] In an attempt to reduce the incidence of congenital infection by encouraging more mothers to undergo treatment, the Public Health Committee decided in 1925 to extend the role of the Child Welfare Centres in the diagnosis and treatment of adult female VD. In 1928, a new clinic was also established in the out-patient department of the Royal Maternity Hospital for the treatment of VD in pregnant women. In addition, from the mid-1920s, the VD Scheme attached a nurse visitor to the female clinics to follow up on defaulters and to perform the functions of a 'social almoner' for patients needing 'moral' or logistical support.[41]

Dundee

For similar reasons, the process of establishing an effective VD Scheme in Dundee proved equally protracted.[42] From 1917, male and female clinics were conducted in the out-patient department of the Royal Infirmary, but the accommodation remained 'hopelessly inadequate' despite lengthy negotiations between the Infirmary and the Public Health Committee. The female centre was only allocated one small room 14 ft by 8 ft and the occasional use of two other very small rooms. Irrigation facilities for gonorrhoea patients were minimal, with some 30–50 patients a day being treated in a room of 11 ft by 4.5 ft,[43] creating delay and congestion and adding to the stress and stigma, and this was duly reflected in the comparatively low attendance levels of female patients.[44] Indoor treatment provisions were equally unsatisfactory with only two beds notionally allocated for male VD patients and six for female patients, all within the ordinary surgical wards. The unsuitability of the premises 'seriously inhibited' the instruction of students in the diagnosis and treatment of VD.

Under pressure from the SBH to establish an integrated treatment centre, Dr W. L. Burgess, Medical Officer of Health, and the Public Health Committee, undertook lengthy negotiations with the Royal Infirmary to try and establish a proper treatment centre either within or adjacent to the Infirmary, but to no avail. The Infirmary pleaded absence of space and funding, but evidence suggests that there was also an underlying reluctance on the part of medical staff to co-operate with local authority initiatives and to recognize the need for the appointment of specialist medical officers for VD work.[45] In 1919, a Special Medical Officer *was* appointed part-time, but due to an escalation in the number of attendances, he was forced to employ two medical assistants at his own expense.

By 1921–2, the Public Health Committee had decided that, whatever the advantages of an integrated centre, it was no longer feasible. It duly appointed a full-time Special Medical Officer, Dr A. C. Profeit. To test the efficiency of a self-contained *'ad hoc'* treatment centre before incurring heavy capital expenditure, the male VD treatment centre was transferred to temporary premises at the Reception House in Fleuchar Street, Polepark.[46] Meanwhile, despite continuing reservations, especially with regard to the lack of in-patient facilities for cases with acute gonorrhoea, the treatment centre for women continued to be attached to the Infirmary, not only for 'reasons of privacy, but also because of the undoubted advantage of being in close touch with a maternity hospital and gynaecological department'.[47] However, an increasing amount of female treatment was also provided at a special clinic established by the Public Health Department in 1922 at the Child Welfare Centre, under the control of a full-time, female Special Medical Officer, appointed to oversee the women's section of Dundee's VD Scheme.

Despite these initiatives, the Scheme continued to suffer from inadequate resources. The Centre at Fleuchar Street was too distant from the city centre and Royal Infirmary for patients and medical students. It suffered from an extremely exposed public entrance and had very limited in-patient facilities. In addition, the lack of proper accommodation for the treatment of female cases at the Infirmary continued to impair the quality of medical care and specialist training, and in 1926, in-patient cases were transferred to King's Cross Hospital.[48] Among other factors, the lack of a properly co-ordinated and resourced VD scheme was clearly affecting the level of attendances and may have contributed to the disturbingly low proportion of patients seeking treatment in the early, acute phases of their infections as well as to the paucity of cases of congenital syphilis receiving treatment.[49]

Nonetheless, by 1924, the Medical Officer of Health was convinced that the Fleuchar Street *'ad hoc'* experiment had succeeded and that 'the Local Authority need have no hesitation in proceeding with a permanent *"ad hoc"* VD treatment centre'.[50] Accordingly, the Public Health Department proceeded to plan for the establishment of a new Public Health Institute in Constitution Road to include a tuberculosis dispensary, VD centres for male and female patients, and a ward for the indoor treatment of male VD patients.[51] The Institute was eventually opened in 1928, with an up-to-date irrigation department divided for privacy into cubicles, and with a room for the application of new techniques such as diathermy for chronic cases of gonorrhoea. The impact of new facilities on the quality and quantity of treatment undertaken and on its uptake by the local community was dramatic. Between 1927 and 1930, out-patient attendances within the VD Scheme rose by nearly 51 per cent and in-patient days by as much as 450 per cent. Contemporary observers certainly viewed these rises as a product of institutional change rather than of any substantive shift in the prevalence of VD.[52]

Aberdeen

The development of VD provisions in Aberdeen suffered from similar constraints.[53] By 1919, the SBH had approved a Joint Scheme for Aberdeen City and the North-Eastern Counties (including the Counties of Aberdeen, Banff, Kincardine, Elgin, and Nairn) to which Orkney and Zetland were subsequently added.[54] The chief treatment centre was housed at Aberdeen Royal Infirmary under the supervision of a Chief Medical Officer, the dermatologist, Dr J. F. Christie, and a sub-centre established at the City Hospital. In no other Scottish city was VD work contracted out to the same degree. In Glasgow, while part of the work was contracted out to the voluntary hospitals, a main municipal centre was also established. In Edinburgh, the VD Centre at the Royal Infirmary was from the beginning very much a municipal centre jointly staffed and controlled by Edinburgh Town Council. In Dundee, the undertaking became almost wholly a municipal one. In contrast, in Aberdeen, the Royal Infirmary and its Directors continued to dominate VD provisions and policy well into the 1920s.[55]

However, the accommodation provided for VD treatment at the Infirmary remained inadequate. Although Christie had been promised a new building with proper in-patient and out-patient facilities, these had still not materialized in 1928.[56] The only addition to the ordinary Skin Out-Patient Department was 'one room and a dark, small one (used as an office)'.[57] Lack of space and apparatus for irrigation meant that 'the main mass of gonorrhoeal infection in Aberdeen women remain[ed] untreated'.[58] Lack of facilities and medical status within the Infirmary led to a high turnover of junior VD medical officers in the early years of the scheme, which undermined the confidence of patients already demoralized by the atmosphere of the general dispensary.[59] As a result, although there was no evidence of a lower prevalence of VD in Aberdeen than in other cities, its treatment centres undertook markedly less work than those elsewhere. In the years 1919–23, an average of 5.9 per 1000 population received treatment in Glasgow, 6.2 per 1000 in Edinburgh, 7.7 per 1000 in Dundee, but only 3.6 per 1000 in Aberdeen.[60]

As in Glasgow and Dundee, from 1922, the Medical Officer of Health for Aberdeen, J. Parlane Kinloch, with increasing support from Thomas Dewar, Medical Officer of the SBH, pressed for a new VD treatment centre to be built outwith the Infirmary within a municipal hospital, as part of a general reform of the city's hospital facilities.[61] Kinloch argued that it was 'the atmosphere and environment of the dispensary of a general hospital' which was 'inimical to successful results':

> The dispensaries of the general hospitals are primarily organised on a charitable basis to provide certain clearly defined and limited curative service for the deserving poor, and in such surroundings, any communal health service, and especially such a communal

service as that relating to venereal disease with its peculiar problems, must almost inevitably languish.[62]

It was evident that, given the physical and ideological constraints of the Infirmary, the major potential for upgrading facilities lay in developing a second major treatment centre at the City Hospital. The Directors of the Aberdeen Royal Infirmary fought a determined rearguard action to abort this proposal.[63] While they conceded the urgent need for new accommodation, they were adamant that given 'the protean nature of venereal infections' and the need for VD medical officers to have access to a range of specialisms, treatment should remain predominantly based at the Infirmary and that the City Hospital should at most remain a sub-centre 'retained for the class of case for which it was originally intended'.[64] Moreover, they clearly viewed Parlane's proposals as indicative of a more general attempt by the public health authorities to undermine the medical and civic status of the Infirmary within Aberdeen.

However, while continuing to contract much of the VD work to the Infirmary, as part of the reform of the statutory hospital services in Aberdeen, the Public Health Department were determined to develop a second main treatment centre to respond to the evident gaps in existing VD provisions under the Scheme, even if this meant 'subvert[ing] a certain section of medical authority within the City'.[65] As a result, the City Hospital's share of both cases and attendances rose from a mere 1 per cent in 1923 to nearly 25 per cent in 1928 along with a significant upgrading of its serological and bacteriological services.

Edinburgh

Although Edinburgh's VD Scheme was widely cited as a role model for co-operation between local authorities and the voluntary hospitals, its development was shaped by very similar impulses and constraints. As elsewhere, the expansion of VD provisions was the outcome of protracted negotiation between public health and hospital authorities, between VD clinicians and other specialties, and between the aims of social hygienists and the financial limitations of public sector economies.[66]

After extensive consultations with the Managers of the Royal Infirmary and the major women's hospitals, with the Edinburgh Committee of the BMA, with the Royal Colleges of Physicians and Surgeons, with the Medical Faculty of the University, and with other interested groups such as the Medical Guild and the Scottish Association of Medical Women, the Corporation's scheme was inaugurated on 1 March 1919.[67] From the start, the Scheme was dominated by the Royal Infirmary which accounted in the early years for *c.*85 per cent of all male and female out-patient attendances and for some 65 per cent of in-patient admissions. Arrangements were made with the Bruntsfield Hospital for Women to treat married women and children and with the Royal Maternity Hospital for the treatment of ante-natal cases.[68] Out-patient clinics for women and children were also opened at the Corporation's child welfare centres at Windsor Street and Grove Street (later removed to Torphichen Street).[69] The Scheme was also made available to patients from Leith and from all local authorities in the Lothians, and reciprocal arrangements concluded with other Schemes in the Borders and in Fife.

The distinguished venereologist, Colonel L. W. Harrison, was appointed as the first Clinical Medical Officer in charge of the Edinburgh Scheme, but before he could take up his duties, he was appointed Special Adviser on VD to the English Ministry of Health. In his place, Dr David Lees was jointly appointed as specialist in VD to Edinburgh Corporation, as honorary consultant to the Infirmary, and (in 1920) as the first University Lecturer in Venereal Diseases. Over the next fifteen years, Lees was to create in Edinburgh one of the foremost centres of venereology in Britain and, as a clinician, teacher and social hygienist, to influence significantly the medical practice and social politics surrounding VD in interwar Scotland.[70]

As in Dundee, Glasgow and Aberdeen, however, the escalation in attendances in the early years of the Scheme, fuelled by the backlog of demand for treatment, created major problems of accommodation and staff resourcing. As late as 1920, at the Royal Infirmary, 'all treatment of men was done in one small theatre adjoining the ward' and overcrowding was such that 'privacy, asepsis, and detailed examination were almost impossible'.[71] Only one patient could use the irrigation facilities at any one time and only then by entering through the operating theatre. One small side room was allotted for the treatment of female out-patients who, in the absence of any waiting room, had to sit on the staircase landing.[72] Conditions were every bit as bad at the Royal Maternity Hospital, where the 'swabbing' and other treatment of venereal cases were carried out in a tiny labour theatre (10 ft by 12 ft) in which deliveries were simultaneously taking place.[73] As the SBH noted, there was an acute shortage of in-patient provisions for women, while the lack of a separate clinic for seamen in Leith put intolerable strain on the out-patient facilities at the Infirmary.[74]

As a result of urgent representations from Lees, a temporary wooden hut was erected for out-patients at the Infirmary adjoining the male ward, with cubicles for examination and treatment and separate rooms for injections, urethral irrigations and microscopic diagnosis, along the lines of Harrison's earlier proposals.[75] Insofar as government expenditure cuts would permit, the existing male and female wards at the Infirmary were upgraded and additional medical, nursing and support staff added to the establishment, including two assistant clinical medical officers and additional staff to cope with the very significant increase in pathological work.[76]

As a means of alleviating the shortage of beds in the female VD wards at the Infirmary and Royal Maternity Hospital, and of reducing the stigma attached to such hospital treatment, Lees also campaigned for additional beds to be allocated in general wards for unspecified 'Diseases of Women and Children'. Accordingly, in 1923, beds were made available at the Municipal Hospital in Pilton. This departure proved especially valuable in treating ophthalmia neonatorum as both mother and child could be hospitalized until cured. It also enabled the syphilitic pregnant woman to have a longer period of hospital treatment than was possible in the maternity hospitals.[77] In 1927, a new ward and additional out-patient clinics were also established at the Elsie Inglis Memorial Maternity Hospital, despite the concern of some of its management committee that this might 'demoralise' ordinary patients.[78] Lees also secured the appointment of a lady almoner to monitor and follow up female patients who discontinued treatment, viewing the appointment as a precursor of the notification and compulsory treatment of defaulters and a means of ensuring a more effective use of public expenditure on the VD clinics.[79]

Another significant addition to the provisions of the Edinburgh VD Scheme was the opening in 1926 of an out-patient treatment centre for seamen at The Shore, Leith.[80] Unfortunately, the clinic was a converted shop on the ground floor of a tenement so that the householders in the flats above could watch patients going in and out, and children frequently played around the entrance and ran into the waiting room. The subsequent opening of a Labour Exchange immediately opposite the clinic further undermined the privacy of patients.[81] However, as with the Broomielaw Centre in Glasgow, the Leith dispensary attracted a large clientele not only from the docks but also from the surrounding communities, and by the mid-1930s was accounting for *c*.15 per cent of all out-patient attendances in Edinburgh.

Despite the international reputation of Lees and the VD

Department, medical facilities for VD treatment in Edinburgh still reflected the low status accorded to the specialty by other clinicians and hospital administrators. The problem of staff resourcing was somewhat eased in 1928 when an honorarium was approved for the hitherto unpaid clinical assistants and house surgeons in the VD wards of the Infirmary.[82] Nonetheless, the 'shoddy reconstructed and badly fitted hut' erected as Ward 45 in 1919 continued to serve as the VD Department despite its cramped and inadequate accommodation[83] *(see Plates 3.3 and 3.4)*. Moreover, despite a five-fold increase in the number of attendances since 1919, no new, paid medical staff had been appointed to the female VD Department.[84]

In 1931, in view of continuing reservations of the Infirmaries' Directors over plans for a new treatment centre, the Public Health Committee seriously considered establishing 'an independent department for the diagnosis and treatment of Venereal Diseases within the City'.[85] However, there were compelling reasons for retaining the centre within the Infirmary. As patients of the Infirmary, those infected with VD could avoid some of the stigma of attending an identifiable clinic and thus 'diminish the risk of loss of employment or damaging of family relationships'. Emphasis was also laid on the fact that many cases were sent in the first place to the medical and surgical out-patient departments of the Infirmary and

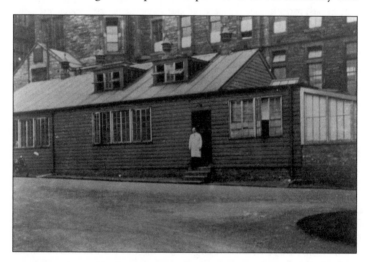

Plate 3.3
Joseph Patterson, outside Ward 45, Royal Infirmary of Edinburgh, 1920s
(courtesy of Lothian Health Services Archives)

were referred from there to the VD Department for diagnosis and treatment, and that an integrated VD Centre could more easily consult with a range of specialists in related fields such as ophthalmology, dermatology and gynaecology. In addition, it was felt that the central location of the Infirmary would continue to facilitate early treatment.[86] Accordingly, a new 'Special Pavilion' was opened in the Infirmary grounds in 1936, funded by the Corporation, 'designed to embrace every modern improvement', and housing both male and female wards and out-patient clinics *(see Plate 3.5)*. At the same time, increasing provision for VD patients was being made at municipal hospitals such as the Western and Northern General.

Provisions for Merchant Seamen

From the outset, Scottish health officials identified merchant seamen as primary victims and vectors of VD and as requiring special treatment provisions. The option of introducing compulsory segregation and treatment for infected seamen was briefly considered but rejected as too disruptive to shipping.[87] Instead, most health authorities, such as in Glasgow and Edinburgh, opted for the provision of clinics within easy reach of the docks, as at Bellahouston and Leith.[88]

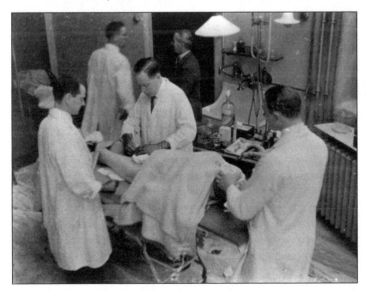

Plate 3.4
Robert Lees operating in Ward 45, Royal Infirmary of Edinburgh, *c.*1935
(courtesy of Dr Lorna Lees)

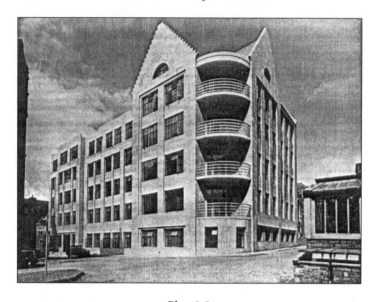

Plate 3.5
The New Dermatology and Venereal Diseases Pavilion, Royal Infirmary of
Edinburgh, 1936 (*Edinburgh Medical Journal* (1936))

In addition, from 1925, Scottish port authorities were party to an
international agreement (the Brussels Agreement) for the treatment
of seamen suffering from VD. Under the agreement, facilities were
established at ports for the free treatment of merchant seamen,
without distinction of nationality. Such facilities included out-
patient treatment, in-patient treatment where necessary, and the
provision of sufficient medical supplies to carry out necessary
treatment during the voyage to the next port of call. Each patient was
issued with a special medical record card registering details of
diagnosis, serological tests and prescribed treatment, and Port
Sanitary Officers were charged with distributing information on
treatment facilities to crews on their arrival.[89] Under the auspices of
the British Social Hygiene Council, initiatives were also taken to try
and encourage Scottish local authorities to develop recreational
facilities for seamen and to ensure adequate and 'decent' on-shore
sleeping accommodation. In addition, a range of propaganda leaflets
was issued designed to impress upon seafarers the serious
repercussions of sexual promiscuity and self-treatment for their
health and that of their families.[90]

In general, provisions at Scottish ports worked tolerably well.

However, major problems remained in ensuring continuity and consistency in the treatment of seamen. Arsenobenzol was rarily administered by ships' medical officers who relied on a policy of 'temporizing' until infected crew reached port. Seamen often concealed their infections from ships' surgeons for fear of victimization from their employers or from other members of the crew. Provisions in overseas ports for British seamen with syphilis were often inadequate and despite the use of record cards, treatment was rarely integrated with previous therapy and serological tests undertaken in the United Kingdom. Treatment of chronic gonorrhoea presented particular difficulties. Seamen were normally in port too briefly to secure systematic examination and a proper course of treatment, and they were not prepared to undergo in-patient therapy for fear of losing their jobs. There were rarely irrigation facilities on board ship and frequent recourse was had to clumsy and damaging attempts at self-disinfection.[91] One Scottish marine officer later claimed that he had cured four of his crew by making them 'drink a glass of gin with as much saltpetre as would lie on a 6d in it, three times a day'.[92]

Provisions for Prisoners

Another area of concern for health officials and social hygiene activists was the provision of adequate diagnostic and treatment facilities for prisoners. This was motivated less by concern for the health of individual prisoners than by the belief that the criminal population harboured some of the most persistent defaulters and sexual recidivists. Their incarceration was viewed as a prime opportunity to administer continuous and effective treatment and to regulate some of the key vectors of VD who were endangering public health.

Prior to 1914, the diagnosis and treatment of VD in Scottish prisons had varied greatly.[93] The prime concern was to try and prevent the spread of infection within the prison population. The most common procedure, endorsed by official circulars in 1907 and 1914, had been to isolate patients with venereal discharges on admission and to give them separate utensils, clothing, and bedding, and where possible, separate toilet and washing facilities. Prison warders had been encouraged to inspect clothing and bedding regularly and to report any 'suspicious stains' to the Prison Medical Officer. Within the prisons, there had been no application of the Wassermann Test or of Salvarsan therapy, in part because Prison Medical Officers lacked the medical expertise, and in part for reasons of expense and prevailing concepts of 'less-eligibility' surrounding the welfare rights of prisoners.[94]

As W. J. H. Sinclair, Medical Officer of HMP Barlinnie, revealed to the Royal Commission on Venereal Diseases in 1914, for most prisoners on shorter sentences, treatment was either non-existent or incomplete, with the result that they were discharged infected back into the community. In his opinion, there was an urgent need for an upgrading of prison medical procedures for VD and for greater integration of prison and local authority provisions.[95] In the event, this proved to be a slow and arduous process. In 1919, the SBH and Prison Commission negotiated for the new VD Schemes to be made available to prisoners under escort. However, evidence would suggest that the bulk of non-surgical treatment continued to be conducted by Prison Medical Officers who remained fiercely protective of their medical authority.[96]

Throughout the 1920s, there was continuing criticism from social hygiene activists and prisoners' welfare groups, increasingly supported by health officials, that prisoners were not receiving adequate treatment in jail and therefore posed, on their release, a potent threat to public health. While prepared to investigate individual complaints, the Scottish Prison Commissioners were primarily concerned to protect the medical autonomy of their Medical Officers against what they viewed as 'ill-informed gossip'.[97] Substantive evidence is lacking of prison facilities for venereal patients in the 1930s. There are indications that, apart from Barlinnie, Scottish prison authorities increasingly relied upon local authority VD clinics.[98] However, there are also indications that for many prisoners with VD, including those whose disease was latent, solitary confinement remained a common experience.[99]

Notes

1   M. W. Adler, 'The Terrible Peril: A Historical Perspective on the Venereal Diseases', *British Medical Journal [BMJ]*, 19 July 1980, 208.

2   Edinburgh Royal Infirmary Clinic dealt with 2,117 new cases in 1919, while 5,724 new cases attended centres in the Glasgow VD Scheme: *Glasgow Medical Officer of Health [MOH] Report (1920)*, 81; *Edinburgh Public Health Department [EPHD], Annual Report (1920)*, 55.

3   'The British Venereal Disease Service 1916–66', *British Journal of Venereal Diseases [BJVD]*, 42 (1966), 223.

4   *Scottish Board of Health [SBH], Second Annual Report, PP 1921 (Cmd. 1319) XIII*, 41; Central Medical Archive Centre [CMAC], SA/BSH/DI/2, Minutes of Medical Committee of National Council for Combating Venereal Diseases [NCCVD], 11 June 1923.

5   See, e.g., Edinburgh City Archives [ECA], Minutes of Edinburgh Corporation VD Sub-Committee, 28 July 1920; Fife Council Archives, 3/40/1, Minutes of Fife and Kinross Venereal Diseases Joint Committee, 8 May 1923.

6   *SBH, Second Annual Report, op. cit.* (note 4), 41.

7   T. Dewar, 'On the Incidence of Venereal Disease in Scotland', *Edinburgh Medical Journal [EMJ]*, 30 (1923), 313–14.

8   *Glasgow Herald*, 3 Dec. 1921; D. Evans, 'Tackling the "Hideous Scourge": The Creation of the Venereal Disease Treatment Centres in Early Twentieth-Century Britain', *Social History of Medicine*, 5 (1992), 424–5.

9   *Scottish Local Government Board, Annual Report for 1918, PP 1919 (Cmd. 230) XXV*, xii; Glasgow City Archives [GCA], C1/3/57, Minutes of Special Committee on the Treatment of VD, 18 June 1917.

10 Dundee City Archives [DCA], Town Clerk's Correspondence, Transcript of Conference, 18 June 1918, 8. For a discussion of the relationship of the VD regulations to the status of venereology as a specialty in interwar Scotland, see below, ch. 4.

11 For a review of this conflict, see I. Levitt, *Poverty and Welfare in Scotland* (Edinburgh: Edinburgh University Press, 1988), 152–9.

12 *SBH, Second Annual Report, op. cit.* (note 4), 41; *Third Annual Report, PP 1922 (Cmd. 1697) VIII*, 24.

13 In Whitehall's view, the issue was not one of individual cure but the wider public health issue of the prevention of the transmission of VD. See, Public Record Office [PRO], MH 55/178, Memo. by F. J. Coutts, 13 Dec. 1920. In May 1920, due to the difficulty of distinguishing between communicable and non-communicable phases of syphilis, local authorities were advised that VD schemes should treat 'all cases requiring anti-syphilitic treatment' with the exception of cases of GPI, (*SBH, Second Annual Report, op. cit.* (note 4), 45).

14 ECA, Minutes of Edinburgh Public Health Committee [PHC], 18 March 1924; *Dundee MOH Annual Report (1920)*, 86.

15 *SBH, Eighth Annual Report, PP 1928 (Cmd. 2881) X*, 112.

16 *SBH, Sixth Annual Report, PP 1924–5 (Cmd. 2416) XIII*, 63; *Ninth Annual Report, PP 1928 (Cmd. 3112) X*, 111.

17 See especially, *SBH, Hospital Services (Scotland) Committee. Report on the Hospital Services of Scotland* (Edinburgh: HMSO, 1926), 29–30. There was particular concern that the expansion of the statutory health services, and the consequent migration of medical provisions for particular diseases such as VD to local authority hospitals, would undermine the training and research of the medical teaching schools.

(*Ibid.*, 36).

18 See especially, *SBH, Ninth Annual Report, op. cit.* (note 15), x, 111–12.

19 *Ibid.*, 113.

20 *SBH, Sixth Annual Report, op. cit.* (note 16), 64.

21 *Ibid.*, 63; *Ninth Annual Report, op. cit.* (note 16), 110–11.

22 *SBH, Sixth Annual Report, op. cit.* (note 16), 63, 67; *Ninth Annual Report, op. cit.* (note 16), 114.

23 *SBH, Annual Reports for 1920–8.*

24 *Glasgow MOH Annual Report (1926)*, 155–8; *EPHD, Annual Report (1920)*, xx; *Dundee MOH Annual Report (1924)*, 116.

25 For details, see below, ch. 5.

26 See, e.g., Royal Infirmary of Edinburgh [RIE], VD Registers.

27 See especially, *SBH, Sixth Annual Report, op. cit.* (note 16), 64–5.

28 *Glasgow MOH Annual Report (1927)*, 142; DCA, City Architect's Office, Sept. 1926, Plans of Public Health Institute.

29 For a fuller discussion of these issues, see below, ch. 5. See also D. Armstrong, *Political Anatomy of the Body: Medical Knowledge in Britain in the Twentieth Century* (Cambridge: Cambridge University Press, 1983), ch. 2.

30 *Dundee MOH Annual Report (1928)*, 131.

31 A. King, 'The Life and Times of Colonel Harrison', *BJVD*, 50 (1974), 395.

32 Unless otherwise specified, the following account is based upon the *Glasgow MOH Annual Reports*; *SBH, Annual Reports*; GCA, C/1/3/57–99, Minutes of the PHC and Sub-Committees, 1917–39; R. A. Cage, 'Sexually Transmitted Diseases and the Economic Historian: Lessons from the Glasgow Experience', University of Queensland, Department of Economics, Discussion Paper 92 (1992).

33 For a detailed breakdown of treatment provisions in Glasgow during the period 1918–28, see Appendix 1.

34 The average number of days' residence for in-patients rose from 32.7 in 1919 to 43.2 in 1925. Over the same period, the average number of attendances of out-patients rose from 9.5 in 1919, to 26.8 in 1925, and the number of pathological examinations undertaken for the VD Scheme doubled.

35 DCA, Town Clerk's Correspondence, File NCCVD 1918. Significantly, the main concern of the conference was to 'stimulate the interest and increase the co-operation of the medical profession in the campaign against VD'.

36 The withdrawal of the Infirmary from the Scheme was partly related to a long-standing dispute with the SBH over the funding of

treatment for non-communicable cases of VD. See especially, GCA, C1/3/66, Minutes of Glasgow PHC, 15 Feb. 1922.

37 During the period 1918–28, over 80% of in-patient treatment was concentrated at the female Lock Hospital, or, for males, at the Royal Infirmary (1917–25) and Belvidere Hospital (1926 onwards).

38 W. G. Clark [Assistant Medical Officer of Health for Glasgow], 'Modern Aspects of Syphilis in Special and General Practice', *GMJ*, 107 (1927), 162–3.

39 VD returns for 1923 reveal that, whereas the ratio of male/female out-patients was 3:1, for in-patients with more chronic symptoms, the ratio was 1:2. While the estimated ratio of gonorrhoea/syphilis in the general population was 3 or 4:1, the ratio amongst new female cases in Glasgow treatment centres was only of the order of 0.5:1.

40 J. F. Fergus, 'The Glasgow Hospitals of a Century Ago', *GMJ*, *Centenary Number 1828–1928*, 173–4.

41 See especially, *Glasgow MOH Annual Report (1925)*, 141.

42 Unless otherwise specified, the following account is based upon *Dundee MOH Annual Reports; SBH, Annual Reports; DCA*, Minutes of PHC; Town Clerk's Correspondence, File 344. For details of the initial scheme, see especially, Minutes of PHC, 5 Feb. 1917, 4 June 1917, 21 Aug. 1917, 28 Aug. 1917, 27 Nov. 1920.

43 *Dundee MOH Annual Report (1919)*, 60.

44 In 1919, male attendances for gonorrhoea were 2275 as compared with 68 for women (*ibid.*, 53).

45 DCA, Minutes of Dundee PHC, 17 July 1919.

46 *Dundee MOH Annual Report (1922)*, 41.

47 *Dundee MOH Annual Report (1922)*, 41; *(1923)*, 132.

48 *Ibid. (1923)*, 132.

49 *Ibid. (1924)*, 123; *(1925)*, 122. It was estimated that only 10% of gonorrhoea patients were attending for early treatment while some 80% of new syphilis cases had either 'well marked secondary syphilis' or its 'late manifestations'.

50 *Ibid. (1924)*, 50.

51 Indoor treatment of female patients was carried out largely at Maryfield Hospital.

52 *Dundee MOH Annual Report (1929)*, 24. The only significant shift in the location of VD treatment provisions in the 1930s was the transfer of all male in-patients in 1934 from the Public Health Institute to Maryfield Hospital (*ibid, (1934)*, 111).

53 Unless otherwise specified, the following account is based upon *SBH, Annual Reports; Aberdeen MOH Annual Reports;* I. Levack and H. Dudley, *Aberdeen Royal Infirmary: The People's Hospital of the*

North-East (London: Bailliere Tindall, 1992); Northern Health Services Archives [NHSA], Box 1/15/6; 1/1/42, Minutes of Aberdeen Royal Infirmary [ARI], Medical Committee.

54   For details of the approved scheme, see *Aberdeen MOH Report for the years 1916–21*, 156–63.

55   During the period 1918–24, the Infirmary accounted for 95% of all attendances under the Scheme.

56   NHSA, 1/15/6, Dr J. F. Christie to ARI Board of Directors, 26 June 1928.

57   *Aberdeen MOH Annual Report (1925)*, 125; NHSA, 1/15/6, J. F. Christie to ARI Board of Directors, 26 June 1928.

58   NHSA, *Aberdeen PHC Minutes*, 31 March 1926; *Aberdeen MOH Annual Report (1924)*, 126.

59   *Ibid., (1922–3)*, 85; NHSA, 1/15/6, J. F. Christie to Chairman of ARI Board, 16 May 1923.

60   *Aberdeen MOH Annual Report (1922–3)*, 83.

61   *Ibid.*, 86; *Annual Report (1924)*, 83–104.

62   NHSA, ARI Admin. Files Misc., Report by J. P. Kinloch on 'Present Requirements and Future Development of the Municipal Health Services', 6 Oct. 1924.

63   For details of this resistance, see NHSA, 1/15/6, Memoranda and Minutes of the Board of Management of ARI with reference to the treatment of Venereal Diseases, 1916–26.

64   NHSA, 1/1/42, Minutes of Medical Committee of ARI, 11 Jan. 1926; *Aberdeen MOH Annual Report (1927)*, 7–9.

65   *Ibid.*, 1.

66   Unless otherwise specified, the following case study is based upon *SBH, Annual Reports*; *EPHD Annual Reports*; ECA, Minutes of the Edinburgh PHC and Special Schemes Sub-Committee; H. P. Tait, *A Doctor and Two Policemen. The History of Edinburgh Health Department 1862–1974* (Edinburgh Public Health Department: Mackenzie and Storrie, 1974); A. Logan Turner, *Story of a Great Hospital: The Royal Infirmary of Edinburgh 1729–1929* (Edinburgh: Oliver and Boyd, 1937); Edinburgh University Library [EUL], Special Collections, Gen 2161, G. H. Percival, 'Some Aspects of the Development of Dermatology with Special Reference to the Contribution of the Edinburgh Medical School'.

67   For details, see ECA, PHC Papers, A. Maxwell Williamson, 'Scheme for the Prevention and Treatment of Venereal Diseases in Edinburgh', 12 July 1917; PHC Minutes, 24 July 1917, 5 Dec. 1917.

68   For a detailed account of the role of Bruntsfield Hospital in Edinburgh's interwar VD provisions, see E. Thomson, 'Women in

Medicine in Late-Nineteenth and Early-Twentieth-Century Edinburgh: A Case Study', University of Edinburgh, Ph.D. thesis (1998), 244–82.

69   For a detailed breakdown of VD provisions in Edinburgh, see Appendices 2–4.

70   For details of his background, ideology and impact, see below, chs 4 and 5.

71   R. Lees, 'The "Lock Wards" of Edinburgh Royal Infirmary', *BJVD*, 37 (1961), 189.

72   ECA, EPHD Files, 15/34, DRT 14, D. Lees to PHC, 25 Nov. 1919.

73   LHSA, LHB 3/30/2, Dr F. J. Browne to Messrs Scott and Patterson, 29 May 1924.

74   ECA, Minutes of Edinburgh Special Schemes Sub-Committee, 25 Jan. 1921, 15 Feb. 1921.

75   ECA, Minutes of Edinburgh PHC, 31 Jan. 1919, 3 Feb. 1919.

76   *EPHD Annual Report (1920)*, 53; ECA, Edinburgh Sub-Committee on VD, 27 Nov. 1919, 4 June 1920. In the closing months of 1919, pathological reports to the VD Department constituted *c.*70% of reports issued to the whole hospital.

77   D. Lees, 'Methods of Securing the Maximum Efficiency of a Venereal Disease Clinic', *Proceedings of the Imperial Social Hygiene Congress* (London: NCCVD, 1924), 142; D. Lees, 'Prevention of Congenital Syphilis: Sociological Problems', *Health and Empire*, Vol. 1, No. 3 (Sept. 1926), 186. See also, Thomson, *op. cit.* (note 68), 259.

78   LHSA, LHB 8/11/1/10, Transcript notes on the History of the VD Department at Bruntsfield Hospital and Elsie Inglis Memorial Maternity Hospital, n.d.; ECA, Minutes of Edinburgh PHC, 11 Oct. 1927.

79   ECA, Minutes of Special Schemes Sub-Committee, 15 April 1924.

80   See especially, *EPHD Annual Report (1926)*, 56. Prior to the amalgamation of Leith with the City of Edinburgh, it had been planned to establish a VD centre at Leith Hospital under the direction of the Port Assistant Medical Officer. However, subsequent negotiations between the Medical Officer of Health and the Hospital Directors proved abortive. ECA, Minutes of Special Schemes Sub-Committee, 23 Sept. 1924.

81   *EPHD Annual Report (1937)*, 102.

82   ECA, Minutes of Edinburgh PHC, 17 Jan. 1928.

83   D. Lees, *op. cit.* (note 77), 136; LHSA, LHB 1/2/48, Royal Infirmary of Edinburgh [RIE], Minutes of Medical Managers' Committee, 6 March 1929.

84 ECA, Public Health Series 10/3, Report by Dr D. Lees on letters from Dr Mary Liston, April 1928.

85 ECA, Minutes of Special Sub-Committee on RIE VD Out-Patient Department, 7 April 1931.

86 'The Royal Infirmary of Edinburgh: The New Dermatological and Special Pavilion', *EMJ*, 43 (1936), 465–9.

87 *Glasgow MOH Annual Report (1914–19)*, 102.

88 Under the Merchant Shipping Acts (Amendment) Act of 1923, shipowners were made liable in law for any medical expenses of masters and seamen suffering from VD.

89 NAS, HH 65/127/17, SBH Circular on International Agreement for the Treatment of Seamen Suffering from Venereal Disease, 17 Dec. 1925.

90 NAS, HH 65/127/15, BSHC, *The Seafarer's Chart of Healthy Manhood* (1925); HH 65/127/25, Minutes of Meeting in Edinburgh on the Problem of the Mercantile Marine, 13 Sept. 1926. For a detailed content analysis of this propaganda material, see below, ch. 6.

91 NAS, HH 65/127/64, Memorandum on the working in Scotland of the Brussels Venereal Diseases Agreement, 29 Sept. 1932; HH 65/127/81, Minute on 'Brussels arrangement of 1924 relating to the facilities to be given to merchant seamen for the treatment of venereal diseases', 30 March 1933.

92 H. P. Taylor, *A Shetland Parish Doctor: Some Recollections of a Shetland Parish Doctor during the past half century* (Lerwick: T. and J. Manson, 1948), 130–1.

93 For details, see NAS, HH 57/566, Prison Commission for Scotland, Treatment of Venereal Diseases in Prisons: General Questions, 1907–23.

94 *Royal Commission on Venereal Diseases, Minutes of Evidence, PP 1916 (Cd. 8190), XVI*, q. 20,091.

95 *Ibid.*, 253–5.

96 See especially, NAS, HH 57/566.

97 *Ibid.*, Prison Commissioners for Scotland to SBH, 7 April 1921; SBH to Scottish Branch of Howard League for Penal Reform, 23 Feb. 1923.

98 See, e.g., the steady rise in prisoners attending the RIE clinic (RIE, VD Registers).

99 NAS, HH 57/567, Treatment of Venereal Diseases in Prison: General Questions, 1930–46.

4

'The Cinderella Service':
Doctors, Patients and Therapies in Interwar Scotland

Patterns of Treatment

Treatment in the Clinics and Hospitals: Syphilis

While treatment regimes for VD in interwar Scotland varied significantly between the different medical centres and even between clinics within the same VD Scheme,[1] some general patterns of therapy can be identified. Already by 1916, the use of Salvarsan or its substitutes (officially designated arsenobenzol compounds) had become standard practice in the treatment of early syphilis. Although it had been anticipated that Salvarsan compounds would entirely replace mercury, in fact in the early 1920s the complementary use of mercury and Neo-Salvarsan (914) was commonly held to be more effective.[2] However, by the mid-1920s, attempts were being made to replace mercury with less toxic and debilitating bismuth preparations.[3]

The need for intensive and prolonged courses of treatment and follow-up to ensure the eradication of the *spirochaete* also became commonly accepted by health administrators and clinicians. In the words of Thomas Dewar, Medical Officer of the Scottish Board of Health [SBH], in 1925, the Salvarsan treatment of syphilis had to be 'pushed with vigour and continued for long'.[4] Thus, a patient with primary syphilis in the Edinburgh and Dundee schemes, however slight the infection, would, unless they defaulted, be kept under observation for at least three years until intensive treatment with intramuscular and intravenous injections had been completed and both Wassermann Tests and lumbar punctures had yielded negative results for at least two years.[5]

The main shifts in treatment regimes for early syphilis in the 1930s focused around the desire to standardize procedures and to reduce the duration and toxicity of the administration of arsenobenzol compounds. Some of the worst immediate side-effects of treatment which had necessitated the provision of a rest room in each clinic had been removed by the mid-1920s, in part due to the replacement of the original Salvarsan (606) by the administration of 'the safer and less formidable' Neo-Salvarsan (914).[6] However, medium- and long-term side-effects such as jaundice and skin diseases continued to plague the VD clinics. Thus, in the Black Street, Broomielaw and Bellahouston Clinics in Glasgow in 1931, some 9 per cent of patients developed jaundice and 5 per cent developed skin diseases.[7] New preparations such as Acetylarsan were explored to try and reduce the incidence of such effects. In addition, in the later 1930s, the major VD schemes gradually adopted more intensive, standardized regimes of treatment based on a series of intermittent rather than continuous courses of Neo-Salvarsan (914) and metallic bismuth. The duration and dosages of treatment continued to vary, often reflecting variance between Scottish venereologists in their definitions of cure and non-infectivity,[8] but there was, in general, a significant reduction in the length of active treatment for early syphilis.[9]

During the 1930s, particular attention was also directed by Scottish clinicians to refining ante-natal 'prophylactic' treatment for pregnant women and developing effective arsenical therapies for children with congenital syphilis which did least damage to their vital organs. Increasingly, maternity hospitals and ante-natal clinics introduced routine Wassermann testing and liaised with the adult VD clinics to identify and monitor children in what were perceived to be high-risk families.[10]

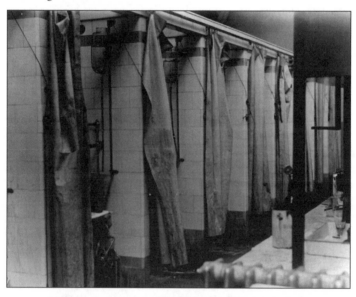

Plate 4.1
Interior of Black Street Clinic in 1929, showing irrigation cubicles
(courtesy of Greater Glasgow Health Board Archives)

Meanwhile, clinicians had extended their use of some of the newer forms of therapy for tertiary and neuro-syphilis. Despite its side-effects, Tryparsamide, an organic arsenic compound, increasingly displaced mercury, iodide of potassium and sedatives in the treatment of syphilitic infections of the central nervous system.[11] In addition, in the major infirmaries and asylums, patients with general paralysis of the insane and locomotor ataxia were increasingly subjected to induced malarial therapy, including the use of monkey malaria, designed to burn out the venereal disease through high-temperature fevers.[12] The proportion of GPI patients admitted to Scottish asylums who were treated solely by means of induced malaria therapy rose from 3 per cent in 1923 to 27 per cent in 1931.[13] While a proper scientific understanding of these therapies was lacking, beyond a vague appreciation that 'one malady sometimes ha[d] the effect of checking another', venereologists claimed that they had transformed the prognosis for patients suffering from neuro-syphilis; their former lot of 'a progressive mental and physical decline through bed-ridden helpless imbecility to inevitable and early death' being replaced in many cases with recovery and rehabilitation into society and employment.[14] According to Dr David Henderson, Physician-Superintendent of Glasgow Royal Asylum, 'astounding and beneficial results' justified malarial therapy 'in every patient suffering from general paralysis who show[ed] a reasonable chance of betterment',[15] and these sentiments were shared by Dr George Robertson at the Royal Edinburgh Asylum.[16]

Treatment in the Clinics and Hospitals: Gonorrhoea

Until the late 1930s, advances in the treatment of gonorrhoea were far less dramatic than those for syphilis. The diagnosis of gonorrhoea was improved by the adoption of new bacteriological and serological techniques, and tests of cure became somewhat more reliable, especially after the introduction of a complement fixation blood test analogous to the Wassermann reaction. But there was no chemo-therapeutic agent comparable with '914' which could ensure the early destruction of the gonococcus and lessen the duration and infectivity of the disease. As a result, for the bulk of the interwar period, gonorrhoea patients in Scotland underwent 'a fearsome series of dilatations, applications of caustic, antiseptic and astringent chemicals, and instrumental investigation of varied types'.[17] Treatment for acute gonorrhoea centred upon urethral irrigation or 'lavage' with strong antiseptic solutions such as potassium permanganate or acriflavin. Irrigation was by syringe and later by gravity from bottles hung two and a half to three feet above the patient's pelvis *(see Plate 4.1)*. In addition, patients were prescribed a strict regime of abstinence from strenuous exercise, alcohol, rich diet, and sexual stimulation.[18]

In cases of chronic gonorrhoea, 'provocative' injections of gonococcus vaccine were also administered, although there was considerable scepticism amongst some clinicians as to its efficacy.[19] In addition, increasing use was made of electro-therapy or diathermy involving the insertion of electrically heated metal bougies and rods. This was a very imprecise medical technology and clinicians freely admitted their ignorance of its precise impact upon the gonococcus or infected tissues.[20] Meanwhile, VD and child welfare clinics were also concerned to implement obligatory procedures laid down by the Central Midwives Board for the prevention and treatment of gonorrhoeal ophthalmia in infants, by the application of a solution of silver nitrate within the eyelids of every child whose birth was attended.[21]

There were no dramatic shifts in treatment regimes for gonorrhoea in the early 1930s. However, there was increasing awareness of the damage done by existing therapies. Irrigation had been 'frequently abused and badly carried out with too much force and too strong antiseptics' and had frequently resulted 'in damage to the lining of the urethra and subsequent stricture formation' along with a range of secondary infections.[22] In an attempt to reduce these side-effects, Scottish clinicians experimented in the early 1930s with new forms of injected gonococcal vaccines and with a wider variety of irrigation solutions. In addition, there was an increasing recourse to surgery in cases which failed to respond to routine irrigation within a reasonable time.[23] Yet, as Dr D. M. Keay, Dundee's VD Medical Officer lamented in 1936, there was still no specific remedy for gonorrhoea; there was 'no royal road to cure and no short cut'.[24] However, over the next three years, the treatment of gonorrhoea was to be revolutionized by the widespread application in Scottish VD clinics and hospital wards of sulphanilamide chemotherapy and in particular the administration, in tablet form, of the sulphapyridine M & B 693. Although irrigation was continued for some time in many clinics, the new therapy quickly dominated treatment regimes with dramatic results. M & B 693 was found to eliminate symptoms and infectivity with amazing rapidity. In Dundee, bacteriological cure was secured in 90 per cent of new acute cases within a week with a very low incidence of complications, and similar results were reported in Glasgow and Edinburgh. Moreover, the new chemo-therapy was also found to be highly effective in the treatment of vulvo-vaginismus in young girls and gonococcal ophthalmia in babies, as well as in the treatment of chronic gonorrhoea.[25] As a result, as early as 1938, a sharp drop in attendances at the VD clinics and in the number of in-patients was being reported.[26]

Prophylactic or Abortive Treatment

The issue of preventive treatment often placed Scottish clinicians and health officials in a moral dilemma. In the early post-war years, the public provision of 24-hour 'ablution' centres for immediate self-disinfection after intercourse was tentatively raised in Scottish public health debate. The experience of such centres in Manchester was monitored with keen interest, but apart from some support from the Glasgow branch of the National Council for Combating Venereal Diseases, they met with a generally hostile response.[27] In line with the Trevethin Committee of Inquiry, appointed by the Ministry of Health in 1922 to investigate 'the best medical measures' for preventing VD, the SBH conceded the possible medical advantages of prompt 'abortive treatment' for gonorrhoea, but it was reluctant to sanction modes of treatment that might act as an incentive to promiscuity and erode the individual's responsibility for venereal infection; a view shared by leading Medical Officers of Health such as A. K. Chalmers.[28]

Nonetheless, while recoiling from the use of public funds to provide Scottish youth with 'a safe exchange with chastity at the nearest ablution centre', the major thrust of the VD propaganda issued by the SBH and the Scottish Committee of the British Social Hygiene Council *was* the need to persuade those exposing themselves to venereal infections to seek professional advice. As the Board's Annual Report noted in 1929:

> It is of real communal importance that persons who may have run the risk of contracting venereal disease should at the earliest possible moment resort to the clinics for expert advice, rather than that they should await the onset of obvious symptoms, too often an indication that the opportunity of rapid cure has passed.[29]

Despite continuing moral reservations, treatment centres undertook *de facto* a significant and increasing amount of such 'prophylactic' diagnosis and treatment,[30] and this was in part reflected in the rising proportion of non-venereal cases among new patients presenting themselves for advice and 'reassurance' at the VD centres, rising from 11 per cent in 1922 to 28 per cent in 1930. As a result, as Dundee's VD Medical Officer noted with some satisfaction, the work of the VD Schemes in Scotland steadily tended 'towards the aspect of preventive medicine'.[31]

VD Treatment by Medical Practitioners

It is impossible to be precise as to the extent of VD treatment undertaken by private practitioners in interwar Scotland. It was widely agreed by medical authorities that the numbers attending the clinics were only a proportion of those infected within the community and that a substantial amount of treatment took place outwith the public treatment centres. Some indication of the degree of involvement of private practitioners can be obtained from their share in the administration of Salvarsan substitutes and in the submission of laboratory specimens. In Glasgow, it appears that only a 'small coterie of medical men', some 9 per cent of local practitioners, administered neo-Salvarsan, accounting for only 5 per cent of doses.[32] Similar participation rates prevailed in other Scottish cities.[33] Meanwhile, the proportion of VD-related specimens sent to medical laboratories by private practitioners in the 1920s ranged from 7 per cent in Glasgow to 10–12 per cent in Aberdeen and Dundee. However, during the 1930s, private practitioners accounted for a mere 3–4 per cent of such specimens.[34]

Even when practitioners made use of facilities provided under the VD Schemes, the medical outcome was often of dubious value. There was widespread evidence that, in cases of syphilis, practitioners awaited the appearance of a secondary rash and positive Wassermann Test before initiating arsenical treatment or referring their patients to a VD clinic, rather than ensuring early action on the basis of microscopic examination of suspected syphilitic sores; procrastination roundly condemned by the SBH as 'in no degree short of malpraxis'.[35] As a result, VD Officers continued to inherit late cases of syphilis 'in which the diagnosis could have been established with certainty during the early phases of the infection'.[36] Similarly, there was ample evidence that practitioners were poorly equipped to diagnose gonorrhoea, especially in women. Consequently, very frequently, symptoms were dismissed as leucorrhoea and treatment delayed until after chronic infection and complications had developed, often necessitating hospitalization.[37]

The treatment procedures of many practitioners were equally suspect, revealing a widespread 'lack of appropriate skills' for the administration of newer techniques in venereology.[38] The SBH were disquieted by reports that some practitioners were still initially treating syphilitic sores with discredited remedies such as black wash and red lotion rather than applying new forms of chemotherapy in the earliest stages of the disease, when they were at their most effective.[39] Dr W. H. Brown, Skin Physician at Glasgow Victoria Infirmary, reported not infrequent cases of secondary syphilis whose genital sores had been initially treated by medical practitioners with local antiseptics and mercury pills, and whose therapy had, in his opinion, been 'tantamount to malpraxis'.[40] Equally serious was the tendency of practitioners to administer a few injections of arsenobenzol rather than systematic courses of arsenobenzol and bismuth over a protracted period. As Dundee's VD Medical Officer lamented as late as 1932:

> to give less than two courses is not only futile but well-nigh malpractice because ... many cases by means of inefficient treatment are not only rendered Wassermann fast, or in other words, resistant to antiseptic treatment, but are exposed to the onset of more serious central nervous system lesions such as Tabes Dorsalis, General Paralysis of the Insane, Cerebro-spinal Syphilis, and the more serious tertiary lesions.[41]

Similar concerns surrounded the treatment of gonorrhoea by private practitioners. There was evidence that some practitioners merely dispensed vague prescriptions for permanganate solutions and vaginal douches for purposes of unsupervised irrigation.[42] According to an Edinburgh Pathological Club inquiry, 'a small syringe and a bottle of lotion for local treatment, and some sandal-wood oil to be taken by the mouth, [seemed] to be the routine, while simple disappearance of the discharge [was] considered sufficient evidence for the pronouncement of a cure'.[43] Intractable cases of gonorrhoea known as 'gleet' frequently presented themselves at the VD clinics having undergone incompetent private treatment for acute infections and having been discharged prematurely.[44]

Unqualified Treatment and Self-Disinfection

Under the 1917 Venereal Diseases Act, only qualified medical practitioners were permitted to treat VD, or to prescribe or advise in connection with venereal infections. In an effort to discourage recourse to 'fallacious and pernicious remedies', commonly obtained at chemists, and to strengthen the position of the clinics, it was also enacted that only drugs or other preparations prescribed by a qualified practitioner might be dispensed for the treatment of VD. Heavy penalties were imposed for the advertisement of all unauthorized consultations or remedies.[45] By 1920, the Act had been applied by order of the SBH to all the major Scottish towns and cities in which VD Schemes had been established and was thereafter gradually extended to the smaller burghs and county areas.[46]

Nonetheless, despite the vigilance of the police and health authorities, a significant extent of unqualified treatment persisted in Scotland throughout the interwar period, and advertisements for 'alternative' therapies continued to appear in the popular press.[47] Such practices were encouraged by the continuing policy of many Approved Societies of withholding health insurance benefits from VD patients on the grounds that their incapacity was due to 'misconduct'.[48] Evidence from prosecutions under the 1917 VD Act and from cases of sexual assault involving the communication of VD reveal a highly organized and lucrative network of unqualified practice. Thus, the self-styled 'Professor' Abraham Eastburn, prosecuted under the Act in the Glasgow High Court in 1920, was shown to be earning thousands of pounds per annum from his consulting rooms in Berkeley Terrace, an income supplemented by selective blackmail of his clients. His charges for a course of treatment, including medication, testified by medical experts to be 'worthless', ranged from £40 to as much as £265. These supported a palatial home in Helensburgh and impressive offices in Glasgow, equipped with fifteen waiting rooms. His services were advertised widely, both in the city and in country districts by means of handbills distributed in the street or posted in public lavatories.[49]

Other quacks operated more modestly, exploiting, as did Eastburn, the social stigma and not infrequent medical negligence surrounding VD. David Lees, the venereologist in charge of Edinburgh's clinics, considered that in the mid-1920s, there were still more people obtaining unqualified and illicit treatment than having recourse to the clinics; a view he reiterated in his annual report for 1930.[50] The amount of infection remaining unprofessionally treated within the community was also reflected in the low ratio of gonorrhoea to syphilis cases attending Scottish clinics.[51] While the known relative incidence of the two diseases was of the order of between 3:1 and 4:1, the ratio experienced in the clinics varied from 0.8:1 in 1921–2 to 1.7:1 by the early 1930s, and was still only 1.9:1 in 1937.

Self-administered treatment for gonorrhoea by urethral syringing and vaginal douching was widely practised in interwar Scotland, reflecting the fact that it remained in the eyes of 'the lay public' a relatively harmless disease compared with syphilis.[52] Not only did such measures delay proper diagnosis and treatment, self-irrigation often produced urethritis and stricture due to the inappropriate solutions injected or instilled.[53] Damaging substances included concentrated solutions of Lysol, undiluted Milton and phenol mouth-wash, and lunar caustic.

The Social Characteristics of VD Patients

Sex

The ratio of male to female VD patients receiving treatment at public clinics in interwar Scotland remained remarkably constant *(see Figure 4.1)*. Throughout the period, VD as witnessed at the clinics was a predominantly male disease, male cases constituting

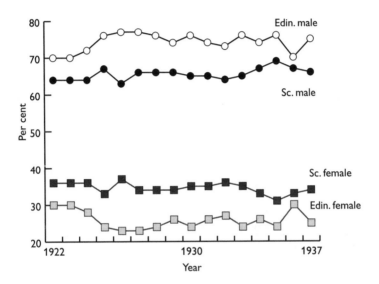

Figure 4.1
Scottish and Edinburgh VD Clinics:
Breakdown of New Patients by Sex
(*Source:* SBH/DHS Annual Reports; EPHD Annual Reports)

between 63 and 69 per cent of all infected cases in Scotland as a whole, and an even higher proportion of cases in specific VD schemes such as Aberdeen and Edinburgh.[54] However, this imbalance was, in the main, a feature of gonorrhoea. Whereas the sex ratio of male/female syphilis patients was in the order of 53:47 for the 1920s and 55:45 for the 1930s, the ratio for gonorrhoea was respectively 75:25 and 73:27. There was compelling evidence that, for a variety of reasons, women were more reluctant to seek treatment for gonorrhoea. In part, this reflected the lack of adequate, accessible, and anonymous out-patient medical facilities for women in many areas,[55] especially in the 1920s. In part, it

85

reflected the asymptomatic nature of the disease in many women in its acute stages and their tendency to view vaginal discharges as part of their natural lot.[56] It also stemmed from a real fear of provoking domestic strife and violence and of being stigmatized by family and neighbours in the event of their disease becoming public knowledge;[57] all too probable within the constricted and inquisitive social world of most working-class women.

Age

Annual returns from VD treatment centres in Scotland reveal that the majority of patients attending the public clinics were in the adolescent and adult age groups. On average, only about 7 per cent of new cases diagnosed as infected were aged under 15 years,[58] some 31 per cent were between 15 and 25, and 62 per cent were over 25. Moreover, on trend, the age distribution of venereal infection shifted towards the over-25s, especially in the 1920s. This age group of patients accounted for 51 per cent of new cases in 1922, for 64 per cent in 1930 and for 67 per cent in 1937.

	1920s		1930s		1931 Census	
	male	female	male	female	male	female
0–1	1.4	7.6	0.8	5.1	1.9	1.7
1–5	0.5	4.3	0.4	2.2	7.3	6.6
5–15	1.5	8.0	1.0	5.2	19.1	17.4
15–25	33.3	31.4	26.2	36.1	18.3	17.3
25+	63.3	48.7	71.6	51.4	53.4	57.0

Table 4.1
Age Breakdown of Patients at Scottish VD Clinics:[59]

However, within this aggregative picture, there were significant variations between the sexes *(see table 4.1)*. A substantially higher proportion of female patients who received treatment were under 15 years of age. In the 1920s, nearly 20 per cent of female patients were under 15 as compared with only 3.4 per cent of male patients, and this six-fold difference continued into the 1930s. Various explanations were advanced by public health officials for this disparity. It was partly attributed to the higher incidence of congenital syphilis in females under 1 year of age, possibly as a result of a higher survival rate *in utero*.[60] More commonly, it was attributed to the incidence of vulvo-vaginitis (often a gonococcal infection) in young girls due to criminal assault or to contamination from infected clothing, bedding and toilet articles in overcrowded and unhygienic homes and institutions.[61]

Another significant feature of the age distribution of VD patients at public clinics was the rising proportion of female patients in the age group 15–25 in contrast to the declining share of their male counterparts *(see Table 4.1)*. Data for gonorrhoea alone revealed an even sharper contrast, with the age-group 15–25 contributing some 45 per cent of female patients during the interwar period as compared with only 34 per cent of male patients receiving treatment. As will be seen in Chapter 5, such evidence was to fuel contemporary fears and proscriptions surrounding female sexuality and, in particular, the 'dangerous sexuality' of the 'problem girl'.

Location

It is difficult to establish with any precision the geographical distribution of VD patients attending public clinics in interwar Scotland as official returns focused on the location of treatment rather than of residence, and it is clear that the major treatment centres attracted patients from many parts of the country. In the 1920s, the centres in Aberdeen, Dundee, Edinburgh and Glasgow accounted for nearly 90 per cent of all new cases, with Glasgow (43 per cent) and Edinburgh (30 per cent) taking the major shares. Aberdeen and Dundee treatment centres accounted for around 6 per cent and 9 per cent of new cases respectively, with the residue fairly evenly divided between the clinics in the Counties of Ayr, Fife, Lanark and Renfrew.[62] Such evidence as is available would suggest that for Scotland as a whole, around 80 per cent of patients attending the treatment centres came from the local area, 18 per cent from elsewhere in Scotland, and 2 per cent from other parts of the United Kingdom and overseas.[63]

However, there were regional variations. Both Aberdeen and Edinburgh drew in the order of 30 per cent of their patients from outwith their city limits, and in the case of Edinburgh, over 10 per cent of patients came from areas quite outside the Joint VD Scheme.[64] In contrast, Dundee's patients appear to have been more localized, with only 13 per cent of patients resident outwith the city.[65] Interestingly, except in Dundee, where female patients were more likely to be local residents, patterns of patient residence were very similar for both sexes.

Occupation and Class

Very little attempt was made by public health officials or by venereologists to estimate the social incidence of VD in Scotland. The Royal Commission on Venereal Diseases had conjectured that in England and Wales there was a relatively high incidence of VD among the upper classes and the semi- and unskilled industrial labour force, but a 'relative immunity' among textile workers, miners and agricultural labourers.[66] However, no comparable observations had been made with respect to Scotland. Scottish clinicians and health officials had merely implied in their submissions that it was the poorer classes who were the most 'syphilised'.[67]

A few scattered references to the social distribution of VD can be found in interwar health reports and medical journals. According to Chalmers in 1921, on the basis of his experience in the West of Scotland, 'the unskilled labourer [had] the highest incidence; the upper and middle classes next. Lowest in the scale [was] the agricultural labourer, and after him the miner'.[68] Dr Madeline Archibald, VD Surgeon at Glasgow Lock Hospital and Victoria Infirmary, considered that the incidence of VD was less common 'among those classes who earn[ed] their livelihood by the expenditure of physical strength and energy', such as miners and boilermakers. In her view, 'adventures in illicit intercourse, in which venereal diseases [were] generally contracted, belong[ed] largely to the sedentary classes, who exploit[ed] their unused energy through sexual channels'.[69] However, given the absence of any information on the social background of private patients and of patients resorting to unqualified or self-treatment, such views remained impressionistic and often reflected powerful fears and assumptions about issues of class and sexual immorality rather than medical reality.

The only piece of systematic research to be published was

Table 4.2
Social Incidence of VD Patients Treated at Aberdeen Royal Infirmary
1921–4 [yearly average per 1000 pop.]

Male:

Labourers	8.7
Artisans	3.8
Commercial	3.0
Professional	1.3

Female:

Housewives	2.8
Domestic Servants	2.1
Factory Workers	1.8
Saleswomen	1.5

Table 4.3

Occupational Breakdown of Sample of Male VD Clinic Patients at
Edinburgh Royal Infirmary and Leith Dispensary in 1936
compared with 1931 Census.[71]

Occupation	% 1936 Sample	% 1931 Census
Agriculture	0.0	2.1
Mining and Quarrying	1.0	1.6
Metal Work	6.0	8.0
Electrical Work	1.0	1.6
Textile Work	0.0	1.5
Food, Drink and Tobacco	3.0	2.7
Workers in Wood	4.0	4.6
Paper Workers	0.0	0.7
Printers	3.0	2.4
Workers in Stone and Brick	0.0	3.8
Painters and Decorators	2.0	2.3
Rubber Workers	3.0	1.4
Transport and Communication	20.0	16.5
Commercial Occupations	8.0	13.2
Public Administration	1.0	2.6
Professional Occupations	0.0	5.1
Personal Services	11.0	4.3
Clerks	5.0	7.6
Warehousemen, Packers	6.0	2.3
Labourers	15.0	11.3
Other Occupations	11.0	4.4

undertaken by Aberdeen's Public Health Department in 1924, in which VD registers were used to estimate the social incidence of patients attending the treatment centre at Aberdeen Royal Infirmary for the years 1921–4 *(see Table 4.2).*[70]

However, systematic random sampling of the surviving VD registers of Edinburgh Royal Infirmary and Leith Dispensary does provide additional information on the occupational and class distribution of male patients in one area of interwar Scotland *(see Tables 4.3 and 4.4).*

It can be seen that the professions and commercial occupations were substantially under-represented in the 1936 cohort of male patients at VD clinics in Edinburgh and Leith, reflecting the fact that

Table 4.4

Class Breakdown of Sample of Male VD Clinic Patients at Edinburgh
Royal Infirmary and Leith Dispensary in 1936,
compared with 1931 Census[72]

Class	% 1936 Sample	% 1931 Census
I. Professional Occupations	0.0	1.4
II. Intermediate Occupations	1.0	9.4
III. Skilled Occupations	47.0	55.9
IV. Semi-skilled Occupations	29.0	11.3
V. Unskilled Occupations	18.0	15.6
Unemployed	2.0	4.2
Students	3.0	2.2

most sufferers within these occupational groups would seek private treatment.[73] In contrast, there was a marked over-representation of transport and storage workers, labourers, and those engaged in 'personal service' (including publicans, barmen, waiters, lodging house keepers, and domestic servants). The high incidence of transport workers is largely due to the disproportionate number of 'water transport workers', especially seamen, seeking treatment between trips. This group of workers accounted for only 3.2 per cent of Edinburgh and Leith's occupied male population enumerated in the Census, but 11 per cent of VD patients. The association of the docks, licensed premises and common lodging houses with prostitution had long figured in the public health and public morality discourse surrounding VD.[74] However, in the absence of case notes and any record of the precise circumstances in which infection was thought to have been contracted, it is impossible to gain any real traction on the linkages between occupation and infection.

While the breakdown of VD patients by social class can only safely be viewed as conveying a rough order of magnitude, it does appear that, for Edinburgh at least, contemporary perceptions of VD as a disease primarily of the casual and unskilled workforce were misplaced. While seamen undoubtedly dominated the waiting room of Leith Dispensary, at the Royal Infirmary it was the skilled and semi-skilled workers rather than the general labourer who predominated, which strongly reflected the socio-economic structure of the city.

The Status of Venereology in Interwar Scotland

It was the social politics surrounding the VD regulations of 1916 and the establishment of a system of public treatment centres that initiated the slow emergence of venereology as a distinct specialty within Scottish medicine. The regulations stressed the technical sophistication and expertise needed for the successful application of 'modern methods of diagnosis and treatment of the venereal infections', and in line with the recommendations of the Royal Commission on Venereal Diseases, advocated the appointment of specialist Medical Officers to head the treatment centres. The intention of the health departments was that, initially, a cadre of army medical officers, with extensive experience in the treatment of VD, would be seconded to public health departments to run many of the new VD Schemes.[75]

Although public health authorities continued to acknowledge the importance of general practitioners in assisting the early diagnosis and treatment of VD, they increasingly viewed this role as one of referral. Thus, in its annual report for 1920, the SBH concluded that: 'The successful treatment of the disease tends increasingly to become specialised, and to be a matter for experts only'.[76] Similarly, in its report for 1924–5, it questioned the competence of general practitioners to deal with cases of gonorrhoea. The 'acquisition of skill in the use of the urethoscope, of bougie, sound and dilator, and in the examination of the prostate' was considered in most cases to be 'beyond the reach of the busy general practitioner', and the treatment of female cases 'so intricate and so protracted that it [was] practically a matter for the specialist alone'.[77] As the VD Schemes became an established part of local health provisions, VD treatment came to be perceived by many public health officials as a function of a select group of venereologists within the clinics and their associated laboratories rather than of primary care.

The specialist status of venereology was also reinforced by the Venereal Disease Act of 1917, limiting all advice and treatment with respect to VD to qualified practitioners and prohibiting the advertisement of 'quack' or 'alternative' remedies. Although the Act was largely an outcome of negotiations designed to reconcile the medical profession as a whole to the introduction of a State medical service for VD,[78] it served to raise the profile of venereology as a specialty. Indeed, in parliamentary debate, the Act was criticized specifically for creating an unprecedented professional monopoly for those empowered to administer Salvarsan and its associated therapies. Several MPs warned that the increased technical sophistication of diagnosis and treatment for VD had shifted the locus of medical power from general practice to the laboratory and the clinic, from where a 'very limited number of specialists' would, with added protection from the Act, impose a new 'orthodoxy'.[79]

Venereology achieved clearest recognition as a specialty in Edinburgh. Both the Royal Infirmary managers and the Faculty of Medicine favoured the appointment as Chief Medical Officer for Edinburgh Corporation's VD Scheme of a specialist 'who had devoted himself to this branch of medicine', and there appears to have been little resistance from other specialties.[80] One medical authority later surmised that, in Edinburgh, the Dermatology Department 'did not wish to be associated with syphilis on the grounds of morality, respectability, or inertia', and that they viewed the intravenous techniques associated with the administration of Salvarsan and the Wassermann Test as 'essentially surgical procedures and outwith their sphere of expertise'.[81]

The first Chief Medical Officer, David Lees had extensive experience of VD work in the Royal Army Medical Corps at military hospitals in Newcastle and Glasgow, and as adviser on VD to Derbyshire County Council. Lees typified an aggressive cohort of social hygiene specialists emerging within the machinery of post-war local health administration and made a powerful contribution to raising the status of venereology as a medical specialty. He was an active member of the newly established Medical Society for the Study of Venereal Diseases and first President of its Scottish Branch, established in 1923; an organization that was to provide a forum for both the medical and professional concerns of the specialty and an influential pressure group in the shaping of VD policy. In addition, until his early death in 1934, Lees was a leading member of the Medical Advisory Committee of the British Social Hygiene Council and of the Venereology Section of the BMA, in which capacities he fought tirelessly for greater recognition, resources and regulatory powers for VD clinicians.[82]

Nonetheless, evidence would suggest that elsewhere in Scotland, venereology was accorded little recognition and remained the 'Cinderella of medicine'. VD patients and clinicians were often held in contempt by hospital committees and medical staff. VD departments were regarded as 'clinical cess pits' and both physically and symbolically located in 'unhygienic cellars' adjacent to boiler houses, kitchens and waste disposal areas. Although prosopographical evidence suggests that doctors employed in hospital VD departments and 'ad hoc' clinics in interwar Scotland possessed a wide range of medical expertise (see Table 4.5), and that compared with control groups from other specialties they were well qualified, they were commonly dismissed by both the medical profession and the public as 'pox doctors' and treated as 'medical and social pariahs'.[83] Junior appointments in the clinics were very poorly paid and 'the number of higher and well paid appointments in venereal work [was] not sufficient to attract the best medical brains to continue at the work'.[84] Moreover, doctors specializing in venereology after taking a Diploma in Public Health lacked the advancement in public health administration accorded to those specializing in tuberculosis or child welfare.[85] According to later practitioners within the specialty, venereology was the 'most neglected and despised of subjects', and 'regarded as highly distasteful and quite unworthy of the attention of anyone who had hopes of becoming more than a medical hack'.[86]

Outwith the Edinburgh Medical School, there was continuing opposition to the creation of a separate specialty. Thus, in Aberdeen, the appointment of Christie as the Chief Medical Officer for the VD Scheme clearly maintained 'the tradition of the syphilides being the province of the dermatologist'.[87] Similarly, despite the fact that David Watson, VD Surgeon at Glasgow Royal Infirmary and Lecturer in VD to Glasgow University, had originated the idea of a Medical

Table 4.5:
Breakdown of Areas of Previous Expertise of Doctors Working in Hospital VD Departments and 'Ad Hoc' Clinics in Interwar Scotland (%)

Career Expertise	All	Male	Female
Asylum	17	17	17
Dermatology	8	9	4
Obstetrics	19	17	25
Ophthalmology	4	4	5
Paediatrics	20	12	50
Pathology	17	21	4
Poor Law	3	2	4
Public Health	58	57	63
TB/Infectious Disease	24	28	8
Urology	2	2	0

Society for the Study of Venereal Diseases,[88] much of Glasgow's medical establishment was resistant to any specialist career structure for venereology, given the wide range of symptoms stemming from venereal infection. Leonard Findlay, Physician to the Royal Hospital for Sick Children, reflected the views of many Glasgow clinicians when he argued in the *Glasgow Medical Journal* in 1925 that:

> There is ... no necessity for the so-called venereal specialist. To classify specialities according to the etiological organism is acting on a wrong principle .... In order to appreciate syphilis in all its manifestations, one would require to be at least a physician, a surgeon, a dermatologist, an ophthalmologist, an aurist and laryngologist, a combination of attributes only met with in some Admirable Crichton. And were our famous syphilologists in truth not just such Admirable Crichtons, to wit, John Hunter, Colles, Lancereaux and Jonathan Hutchinson, whose versatility and wide knowledge of general medicine and surgery enabled them to leave their mark on the history of syphilis.[89]

As a result, in Glasgow, VD work was farmed out among a number of specialties. Male clinicians in the '*ad hoc*' clinics were recruited on a part-time basis from the visiting staffs of the voluntary hospitals and included a mix of physicians, dermatologists, and genito-urinary surgeons, who regarded work in the treatment centres as a valuable supplementary source of income.[90] The widespread practice of rotating junior posts in the hospital VD clinics at frequent intervals also discouraged specialization.[91]

As in England, there was a widespread use of general practitioners to staff the clinics.[92] Private practitioners had been reluctant to acknowledge the expert status and municipal powers of VD Medical Officers and the possibility of a small group of specialist clinicians and serologists monopolizing the market in clinical venereology to the detriment of general practice. From the outset, public health departments were keen to employ general practitioners as clinical assistants within the VD Schemes, partly as a means of placating such fears, but more importantly as a cheap means of resolving chronic staff shortages due to the low prestige of the work.[93] In addition, in many areas, Assistant Medical Officers of Health and Infectious Diseases Officers were reluctantly drafted in to run local clinics as part of the '"any other duties" that a Medical Officer of Health might devolve'.[94] While aware of the epidemiology and public health implications of VD, their Diplomas of Public Health furnished them with limited expertise in recent developments in venereology, and the burden of routine diagnosis and treatment often fell upon ward orderlies and nurses.[95]

Moreover, the heavy representation of women within the specialty (22 per cent), who were frequently discriminated against in terms of pay and promotion,[96] served to perpetuate its 'Cinderella' image. As Elaine Thomson has documented, VD work, with its emphasis on hygiene and moral regeneration, was perceived as peculiarly suited to the role of medical women in the public sphere.[97] Furthermore, given that they suffered from restricted access to clinical appointments, they inevitably congregated in areas of medicine such as venereology and maternal and infant welfare which were considered to be marginal to the main interests of the medical profession, and thus lacking in prestige.[98]

The low status of venereology within interwar Scotland both reflected and reinforced the lack of provision for medical training in the specialty. Particular concern was attached to practitioners who had qualified prior to the First World War. Although Scottish medical authorities claimed that VD was adequately taught and examined, the Royal Commission on Venereal Diseases had concluded that pre-war medical training in the diagnosis and treatment of VD was seriously deficient.[99] According to the evidence of Carl Browning, Director of Clinical Pathology in the University of Glasgow, despite the existence of a Lectureship in Syphilis at Glasgow Royal Infirmary, medical students lacked 'systematic practical instruction'.[100] Mary Liston, Assistant VD Medical Officer for Edinburgh during the period 1922–37, who had qualified M.B. Ch.B. (Glasgow) in 1900, recalled that:

> All the teaching I got on the subject [VD] was contained in one and a half lectures, and I was certainly led to believe that the disease affected the sinner .... No stress was paid on the difficulty of cure, nor were we ever led to believe that disastrous results would follow imperfect treatment.[101]

Certainly, the Royal Army Medical Corps experienced an acute shortage of civilian medical expertise in VD upon which it could draw during the First World War.[102]

Under pressure from the General Medical Council and Licensing Authorities, the Royal Commission on Venereal Diseases reluctantly refrained from recommending that a separate course of instruction on VD should be made compulsory for every medical student. It did, however, stress the need for a substantive improvement in clinical instruction, and the provision of adequate training facilities was subsequently enshrined in the 1916 Venereal Diseases Regulations as a condition of approval of VD Schemes by the SBH.

Thereafter, local health authorities pressed for alterations to the curricula of the medical schools so as to bring VD 'within the competence and skill of the general practitioner'.[103] In Edinburgh, the Corporation's VD Medical Officer, David Lees, was appointed to a University Lectureship in Venereology in 1920 and VD was made a compulsory part of the medical curriculum. A three-month course of 25 clinical lectures was given to final-year students with detailed information on new developments in diagnosis and therapy.[104] Similar developments took place in Glasgow with clinical instruction in VD at the Royal and Western Infirmaries. In addition, the Lock Hospital became a major teaching centre with the University Lecturer on Venereal Diseases, who also acted as its Chief Medical Officer, conducting 'large classes of 130 or more students'.[105] Meanwhile, in Aberdeen, attendance at a course of instruction in VD at a 'recognised hospital or clinic centre' had been made compulsory for all medical students in 1918.[106] In addition, in response to a recommendation from the Central Midwives Board for Scotland, arrangements were made to give pupil midwives some practical experience of VD cases in ante-natal departments.[107] Increased provision was also made in many teaching centres for postgraduate training in venereology for general practitioners. For example, by the mid-1920s, David Lees was running a summer course of eighteen lectures for practitioners at Edinburgh Royal Infirmary designed to coincide with his VD clinic in the hope that actual cases might be used.[108]

Nonetheless, the amount and quality of training in venereology remained limited. There was a chronic lack of adequate funding. After 1920, the SBH, faced with the need for public economy cuts, refused to refund expenditure incurred in VD teaching against the VD Grant, and its financing became, in some areas, a lasting bone of contention between public health, university, and hospital authorities.[109]

Secondly, undergraduate courses often lacked a worthwhile clinical component. Thus, according to one of the students who attended at Edinburgh Royal Infirmary:

> The lectures were not illustrated, apart from showing one or two casts of late nodular lesions borrowed from the skin department [and] ... in the absence of clinical instruction were of little practical value. The clinics were mainly held in the evenings, and as secrecy

was regarded as being of prime importance, students were not encouraged. Attendance was more or less limited to one evening per three months per student, and all that could be guaranteed was the demonstration of an intravenous or intramuscular injection, the withdrawal of blood for a Wassermann Test and possibly a lumbar puncture. In spite of the fact that Parliament, Public Health Committees, the medical profession and in particular the lecturer on venereology were unanimous in realising the extreme importance of the subject, at that time a student would have been lucky to see a chancre, a secondary cutaneous or mucous membrane lesion, or an acute gonorrhoea during his medical course.[110]

Finally, there was continuing resistance from other clinicians and medical authorities to the provision of discrete training in venereology. This stemmed from concern at adding to an already overcrowded medical curriculum, and from a belief in some medical centres that, as VD affected so many organs of the body, its study should remain integrated within general medical instruction. It also stemmed from the low priority accorded by both students and Faculty to this aspect of medical training. Even David Lees had to struggle to maintain the integrity of his course within the Edinburgh curriculum, being compelled on more than one occasion to make additional provisions for students whom the Medical Faculty had permitted to graduate despite having failed to secure a class certificate in VD.[111]

Notes

1   See, e.g., *Glasgow Medical Officer of Health [MOH] Annual Report (1930)*, 192; Medical Society for the Study of Venereal Diseases, Scottish Branch [MSSVDSB], Minutes, 19 Dec. 1928, 25 March 1931.

2   Lees, 'Remarks on the Treatment of Syphilis', *Journal of State Medicine, XXXI* (1923), 255–6; I. Mackenzie [Visiting Physician, Victoria Infirmary, Glasgow], 'The Treatment of Syphilis', *Glasgow Medical Journal [GMJ]*, 91 (1919), 332–41.

3   W. R. Snodgrass [VD Medical Officer, Western Infirmary, Glasgow], 'The Treatment of Syphilis', *GMJ*, 101 (1924), 330; Scottish Board of Health *[SBH], Seventh Annual Report, PP 1926 (Cmd. 2674) XI*, 68.

4   *Ibid.*, 68.

5   *Dundee MOH Annual Report (1924)*, 58; *Edinburgh Public Health Department [EPHD] Annual Report (1924)*, 58.

6   *SBH, Sixth Annual Report, PP 1924–5 (Cmd. 2416) XIII*, 66.

7   *Glasgow MOH Annual Report (1930)*, 192; *(1931)*, 123–4.

8 See especially, MSSVDSB Minutes, 29 March 1933.

9 *EPHD Annual Report (1935)*, 80; *Dundee MOH Annual Report (1935)*, 107–8. In Edinburgh, where the VD Scheme adopted the recommended treatment regime of the Health Organization of the League of Nations, active treatment was reduced from 104–120 weeks to 60–90 weeks.

10 See, e.g., *Dundee MOH Annual Report (1936)*, 113–14; *EPHD Annual Report (1935)*, 76–7.

11 *SBH, Seventh Annual Report, op. cit.* (note 3), 68–9; *Glasgow MOH Annual Report (1925)*, 151–3; *Dundee MOH Annual Report (1932)*, 111; *EPHD Annual Report (1925)*, 56; *(1926)*, 60; *(1935)*, 80.

12 For details of this therapy, see *Dundee MOH Annual Report (1935)*, 108; *EPHD Annual Report (1932)*, 68; *(1935)*, 80; *(1936)*, 85; R. Lees, 'The Treatment of General Paralysis of the Insane', Edinburgh M.D. thesis (1938). On the history of malarial therapy, see E. S. Valenstein, *Great and Desperate Cures: The Rise and Decline of Psychosurgery and Other Radical Treatments for Mental Illness* (New York: Basic Books, 1986), 29–31. For a detailed examination of treatment regimes within the Scottish asylums, see G. L. Davis, 'The Cruel Madness of Love: Syphilis as a Psychiatric Disorder, Glasgow Royal Asylum 1900–1930', University of Glasgow, M.Phil. thesis (1997), 45–55. In some medical centres, the inoculation of GPI patients with benign tertian malaria also played a significant role in experimental research into anti-malarial drugs and afforded an opportunity for maintaining strains of malaria parasites in man. See H. Power, 'Malaria, Drugs and World War II: The Role of the Liverpool School of Tropical Medicine in the Development of Paludrine', *Medical History* (forthcoming).

13 *Report of General Board of Control for Scotland for 1931, PP 1931–2 (Cmd. 4163) XI*, xxiii.

14 *EPHD Annual Report (1935)*, 80; *Report of General Board of Control for Scotland for 1935, PP 1935–6 (Cmd. 5124) XIII*, xxvi; *for 1937, PP 1937–8 (Cmd. 5715) XIII*, xxii; Lothian Health Services Archives [LHSA], *Royal Edinburgh Asylum, Physician Superintendent's Annual Report (1922)*, 22.

15 Cited in Davis, *op. cit.* (note 12), 50.

16 LHSA, LHB 7/7/14, *112th Annual Report of the Royal Edinburgh Asylum (1924)*, 19.

17 R. Lees, 'Some Random Reflections of a Venereologist', *British Journal of Venereal Diseases [BJVD]*, 26 (1950), 158.

18 *SBH, Seventh Annual Report, op. cit.* (note 3), 74–5; *EPHD Annual Report (1924)*, 57; *Glasgow MOH Annual Report (1925)*, 152;

Dundee MOH Annual Report (1924), 124.

19 SBH, Seventh Annual Report, op. cit. (note 3), 75; *EPHD Annual Report (1924),* 57; *Dundee MOH Annual Report (1924),* 125.

20 *EPHD Annual Report (1924),* 57; *Dundee MOH Annual Report (1928),* 132, 134; MSSVDSB Minutes, 30 Jan. 1929. Typically, diathermy would be administered twice a week for 5–10 minutes at a temperature of *c.*112 degrees. See also, E. Mackenzie, 'Chronic Gonorrhoea in Women and its Treatment', Edinburgh M.D. thesis (1927).

21 SBH, Seventh Annual Report, op. cit. (note 3), 78.

22 *EPHD Annual Report (1938),* 131; *Glasgow MOH Annual Report (1929),* 149. At some clinics, in excess of 20% of patients receiving urethrovesical irrigation developed complications. See, *Glasgow MOH Annual Report (1925),* 152.

23 *Dundee MOH Annual Report (1932),* 108, 124; *EPHD Annual Report (1935),* 81; *Glasgow MOH Annual Report (1932),* 138; *(1934),* 140.

24 *Dundee MOH Annual Report (1936),* 112.

25 *Dundee MOH Annual Report (1937),* 126; *(1938),* 13, 122; *EPHD Annual Report (1937),* 94; *(1938),* 127, 130–1; *Glasgow MOH Annual Report (1937),* 130–1; *GMJ,* 130 (1938), 123; MSSVDSB Minutes, 12 Jan. 1938, 22 Feb. 1939.

26 By 1940, the decline in in-patients had led the Directors of the Glasgow Lock Hospital to conclude that its 'usefulness was coming to an end' (*GMJ,* 133 (1940), 184).

27 Glasgow City Archives [GCA], Glasgow Public Health Committee [PHC] Minutes, 21 Sept. 1921; Glasgow Public Health Department newscuttings, 1920–1; A. K. Chalmers, *The Health of Glasgow 1818–1925: An Outline* (Glasgow: Glasgow Corporation, 1930), 394–6; Contemporary Medical Archives Centre [CMAC], SA/BSH/A2/5, National Council for Combating Venereal Diseases [NCCVD] Executive Committee Minutes, 1 May 1922.

28 *Ministry of Health, Report of the Committee of Inquiry on Venereal Disease* (London: HMSO, 1923); SBH, Seventh Annual Report, op. cit. (note 3), xi, 73; Chalmers, op. cit. (note 27), 404; *EPHD Annual Report (1921),* 41. Sadly, the Scottish evidence to the Trevethin Committee does not appear to have been preserved. See below, ch. 5 for a discussion of the moral discourse underpinning contemporary attitudes to prophylactic and other treatment regimes.

29 *Department of Health for Scotland [DHS], First Annual Report, PP 1929–30 (Cmd. 3529) XIV,* 101.

30 *EPHD Annual Report (1924),* 55; *Dundee MOH Annual Report*

(1928), 133; DHS, First Annual Report, op. cit. (note 29), xiv, 101.

31 Dundee MOH Annual Report (1936), 109.

32 Glasgow MOH Annual Reports.

33 DHS, Fourth Annual Report, PP 1932–3 (Cmd. 4338) XII, 82. Under the 1916 VD Regulations, Salvarsan and its substitutes were to be supplied only to practitioners who could 'show satisfactory evidence of training or experience in the administration of these drugs'.

34 EPHD and Dundee MOH Annual Reports.

35 EPHD Annual Report (1919), 56; SBH, Seventh Annual Report, op. cit. (note 3), xi, 70, 79; Dundee MOH Annual Report (1930), 116; see also comments of David Lees at the 1921 BMA Conference Session on the Treatment of Syphilis, British Medical Journal [BMJ], 24 Sept. 1921, 479.

36 Dundee MOH Annual Report (1932), 110–11, 122.

37 See, e.g., Dundee MOH Annual Report (1932), 112; Mackenzie, op. cit. (note 20), 2. Diagnosis of gonorrhoea was also frequently complicated or delayed by 'faulty swabbing' by general practitioners.

38 SBH, Ninth Annual Report, PP 1928 (Cmd. 3112) X, 107, 115; Lees, op. cit. (note 2), 250.

39 SBH, Seventh Annual Report, op. cit. (note 3), 79; Ninth Annual Report, op. cit. (note 38), x, 115.

40 W. H. Brown, 'Modern Aspects of Syphilis in Special and General Practice', GMJ, 107 (1927), 130–2.

41 Dundee MOH Annual Report (1932), 111. See also L. W. Harrison, 'Education of Students in Venereal Diseases', in Edinburgh Pathological Club, An Inquiry into the Medical Curriculum (Edinburgh: W. Green and Son, 1919), 267.

42 SBH, Seventh Annual Report, op. cit. (note 3) xi, 75–6; M. Archibald, 'The Position of the General Practitioner in Anti-Venereal Disease Schemes', Proceedings of the Imperial Social Hygiene Council (London: NCCVD, 1924), 192.

43 Harrison, op. cit. (note 41), 267.

44 SBH, Ninth Annual Report, op. cit. (note 38), 115; Dundee MOH Annual Report (1932), 111.

45 Hansard [HC] 92, cols 2071–2127, 23 April 1917; 7 & 8 Geo. 5, ch. 21, Venereal Disease Act, 1917.

46 SBH, Second Annual Report, PP 1921 (Cmd. 1319) XIII, 45.

47 Report from the Joint Committee on the Criminal Law Amendment Bill and Sexual Offences Bill, PP 1918 (142) III, q. 3051; EPHD Annual Report (1922), 43; T. F. Dewar, 'On the Incidence of Venereal Disease in Scotland', EMJ, XXX (1923), 330; SBH, Eighth Annual

Report, PP 1927 (Cmd. 2881) X, 82. Fraudulent advertising of cures for ailments arising from 'sexual indulgence' was still the subject of parliamentary concern in 1936. See *PP 1935–6 (Bill 33) II, Medicines and Surgical Appliances (Advertisement) Bill.*

48 *Report on the Administration of National Health Insurance in Scotland, PP 1920 (Cmd. 827)* XXII, 20; *GMJ*, 91 (1919), 53–4.

49 NAS, AD15/20/62, Precognitions against Abraham S. Eastburn, Glasgow High Court, Feb. 1920; *Glasgow Herald*, 25 Feb. 1920.

50 Dewar, *op. cit.* (note 47), 330; *EPHD Annual Report (1930)*, 74.

51 *SBH, Eighth Annual Report, PP 1927 (Cmd. 2881) X*, 82; *Tenth Annual Report, PP 1928–29 (Cmd. 3304) VII*, 218; *EPHD Annual Report (1921)*, 40; *(1930)*, 74; *(1933)*, 80.

52 *Glasgow MOH Annual Report (1921)*, 80; *(1932)*, 134; *EPHD Annual Report (1919)*, 56; *(1933)*, 80.

53 See, J. A. Burgess, 'Primary Non-Gonococcal Urethritis', Edinburgh M.D. thesis (1935), 28–31, 67.

54 Throughout the interwar period, the ratio of male to female cases treated at treatment centres in Edinburgh and Aberdeen was markedly more skewed than in Glasgow and Dundee. Their respective ratios were Edinburgh 74:26, Aberdeen 74:26, Glasgow 67:33 and Dundee 60:40. The substantially greater number of female cases in Dundee was arguably in part a function of its demographic structure and distinctive labour market.

55 See above, ch. 3.

56 See, e.g., *SBH, Ninth Annual Report, op. cit.* (note 38), x, 108; *EPHD Annual Report (1935)*, 77.

57 See, e.g., *SBH, Ninth Annual Report, op. cit.* (note 38), x, 118.

58 There were local variations. Patients under the age of 15 constituted 9% of the case-load in Dundee but only 4% of the case-load in Edinburgh.

59 Source: *SBH/DHS, Annual Reports; Report of the Fourteenth Decennial Census of Scotland, Vol. 2* (Edinburgh: HMSO, 1933), Table 31.

60 See, e.g., *Glasgow MOH Annual Report (1931)*, 122–3.

61 See, e.g., *SBH, Seventh Annual Report, op. cit.* (note 3), xi, 77; *EPHD Annual Reports (1924)*, 56; *(1929)*, 73; *(1936)*, 84.

62 *SBH, Tenth Annual Report, op. cit.* (note 51), 222.

63 *DHS, Fifth to Ninth Annual Reports.*

64 *EPHD Annual Reports; Aberdeen MOH Annual Reports.*

65 *Dundee MOH Annual Reports.*

66 *Final Report of Royal Commission on Venereal Diseases [RCVD], PP 1916 (Cd. 8189) XVI*, 19–20, 74–5, 79.

67 RCVD, *Minutes of Evidence of Dr J. Kerr-Love and Dr A. K. Chalmers, PP 1914 (Cd. 7475) XLIX*, qq. 4405–6; *PP 1916 (Cd. 8190) XVI*, qq. 17962–6.

68 *Glasgow MOH Report (1921)*, 109–10.

69 M. Archibald, 'Modern Aspects of Syphilis in Special and General Practice', *GMJ*, 107 (1927), 137.

70 *Aberdeen MOH Annual Report (1924)*, 125–7.

71 n=100. VD Registers for RIE and Leith Dispensary; *Fourteenth Census of Scotland, Preliminary Report*, Vol. 1 (Edinburgh: HMSO, 1931), 9, 12, 28–30. In order to achieve a meaningful comparison with the Census, the sample was of patients with addresses in Edinburgh and Leith. Random sampling could not be undertaken for earlier years as details of occupation were not recorded in the registers. Occupational details of female patients were not systematically recorded prior to the Second World War. Unfortunately, the case notes have been destroyed. The author is not aware of any other surviving VD registers from this period that recorded the occupation of patients.

72 n=100. It should be noted that information in the VD registers enabled only a very rough social class allocation of the occupational data.

73 It is interesting to note that at Gartnavel Asylum, a private institution, it is estimated that 53% of neuro-syphilitic patients during the period 1900–30 were from these occupational groups. See Davis, *op. cit.* (note 12), 37.

74 See above, ch. 2.

75 *Local Government Board for Scotland, Public Health (Venereal Disease) Regulations and Memorandum on Schemes for the Diagnosis, Treatment, and Prevention of Venereal Diseases* (Edinburgh: HMSO, 1916), 3, 7.

76 *SBH, Second Annual Report, PP 1921 (Cmd. 1319) XIII*, 42.

77 *SBH, Seventh Annual Report, op. cit.* (note 3), 80–1.

78 D. Evans, 'Tackling the "Hideous Scourge": The Creation of the Venereal Disease Treatment Centres in Early Twentieth-Century Britain', *Social History of Medicine*, 5 (1992), 422–3.

79 *Hansard [HC] XCII*, 23 April 1917, cols 2114, 2123; *[HC] XCIII*, 15 May 1917, cols 1514, 1521–2.

80 LHSA, LHB1/1/55, Minutes of Board of Managers of Royal Infirmary of Edinburgh [RIE], 2 April 1917; Edinburgh University Library [EUL], DA 443, Faculty of Medicine Minutes, 18 June 1918.

81 EUL, Special Collections, Gen. 2161, G. H. Percival, 'Some Aspects of the Development of Dermatology with Special Reference to the

Contribution of the Edinburgh Medical School' (1982), 340.

82   *BJVD*, 10 (1934), 79–81; *BMJ*, 7 April 1934; *Lancet*, 7 April 1934.
     See also below, ch. 8. In 1925, David Lees was responsible for
     drafting a British Social Hygiene Council [BSHC] resolution calling
     for the immediate appointment of trained specialists to all VD
     treatment centres. CMAC, SA/BSH/A1/4, Minutes of Council, 23
     Nov. 1925.

83   Compared with a control group of ophthalmologists, a larger
     proportion of male venereologists had only basic medical
     qualifications and a further 20% only a Diploma of Public Health at
     postgraduate level. However, some 16% of male venereologists,
     double that of the control group, had three or more postgraduate
     qualifications. Meanwhile, some 67% of female doctors involved in
     VD work in Scotland had postgraduate qualifications (primarily the
     DPH) compared with only 38% of female ophthalmologists. These
     findings are based on a computer-based prosopographical study of
     Scottish venereologists (1918–39) undertaken by Ann McCrum,
     University of Edinburgh.

84   D. Lees, 'Methods of Securing the Maximum Efficiency of a
     Venereal Diseases Clinic', *Proceedings of the Imperial Social Hygiene
     Congress* (London: NCCVD, 1924), 137–8.

85   *Ibid.*, 138.

86   Lees, *op. cit.* (note 17), 157–8; A. King, 'Venereology – A Backward
     Look', *BJVD*, 48 (1972), 412; A. S. Wigfield, 'The Emergence of
     the Consultant Venereologist', *BJVD*, 48 (1972), 549–50; Transcript
     of interview with retired consultant venereologist, 24 May 1996.

87   T. E. Anderson, 'The Development of Dermatology in Aberdeen',
     Aberdeen Post-Graduate Medical Bulletin (Sept. 1973), 39.

88   R. S. Morton, 'A Short History of the Medical Society for the Study
     of Venereal Diseases on its 75th Birthday', *Sexually Transmitted
     Infections*, 74 (1998), 155–8.

89   L. Findlay, 'The Ravages of Congenital Syphilis – How to Combat
     Them: A Plea for Notification', *GMJ*, 95 (1921), 280–1. See also,
     D. Newman, 'The History and Prevention of Venereal Disease',
     GMJ, 81 (1914), 175; A. D. MacLachlan, 'Modern Aspects of
     Syphilis in Special and General Practice', *GMJ*, 108 (1927), 156. For
     the broader implications of this tension between an élite medical
     generalism and the emergence of a new laboratory-oriented specialty,
     see S. Sturdy and R. Cooter, 'Science, Scientific Management, and
     the Transformation of Medicine in Britain c1870–1950', *History of
     Science*, XXXVI (1998), 427–9.

90   *Glasgow MOH Annual Report (1931)*, 125.

91 See, e.g., GCA, C1/3/79, Glasgow Corporation, Minutes of Sub-Committee on the Treatment of VD, 19 Oct. 1928.

92 J. M. Eyler, *Sir Arthur Newsholme and State Medicine: 1885–1935* (Cambridge: Cambridge University Press, 1997), 291.

93 See, e.g., DCA, Town Clerk's Correspondence, File NCCVD, 1918, Transcript of NCCVD Conference, 18 June 1918, 17.

94 Transcript of interview with retired consultant venereologist, 4 Aug. 1994.

95 *Ibid.*; Wigfield, *op. cit.* (note 86), 549.

96 For example, the Royal Infirmary of Edinburgh refused to sanction the appointment of Mary Liston as a Junior Clinical Medical Officer in 1919 and restricted her status to that of Clinical Assistant in the female VD department. Despite a prolonged campaign, backed by the Scottish Union of Medical Women, they subsequently maintained her salary at £400 p.a., £100 lower than the salary of the Male Assistant (LHSA, LHB 1/1/56, Minutes of Board of Managers, 24 Feb. 1919, 7 April 1919; ECA, Public Health Series, 10/3, Report by Dr Lees on Letters from Dr Mary F. Liston).

97 E. Thomson, 'Women in Medicine in Late Nineteenth and Early Twentieth-Century Edinburgh: A Case Study', University of Edinburgh Ph.D. thesis (1998), 103, 165, 246–7, 264.

98 *Ibid.*, 207–11.

99 *RCVD, Final Report, op. cit.* (note 66), 59–60, appendix xxvi; *Minutes of Evidence, PP 1916 (Cd. 8190) XVI*, q. 19228.

100 *RCVD, Minutes of Evidence, PP 1914 (Cd. 7475) XLIX*, qq. 7014–5, 7098. For a later endorsement of this view, see *Glasgow MOH Annual Report (1921)*, 80.

101 University of Reading Library, Nancy Astor Papers, MS/1/1/229, Liston to Lady Astor, 12 Feb. 1928.

102 CMAC, SA/BSH/D1/1, BSHC Medical Committee Minutes, 25 June 1917.

103 *EPHD Annual Report (1919)*, 56; *Glasgow MOH Annual Report (1921)*, 80–1.

104 D. Lees, *BMJ*, 24 Sept. 1921, 479.

105 *GMJ*, 108 (1927), 230; *Centenary Number* (1928), 174.

106 Northern Health Services Archives [NHSA], E1/5/37, Aberdeen Public Health Committee [PHC] Minutes, 22 Sept. 1920.

107 CMAC, SA/BSH/D3, BSHC Medical Committee Minutes, 25 Nov. 1932.

108 *Ibid.*, 5 July 1929.

109 See, e.g., NHSA, 1/15/6, VD file, SBH to MOH Aberdeen, 22 Oct. 1920; E1/5/37, Aberdeen PHC Minutes, 22 Sept. 1920.

110 Percival, *op. cit.* (note 81), 342.

111 EUL, Special Collections, DA/43, Faculty of Medicine Minutes, 21 Nov. 1921, 17 July 1925.

5

Sin and Suffering:
The Moral Agenda of VD Administration, 1918–39

The Ideology of Social Hygiene

Shaping venereal disease policy in interwar Scotland was a powerful cohort of public health administrators and clinicians who embraced the social and medical ideology of the Social Hygiene Movement.[1] The majority of the more influential Medical Officers of Health and Venereal Disease Medical Officers were active members of the National Council for Combating Venereal Diseases [NCCVD], renamed the British Social Hygiene Council [BSHC] in 1925. Many, such as A. Maxwell Williamson and John Guy (Medical Officers of Health for Edinburgh), A. K. Chalmers and A. S. M. Macgregor (Medical Officers of Health for Glasgow), W. L. Burgess (Medical Officer of Health for Dundee), and David Lees and R. J. Peters (Chief VD Medical Officers for Edinburgh and Glasgow) were members of their Scottish Executive Committee. Other members included Thomas Dewar, Medical Officer in charge of the Infectious Diseases Section of the Scottish Board of Health (later, Department of Health for Scotland) [SBH/DHS] and H. L. F. Fraser, its Principal Assistant Secretary. David Lees, one of the major architects of VD policy in the East of Scotland, was Chairman of the Council's Medical Advisory Board. Moreover, local committees of the NCCVD/BSHC were commonly administered by local authority health officers from within Public Health Departments.[2]

Scottish VD administrators shared the BSHC's commitment to a moral as well as medical strategy towards public health and its association of national health and efficiency with sexual discipline. 'Promiscuity', broadly defined as non-marital intercourse, was viewed as a form of 'sexual atavism' that undermined racial 'fitness' and evolution. Thus for Guy, a 'healthier race' was contingent upon 'the adoption and practice of a strict moral code of ethics', while for Lees the 'one sure method' of prevention and 'the production of a healthy stock' remained 'the attainment of a higher moral standard in the community, and the avoidance of promiscuous sexual intercourse'.[3]

Consistent with the medico-moral ideology of the Social Hygiene Movement, Scottish VD administrators viewed VD not just as a physical pathology but as the stigmata of the transgression of moral norms. They subscribed to an aetiology that incorporated an explicit taxonomy of guilt and blame. Thus, although David Lees sought 'to heal the sick, not to judge sin',[4] he clearly differentiated between patients according to the moral culpability of their condition.[5] A similar calibration informed the medical ideology of many Public Health Departments and the SBH.[6] Disease 'venereally' acquired remained synonymous within the minds of most practitioners with moral turpitude and sexual intemperance. For William Robertson, Medical Officer of Health for Edinburgh (1923–30), infection was the 'noose' into which 'licentious and immoral people' ran their heads.[7]

Those shaping VD policy in Scotland therefore sought preventive and curative strategies that accommodated both the moral and the physical agenda of Social Hygiene. Thus, although some Scottish venereologists such as David Lees supported the selective introduction of closely monitored ablution centres for post-coital 'abortive' treatment,[8] the majority of Medical Officers of Health resisted the issue of prophylactic packets and the establishment of public ablution centres on the grounds that, irrespective of their medical efficacy, they might legitimize 'irregular' and promiscuous sex and thus actively promote immorality by removing the natural penalties associated with promiscuity.[9] Typical was the view of Chalmers that 'the developing manhood of the population' would come to view them as provisions 'for compromising with chastity'.[10] Even where a Medical Officer of Health such as Robertson *was* prepared to advocate prophylaxis and self-disinfection, underpinning his medical philosophy was a set of powerful moral assumptions. For Robertson, while the 'clean section of society' might prove responsive to 'propaganda', there existed a dangerous residuum of 'sensually minded', irredeemable sexual degenerates for whom prophylactics were essential in the interests of racial health.[11]

The moral surveillance and regeneration of patients came increasingly to be perceived as part of the remit of the VD treatment clinics in Scotland. Although venereologists were broadly agreed that there was 'no place for preaching within the clinic',[12] many accepted the need to 'alter and direct into right lines the moral outlook of patients'.[13] Their operational philosophy therefore envisaged a pro-active role based upon the registers and case notes of the clinics that would deploy nurse almoners and existing lay and religious social work agencies to identify and reform dangerous sexualities: pre-eminently 'defaulters' from treatment who remained sexually active, parents of infected children who refused treatment, and 'problem girls'.[14] In the final analysis, where moral exhortation proved abortive and where women and children were at risk of innocent infection, most health officials were prepared to proscribe such deviants by law by means of compulsory notification and/or treatment. The loss of civil liberties was viewed as a legitimate stigma for those 'libertines' whose behaviour endangered the sexual health and social efficiency of the nation.[15]

The Moral Taxonomy of Treatment

The Innocent Patient

Accordingly, the administration of VD provisions in interwar Scotland remained firmly underpinned by a set of moral assumptions and categories in which 'innocent' and 'guilty' patients were clearly differentiated. Within the reports of the SBH/DHS and Public Health Departments, clinical and moral taxonomies were juxtaposed. Gradations of blame were reflected in a hierarchy of recommended treatment and controls for VD, with conventional principles of 'less eligibility' shaping attitudes to medical treatment, welfare support, and civil liberties.

At one end of the spectrum, there were what were described as the 'innocent patients' suffering from 'innocent infections': children and *married* women who were 'in no wise associated with guilt or blame' and 'against whom there [was] no suggestion that they [had] transgressed any moral or other law'.[16] For these deserving patients, Medical Officers advocated a range of special provisions designed to minimize stigma. Thus in Edinburgh, Glasgow, and Dundee, from the mid-1920s onwards, the diagnosis and out-patient treatment of mothers and children with VD were removed from the VD centres, and clinic facilities were increasingly provided as part of the Maternity and Child Welfare Services, especially at ante-natal clinics.[17] Furthermore, 'in order to provide hospital treatment for innocent patients without attaching a stigma to them', an increasing number of hospital beds were allocated for unspecified 'Diseases of Women and Children'. It was considered as 'obviously unfair to label these patients as cases of venereal disease or at any rate as cases of disease venereally acquired'. The extension of such facilities under the Child Welfare Schemes, and the need to treat 'innocently infected' women in gynaecological or ante-natal departments, remained an important objective of Medical Officers of Health and VD Clinical

109

Medical Officers in Scotland's major cities.[18]

In addition, in the interests of treatment, this 'deserving' category of 'innocently infected mothers and children' was, by the late 1920s, being increasingly accorded a range of welfare support denied to other sufferers. Philanthropic funding was mobilized to provide clothing, fuel and 'extra nourishment' for poorer patients.[19] Short holidays were arranged for children requiring 'fresh air and sunlight'. 'Housing conditions were brought to the notice of the Sanitary Authority, and public assistance was obtained for many who through unemployment were unable to provide sufficient nourishment for their children.' Efforts were even made to reinstate innocent patients whose attendance at VD clinics had resulted in dismissal from employment.[20]

The Defaulter

At the other end of the spectrum of blame were the defaulters, particularly infected married men and 'problem girls'. In terms of the medico-moral ideology of interwar health administrators and clinicians, this group of patients was doubly guilty. Not only had they contracted VD wilfully and 'venereally' by means of 'illicit' and 'promiscuous sexual intercourse', they also remained major vectors of disease within both their own families and the community at large, by virtue of their failure to sustain treatment until cured and to modify their sexual behaviour. It was this category of defaulter who came to dominate interwar debate over VD policy, and who fuelled the Scottish campaign for controls, including compulsory notification and treatment.[21] It was upon the defaulters that the burden of guilt for the continuing incidence of VD, despite the introduction of new medical therapies and facilities, was placed, and their identification and condemnation by clinicians and health officials within central and local government were a potent example of the process of stereotyping in the social construction of 'dangerous sexuality'.[22]

Within public health debate, defaulters were increasingly viewed as sexual offenders whose alleged venereal recidivism rendered them a prime source of infection within the community and threat to the success of the VD medical services.[23] According to the SBH, in the 1920s, one-third of patients attending VD clinics failed to complete a course of treatment, while another one-fourth withdrew before a final test for cure.[24] Defaulters were regularly depicted by health officials and practitioners as promiscuous 'libertines'; as 'hardened', 'incorrigible', 'intemperate' and 'habitual offenders' whose penchant for 'sexual indulgence' rendered them unresponsive to the necessary discipline of medical therapy.[25] In the view of Chalmers, Medical Officer of Health for Glasgow and an influential adviser to the SBH, 'being recessive towards the period of phallic worship, [the defaulter] will practice his cult directly a fresh opportunity offers and get reinfected'.[26]

Such behaviour not only offended public and professional opinion because of its implications for the spread of disease and its threat to 'social hygiene'. It also undermined the moral agenda of social reform in early twentieth-century Britain which sought in part to render welfare benefits contingent upon individual behaviour consistent with the 'social good'.[27] The alleged propensity of defaulters to accept repeated but incomplete courses of free treatment at the VD clinics, without modifying their sexual habits, ran directly counter to this agenda. Indeed, in the opinion of many Scottish medical officials, it posed as serious a risk of reducing the VD services to 'a convenient aid to further promiscuity' as had the proposed issue of prophylactic packets or the establishment of ablution centres during the immediate post-war years.[28] According to this viewpoint, the 'sexual intemperance' of defaulters was breeding 'just that casual outlook on venereal disease' which the treatment centres had been established to eliminate.[29]

Contemporary protest by Scottish local authorities and VD Medical Officers at the impact of default upon the cost-efficiency of VD clinics also harboured moral concerns. In a period of public expenditure cuts and increasing awareness of the health costs associated with venereal infections, the free provision of treatment to 'habitués' was regarded as a subsidy to vice. It offended against the principles of less eligibility that health expenditure on those venereally infected through wilful promiscuity should be permitted to enjoy 'a free and unfettered regime' in the use of State-subsidized facilities.[30]

The married male defaulter was increasingly singled out by public health authorities as a social and sexual pariah. In part, the concept of male responsibility for the spread of VD had been inherited from the feminist campaign of the Edwardian period. 'It was men, through their sexual licentiousness, who had brought disease into marriage; this was the main cause of women's sterility and infant mortality and morbidity.'[31] The guilty sufferer had come more often to be perceived as 'a male, conveying disease to the innocent women and children of his family, as opposed to a contaminated prostitute infecting healthy young male bodies'.[32] After the war, such views were reinforced by growing evidence and awareness of the repercussions of male infection for congenital syphilis and ophthalmia neonatorum, and the impact upon family and racial health of male promiscuity became a leading item on the agenda of the health reform ideologies of the period. Although the gender distribution of default varied markedly between Scottish cities, aggregate Scottish data revealed significantly higher rates for men after 1925.[33] The problems of default and reinfection were increasingly depicted in public health reports as a male pathology, with morally hygienic, married women requiring protection from the sexual whim of their carnal menfolk.[34] In addition, men were often held responsible for the default of innocently infected women either through 'direct domestic pressure' and intimidation or through their own refusal to seek or sustain treatment. Women were disinclined to attend VD clinics regularly if they faced the prospect of early reinfection from a defaulting partner.[35]

In important respects, the problem of the defaulter was a construct of the social fears and moral assumptions of medical practitioners and health officials within interwar Scotland. Opponents of the Scottish campaign for the compulsory notification and treatment of VD, most notably the Ministry of Health, claimed that the Scottish default statistics greatly exaggerated the threat of VD to public health. It was widely argued that many cases of syphilis attending clinics were already past the infectious stage, that the standard of cure was so high that many cases of gonorrhoea were non-infective well before the completion of treatment, and that many so-called defaulters moved to other clinics or opted to continue treatment under private practitioners.[36] Crude measures of default also failed to take account of patients who resumed treatment as a result of follow-up procedures. Moreover, given the dramatic rise in the interwar period of standards of cure prior to medical discharge, and the equally marked increase in average attendances per patient, the apparent crisis in commitment to treatment regimes was, in reality, largely a statistical illusion produced by changes in venereology and clinical practices.[37]

The behavioural stereotype of the defaulter deployed within Scottish public health debate was similarly lacking in empirical support. As Chalmers had to admit to the Society of Medical Officers of Health in 1928, despite the fact that the defaulter's supposed sexual habits had underpinned much of the campaign for VD controls, little research had been undertaken into 'the causes of default, and the social and civil status of the defaulter'.[38] Fragmentary evidence suggests that default from treatment was a complex phenomenon influenced by a range of economic, social, and cultural factors. A prime factor was the patient's fear of 'social ruin' should his or her venereal infection become public knowledge, and the difficulty of sustaining effective treatment over a lengthy period without alerting family or workmates. Other deterrents included the cost of travel to VD clinics, 'judgmental and unsympathetic staff', and the incompatibility of regular employment with therapy involving daily treatment at unsuitable surgery hours over a period of weeks or, in some cases, at regular intervals for years.[39] Moreover, as we have seen, the treatment regimes for syphilis and gonorrhoea were extremely invasive and unpleasant and not infrequently accompanied by faulty injections and lumbar punctures as well as highly toxic side-effects.[40] Many patients, especially those who were mentally deficient, were simply incapable of comprehending the importance of protracted treatment when the symptoms of their venereal disease were dormant.

The allegation that defaulters from treatment at the VD clinics were, as a group, more promiscuous and major vectors of VD within the community, was equally tenuous. Research on the case records of selected male clinics within Glasgow in 1928–9 appeared to indicate that the defaulter was a 'much less temperate individual, as far as sexual indulgence [was] concerned, than the rest of the population' and therefore more liable to contract and to transmit VD. However, as the investigator, R. J. Peters, conceded, given the clinical problems of distinguishing between relapse and reinfection and the impressionistic nature of much of the data, these conclusions could only be speculative. Significantly, no other serious study of the sexual behaviour of defaulters was undertaken in Scotland until the Second World War, when the issue of additional VD controls re-emerged. Investigation of sexual 'contacts' under Defence Regulation 33B then revealed no clear correlation between reported vectors of the disease and patients defaulting from treatment.[41]

There are interesting parallels between the identification and proscription of defaulters as a sexual sub-culture in interwar Scotland and the preoccupation with recidivism amongst penal reformers before the First World War.[42] Although some limited research into the problem of default was undertaken, like recidivism, its prominence reflected very much the orchestration of social fears by experts and officials informed by ill-disguised Social Darwinism. It too rested upon displaced anxieties about social disorder and moral decline, as well as bureaucratic self-interest. Similarly, it is arguable that the 'crisis of default', as with the panic over criminal recidivism, in part articulated 'the subliminal need' of specialists 'to demonstrate their professional credentials and utility'.[43] Certainly, there are similarities in the way that the identification of a new category of seasoned sexual offender fuelled the kinds of anxiety that justified more stringent controls over those who failed to comply with the moral dictates of middle-class professionals within central and local government.

The 'Problem Girl'

Meanwhile, as in many other countries, a distinct set of strategies was advocated to deal with young, infected girls and single women – officially described as 'problem girls' – who were allegedly responsible for a large proportion of default and who were viewed as major vectors of venereal disease through their sexual promiscuity and frequent recourse to amateur prostitution.[44] While the age-group 15–25 represented under 20 per cent of the female population in interwar Scotland, it accounted for over 30 per cent of female VD cases at the clinics and some 45 per cent of gonorrhoea cases.[45] Throughout the interwar period, Medical Officers of Health and VD clinical medical officers in the major Scottish cities pressed for more dedicated institutional provisions for young female patients, on both medical and socio-moral grounds. Concern was expressed that, while rescue workers often persuaded adolescent girls and young women to seek treatment, on discharge from hospital there was a lack of support and control mechanisms to ensure that treatment was sustained and that they did not 'return to the gutter'.[46] The loss of accommodation (frequently due to 'disgrace at home') and of employment (especially domestic work) due to infection and hospitalization, and the consequent recourse to prostitution and default from treatment, was viewed as a central factor in the continuing spread of venereal disease.[47]

The most common proposal, especially in the 1920s, was that public health and police authorities should have powers to detain 'girl' patients until they were both medically cured and employable. For this purpose, a new system of hostels was advocated in which medical treatment could be dispensed and occupational training provided. Thus, in his annual report for 1921, Lees argued that:

> The establishment of hostels or homes, where these girls could earn their living and yet be under medical observation until they are cured, seems the only method of dealing with this difficulty, and there is great need for such an institution as an annex to the work of

114

a venereal clinic .... There is no reason why such a Home under tactful management should not be run on self-supporting lines. It would give these girls a chance to make good, and enable them to feel that they were doing something to help themselves while still in touch with a clinic and under medical supervision.[48]

Lees and his successor, R. C. L. Batchelor, along with the nurse almoners, continued to advocate such proposals throughout the 1920s and 1930s, as did their opposite numbers within the Glasgow Public Health Department.[49]

The moral agenda underpinning such schemes is evident. The role of 'problem girl' patients as vectors of VD was consistently identified with their moral 'deficiency' and depravity and the aims of the hostels calibrated accordingly.[50] In the view of public health officials and clinicians, the function of homes and hostels was to provide not only an institutional base for continued and, if necessary, compulsory treatment, but also a means to 'direct into right lines the moral and mental outlook of patients' and to commence the 'work of reclamation'.[51] Occupational training was not merely designed to impart skills for use in the labour market, thus reducing dependency on casual prostitution, but to instil norms of regularized sexual and work behaviour consistent with middle-class ideals. In the words of the conference 'on the role of hostels in the campaign against VD' held in Edinburgh City Chambers in late 1918, 'hostels were vital to put an end to the moral and spiritual diseases' upon which VD fed, in order that single women patients 'may be brought to a normal and profitable form of existence' and thus 'redeem and restore their characters'.[52] Certainly, clinicians such as Lees, however aggressive in their medical strategies, perceived a continuing role for moral agencies and religious bodies.[53]

Although contemporary social hygiene debate in Scotland was critical of existing institutions such as the Magdalene Asylums and Church Homes for being too repressive,[54] for failing to differentiate between the needs of inmates, and for focusing on forms of employment such as laundry and domestic work whose tedium allegedly predisposed young women to seek sexual diversions,[55] in many respects the value system shaping the proposals of VD administrators and clinicians was little different. In the quest for the 'hostelization' of defaulters there lay the same desire as articulated by the Magdalene Asylums for a 'control apparatus for the surveillance, sexual and vocational control, and moral reform of a section of the female working-class population who defied middle-class standards of sexual and vocational propriety'; a similar concern to ensure the confinement of female homeless and jobless in order to reduce the level of hardened prostitution and 'to protect society from the spread of corruption and contagious disease'; and a similar set of strategies for moral regulation involving a disciplined regime of moral education and industrial training.[56]

Indeed, in Edinburgh, there was an early post-war attempt to build on the traditional complementary roles of the lock hospitals and Magdalene Asylums in Scotland when, in 1920, the Public Health Committee proposed to the Edinburgh Asylum that they should cooperate over monitoring 'problem girls' discharged from hospital after treatment for venereal disease. Doctors M. Liston and M. H. Macnicol, in charge of the female VD clinics at Bruntsfield Hospital and the Royal Infirmary, urged supervision of such inmates 'by a special visiting nurse, occasional visits of inspection to Infirmary or Hospital, and a special room which would be fitted up at the expense of the Public Health Committee'.[57] Ever jealous of their independence, the Directors of the Asylum declined the overture.

For a brief period, 1926–9, in Edinburgh, the VD service collaborated with the Moral Welfare Committee of the Council of Social Service in order to provide voluntary social workers to befriend and monitor the out-patient welfare and treatment of young female patients. Under this scheme, the Committee attempted to pursue a more 'scientific' strategy towards this high-risk default group with greater specialization of institutional provisions. According to the social work report for 1926:

> It [was] now felt that classification [was] essential, that all measures should be positive rather than negative, dangerous and unwholesome interests being effectively displaced only by wholesome and absorbing occupation for the mind as well as the body, and that the methods of government should be such as to fit rather than unfit the subject for life in the world.[58]

However, this intrusion into rescue and preventive work appears to have ended by 1930 and, along with Salvation Army Homes, Church of Scotland Homes, and shelters such as The Edinburgh Rescue Shelter, dedicated to supervised 'spiritual and temporal welfare', Scottish VD authorities continued to use the Magdalene institutions in an attempt to regularize the behaviour of 'girl' patients and to reduce levels of default and reinfection.[59]

The official response towards infected girls and young women has

116

to be placed in the general context of female sexuality and its regulation in early twentieth-century Britain. In many respects, the concept and treatment of 'problem girls' adopted by Scottish VD authorities in the interwar period perpetuated a wartime ideology of VD and its transmission, what Lucy Bland has termed the 'militarization of venereal disease'.[60] Concern for the institutional and social control of infected 'problem girls' echoed the fear and rhetoric associated with casual promiscuity and prostitution during World War I and served to sustain the epidemiological model of VD in which such groups were seen as the 'source' of infection contaminating the manhood and efficiency of the race.[61]

Thus, views such as those of Robertson and Chalmers, Medical Officers of Health for Edinburgh and Glasgow, that young females were the 'infecting agents ... abroad in our midst' who were insinuating a 'lower moral code ... sapping the vigour of our youth' carried on the operational philosophy of wartime venereologists into the 1920s.[62] Even where medical officials advocated a deeper analysis of the 'social epidemiology' of VD, it was predominantly the social and economic variables, such as low pay and inadequate housing, shaping *female* sexual habits that were identified. The factors determining *male* sexual proclivities were notably absent from the agenda.[63] Likewise, even David Lees, who always protested the absence of sexual discrimination from his proposals for VD controls, retained the view of women being the basic 'reservoir' of venereal infection in Scottish society.[64]

In their preoccupation with 'problem girls', health authorities in interwar Scotland were also perpetuating the growing orthodoxy that it was 'amateur prostitutes' with their disregard for precautions and/or effective treatment, rather than 'deliberate courtesans', who were the real focus of venereal infection.[65] At the same time, the treatment of infected girls and single women by VD authorities was also strongly informed by the sexual ideology of the Social Hygiene Movement. Their default and reinfection offended both the Movement's concern with social purity deriving from religious conceptions of self-control, willpower, and morality, and its medical preoccupation with public health. The 'unnatural' promiscuity of 'problem girls' that had engendered infection was both immoral and unclean. It threatened not only the health and stability of family and community relationships but also the essentially masculine authority of medical science.[66]

In addition, there were powerful strands of continuity between pre-war evangelical rescue work, wartime mechanisms designed to

contain the sexual behaviour of females 'of loose behaviour' such as
the Women Patrols Scheme, and interwar efforts to regulate infected
'girls'.[67] Attempts in interwar Scotland to control the 'sex delinquency'
of 'problem girls' by institutionalization and 'reconstruction' displayed
the same ambivalent mix of protective rhetoric and repressive aims
and a similar middle-class philanthropic view of young working-class
women as requiring 'custodial' surveillance to ensure a material and
moral environment in which norms of sexual passivity might be
instilled.[68]

Follow-Up Work and Contact Tracing

A range of procedures was initiated to try and reduce the level of
default at the VD clinics. The degree of intervention varied, in part
according to the degree of 'venereal offence'. After initial,
unsuccessful attempts to contact defaulters by confidential
correspondence, both Edinburgh and Glasgow Public Health
Departments addressed the problem of married female default in
1925 by the appointment of lady almoners attached to the female
and child welfare clinics who were empowered to follow up on
defaulters by domiciliary visits.[69]

From the start, the role of the 'default nurse' was defined broadly
as one of 'social almoner', who would, by a series of visits, thoroughly
familiarize herself with the patient's background and moral proclivities
and in liaison with other social workers 'induce a return to
treatment'.[70] As part of their efforts to reduce financial and logistical
constraints upon regular attendance, the nurse almoners became
increasingly involved in the provision of welfare facilities and family
counselling to 'innocent' patients. Visits 'for sociological purposes'
became the norm in the 1930s, with growing collaboration with other
medical and social work agencies such as the Child Welfare
Departments, Hospital Almoner Services, the Society for the
Prevention of Cruelty to Children, the Salvation Army, and Public
Assistance Departments.[71] The provision of charitable benefits
targeted by the nurse almoners became a potent inducement for
mothers to remain in contact with the clinics. In his report for 1937,
Edinburgh's VD Clinical Medical Officer well captured the role of the
almoner in bringing philanthropy to bear on the problem of default:

> an interesting innovation this year has been the presentation of
> Christmas stockings and gifts to children who are patients. These
> seasonable presents were provided by the Candlish Church and
> Warrender Park Church companies of Girl Guides and Brownies,

who, themselves, also carried out the presentation. The meeting of the Guides and Brownies and the children who came to receive the gifts took place at an interesting little ceremony arranged by our nurse almoner. This piece of practical social service, and the Christmas treats arranged for the Royal Infirmary and Corporation hospital and clinics are of great assistance in keeping in touch with families and of value in ensuring co-operation and regularity of attendance.[72]

However, especially in Edinburgh, the disciplinary element of visitation remained an overriding concern. The Public Health Department had explicitly viewed the appointment of a default nurse in 1924 as part of a future system of notification and controls. In their view, 'her work would be educational and preventive and would anticipate the very step forward we are anxious to see carried out; namely compulsory continuance of treatment'.[73] Thereafter, despite evidence that follow-up work was proving extremely effective,[74] the Nurse Almoner's annual reports echoed similar sentiments, with a regular call for legal controls upon 'recalcitrants' who resisted follow-up procedures.[75]

The process of follow-up was highly gender-specific. Men were not normally subjected to domiciliary visits nor the target of the same investigation and socio-medical surveillance. In the 1920s, reliance was placed on letters issued by the VD Medical Officer to male defaulters, inviting them to resume treatment but phrased so vaguely as to 'avoid causing domestic unhappiness'.[76] Although the effectiveness of such correspondence was limited,[77] other forms of follow-up were not employed. As Lees observed in 1929, 'it is difficult to send a visitor to the home of a male patient with any hope of finding him in except after his hours of work. A visit at this time by a hospital official would undoubtedly create suspicion in the case of both married and single men'.[78] In the view of Edinburgh Public Health Department, the application of a system of home visitation to men would 'almost certainly lead to exposure of the individual' and to a failure to uphold the pledge of confidentiality.[79] In contrast, in the case of married women, visitation could normally be disguised as part of generic child and maternity health care. The prevailing view of Scottish public health and clinical opinion was that there seemed 'to be no alternative to cope with the defaulter rate in the case of male patients other than to give the Medical Officer of Health some administrative controls over known infective cases'.[80]

However, faced by a continuing rise in the incidence of

gonorrhoea in the 1930s, nurse almoners in the major VD Schemes began to develop informal systems of contact tracing within the community as part of their regular follow-up work. Given the sensitivity of such work, not least the vulnerability of health officials under Scots Law to charges of defamation, few details were published. However, from 1932, the annual report of Dundee's Public Health Department did record the number of patients referred to its Public Health Institute, based upon information received in the male and female clinics. In the period 1932–8, some 5 per cent of male cases and 4 per cent of female cases treated at the Institute were identified through tracing. According to W. L. Burgess, Medical Officer of Health, 'all the resources at our disposal are utilised to get in touch with all consorts and contacts with a view to eliminating the source of infection and preventing spread'.[81] Other centres remained silent on the issue, but in subsequent wartime discussions it was admitted that regular contact tracing by letter and 'almonery visits' were by the late 1930s 'a normal procedure of any well run centre to get hold of sources of infection'.[82] The VD Medical Officer for Glasgow recalled that:

> The contacts of both male and female patients, when known, [were] followed up by male and female staff respectively, and where the patient [was] unwilling to provide the name and address of the infecting person or [did] not know accurately who the person was, he or she [was] asked to give, if possible, their contact a note of the times and places of the treatment centres and a letter which the contact should present to the doctor at the centre.[83]

The letter typically contained details of the patient's dates of exposure and the onset of symptoms along with the medical diagnosis and the results of serological tests, expressed in medical notation. The term VD was not mentioned and the patient was expressly warned not to make accusations against his/her alleged contact.[84]

Morals and Medical Therapy

Methods of treatment for VD in interwar Scotland reflected the medico-moral aetiology subscribed to by clinicians and health officials. While treatment regimes varied even between clinics within the same VD Scheme,[85] the official reports of the VD Medical Officers along with the treatment handbooks of leading Scottish venereologists reveal them to have been shaped to a significant extent by the social values and moral imperatives of the medical profession.

Thus, as we have seen, most Scottish health officials and

practitioners resisted prophylactic treatment such as the provision of disinfection packets or ablution centres (for 'abortive' treatment after exposure) on the grounds that, irrespective of their therapeutic effects, they might serve to further undermine chastity and sexual self-restraint. Typical was the view of Chalmers that the 'libertine' and venereal recidivist would merely exploit them to alleviate acute symptoms at the public expense.[86]

The lingering belief, despite protestations to the contrary, that VD was the penalty for vice and sexual irresponsibility, and that treatment for venereal infection should be neither too easy nor too accessible, also explains in part the penitential regime operating in the clinics of interwar Scotland. No doubt solid therapeutic considerations prevailed, but one is struck by the moral overtones of contemporary treatment; not only the predictable prohibition on alcohol, but also on dancing, masturbation, and 'everything which [tended] to stimulate the sexual sense'.[87] Likewise, at a time of acute uncertainty over the duration of infectivity in sexually transmitted diseases, the proscription on intercourse for four years for patients treated for syphilis appears to have been motivated as much by the desire to purge the sin as the disease.[88] That irrigation treatment for gonorrhoea was continued in many clinics until the Second World War as a 'balm to conscience', despite clear evidence of its damage to the urethra and the availability in the late 1930s of M. and B. 693 chemotherapy, has arguably similar implications.[89]

Equally suggestive is the contrast between the lack of scientific consensus over treatment and the rigidity of regimes laid down by local clinicians. Throughout the interwar period, therapy for syphilis in particular remained subject to considerable debate and conflict over correct dosages, length of treatment, and definitions of infectivity and cure.[90] Yet the treatment regimes laid down in many Scottish clinics continued to be shaped by moral absolutes as well as medical imperatives. In the official reports, the conflation of middle-class morality and professional expertise in defining norms of patient compliance is again apparent. According to the SBH, only the 'virtues' of 'regular, unremitting and persistent' attendance would 'have their sure reward', while defaulters would return 'in penitence and regret'.[91]

Both moral and medical regeneration were viewed as a function of submission to the controlled, asexual regime of the treatment room with its daunting irrigation equipment, probes and bougies, and to the regular surveillance of the medical records and attendants. Thus, clinicians frequently opted for intramuscular or intravenous medication with bismuth or mercury rather than oral medication, or persisted with injections of arsenobenzol compounds regardless of negative Wassermann Reaction in order to ensure the continued attendance and surveillance of patients until they were deemed socially hygienic.[92] For similar reasons, many clinics continued lavage treatment for gonorrhoea for some time after the efficacy of sulphanilamide drug therapy had been established.[93]

Indeed, as in the United States, the new chemotherapy of the late 1930s, in enabling self-administered medication with a minimum of contact with the clinic, posed a fundamental threat to the established role of medicine in sexual prescription.[94] In interwar Scotland, treatment was perceived and articulated within a discourse that assumed a symmetry between medical and sexual health and reclamation.[95] In the words of David Lees, the patient could only 'resume his place in society' once a professionally monitored and certified cure had been attained and 'the ordinary [sexual] rules of civilised life' conformed to.[96] Along with other leading venereologists, his concept of 'scientific' treatment was laden with the values of Social Hygiene. Cure implied a social as well as therapeutic response to treatment which would enable safe rehabilitation into the world of clean and socially acceptable marital sex. It was for the medical adviser to determine the point of re-entry, and to counsel abstention from intercourse and, if necessary, delay in marriage and conception.[97]

The Implications

The development of venereology and of the VD services in interwar Scotland was clearly shaped by a powerful set of moral fears, assumptions and objectives. Despite the assertion of some politicians and medical practitioners that VD should be treated as purely a medical issue, the provision of a comprehensive system of State-funded diagnostic and treatment facilities did not 'mean the end of moralistic service or the demystification of the diseases'.[98] On the contrary, moral issues and taxonomies continued to inform the aetiology and epidemiology and the treatment and follow-up of VD. For Scottish health administrators, inspired by the ideology of Social Hygiene, medical treatment and moral instruction were mutually interdependent solutions to the 'hideous scourge', both strands heavily defined by prevailing concerns over the apparent breakdown in social and sexual controls.

Equally, the evidence suggests that in Scotland, as in many other countries, the articulation of VD as a public health issue provided a powerful legitimation for the social construction and regulation of 'dangerous sexualities'.[99] One witnesses the same stereotyping and proscription of risk groups such as 'defaulters' and 'problem girls', the same confusion of clinical aetiology and moral accountability in confronting sexually transmitted diseases, and a similar use of treatment agencies and a judgemental epidemiology to define and reform unhygienic habits and 'anti-social sexual practices' that endangered fertility and racial health.

Certainly, the ideology of the treatment regimes prevailing at Scottish VD clinics and of their associated follow-up and tracing strategies conforms with the Foucaultian view of the rise of a medico-sexual regime, advancing a pathology of 'unproductive' sexual practices and a discourse in which the implications of the private world of sexuality for social health and efficiency sanctioned new forms of surveillances and controls.[100] This study also supports a related thesis that the interwar VD clinics formed part of 'the new hygiene of the dispensary' in which the focus of concern and controls in public health shifted from issues of sanitation and the natural environment to patterns of social contact and transmission.[101] As Armstrong observes, 'the national outcry against the spread of venereal disease was not only a manifestation of moral outrage but also of latent surveillance possibilities. The path of venereal disease throughout the community traced the threads which linked one person intimately with another. The dangers of venereal disease could be used as a means of observing behaviour, educating thoughts and teaching contacts.'[102] In these respects, one might question the view that the interwar period in Britain witnessed a 'wider laissez-faire policy by government' towards sexual issues.[103] Evidence would suggest that, in Scotland, the VD service and its clinicians were heavily involved in strategies of moral reform and that the local State remained highly interventionist on socio-sexual issues throughout the period.

Contemporary discourses surrounding the treatment of VD advanced taxonomies of innocence and guilt, of 'default' and 'sex delinquency' that appeared class-free. However, closer examination of the ideology and operation of the VD service in Scotland reveals that it articulated essentially middle-class values of moderation, self-restraint, abstinence, and hygiene as a means of remoralizing the poorer classes who attended the clinics. As D. Evans has rightly speculated: 'Even when treatment was effective, the experience of patients may have been stigmatizing and disempowering. Patients were likely to be working class and may have experienced the treatment and education they received as a form of social control.'[104] Implicit in the categorization of patients and 'defaulters' was an assumed correlation between class and 'wantonness'. As elsewhere,[105] it was predominantly working-class sexual behaviour that was scrutinized and appraised (or, more accurately, stereotyped) by the health authorities. Similarly, despite the absence of any reliable data on the social distribution of venereal disease, it was the 'libertines' and 'intransigents' within the working class who were identified as the major vectors. As Armstrong has demonstrated, the 'deference' of patients to the medico-moral behavioural prescriptions of middle-class health clinicians and administrators, including the need for 'rational' and 'temperate' habits, was central to the 'new hygiene of the dispensary'.[106]

Significant aspects of the campaign against VD in interwar Scotland were not only class-specific but also gender-specific. Despite the vigorous attack of health administrators and medical officers upon married male recidivists as vectors of disease within the family, they still perceived sexually active working-class women as the fundamental 'reservoir' of VD. As in many other countries, such as Australia, New Zealand, Canada, and the USA, female default due to medical or logistical reasons was often presented as wilfulness or viciousness peculiar to female sexual proclivities. In addition, as eugenic ideology gained currency, women who evaded treatment were increasingly stigmatized as 'moral imbeciles' whose alleged mental deficiency posed a major threat of racial degeneration.[107] Even where a proper 'social epidemiology' was called for, it was the dynamics of the *female* labour market that were targeted for investigation. The thrust of the more coercive strategies associated with the clinics, such as the use of hostels and other reformatories, was directed at 'problem girls', their protective surveillance designed to ensure a moral environment in which middle-class norms of sexual passivity might be instilled. Contemporary constructions of 'sex-delinquency' rarely addressed male sexuality.[108] It is therefore arguable that, despite its innovatory features, the ideology and procedures shaping the new VD service were to a significant extent repressive and discriminatory and that the 'discourse' shaping medical practice and policy towards VD both reflected and reaffirmed patterns of social and sexual subordination in interwar Scotland.

Notes

1   For an overview of the Social Hygiene Movement and the ideology of the National Council for Combating Venereal Diseases/British Social Hygiene Council [NCCVD/BSHC], see especially, G. Jones, *Social Hygiene in Twentieth Century Britain* (London: Croom Helm,

1986); E. J. Bristow, *Vice and Vigilance: Purity Movements in Britain since 1700* (London: Gill and Macmillan, 1977), ch. 6.

2   For these close institutional links, see *Royal Commission on National Health Insurance, Mins of Ev.* (London: HMSO, 1926), q. 20847; Edinburgh City Archives [ECA], Edinburgh Public Health Department [EPHD] Papers, Box 8, Files 15/1, 15/5, 15/11, Minutes of Scottish Executive Committee of BSHC.

3   *EPHD Annual Report (1930)*, viii; D. Lees, 'VD in City Life', *Journal of State Medicine*, 40 (1932), 87, 93. For expressions of similar views employing the rhetoric of Social Darwinism and National Efficiency, see also *Glasgow Medical Officer of Health [MOH] Annual Report (1920)*, 9; *(1923)*, 21; A. K. Chalmers, *The Health of Glasgow 1818–1925: An Outline* (Glasgow: Glasgow Corporation, 1930), viii.

4   *Scotsman*, Obituary, 28 March 1934.

5   See, e.g., Lees, *op. cit.* (note 3), 94–5.

6   See especially, *EPHD Annual Report (1920)*, xxii; *Aberdeen MOH Annual Report (1935)*, 51; *Scottish Board of Health [SBH], Seventh Annual Report, PP 1926 (Cmd. 2674) XI*, 66.

7   W. Robertson, 'The Controversy Regarding the Prevention of Venereal Diseases', *Edinburgh Medical Journal [EMJ]*, 28 (1922), 123.

8   Contemporary Medical Archives Centre [CMAC], SA/BSH/G3, Minutes of Manchester (Ablution Centres) Enquiry Committee, 13 Feb. 1922.

9   For an overview of contemporary debate over this issue, see especially, B. A. Towers, 'Health Education Policy 1916–1926: Venereal Disease and the Prophylaxis Dilemma', *Medical History*, 24 (1980), 70–87.

10 *Glasgow MOH Annual Report (1920)*, 9. See also, *SBH, Seventh Annual Report (1925)*, *op. cit.* (note 6), 73.

11 W. Robertson, *op. cit.* (note 7), 123–31, and 'The Administrative Control of Venereal Disease', *Transactions of the Incorporated Sanitary Association of Scotland (1919)*, 59–68.

12 David Lees in *Glasgow Herald*, 3 Dec. 1921.

13 *EPHD Annual Report (1931)*, 76. For Mary Liston, Assistant VD Medical Officer for Edinburgh, who advanced the somewhat unorthodox aetiology that 'passions excessively indulged in' upset the balance of the endocrines creating the localization of toxins and bacteria in the genital region, 'godliness and cleanliness, and nothing else, [were] the rules of health' (National Archives of Scotland [NAS], HH 104/35/28, M. Liston, 'The Prevention of Venereal Diseases').

14 For an excellent overview of this 'new hygiene of the Dispensary', see D. Armstrong, *Political Anatomy of the Body: Medical Knowledge in Britain in the Twentieth Century* (Cambridge: Cambridge University Press, 1983), 7–18.

15 See below, ch. 8.

16 *SBH, Seventh Annual Report, op. cit.* (note 6) 66; *Ninth Annual Report, PP 1928 (Cmd. 3112) X,* 110; *EPHD Annual Report (1923),* 48.

17 *EPHD Annual Report (1925),* 57; *Glasgow MOH Annual Report (1924),* 124; *(1925),* 145; *(1926),* 158; *Dundee MOH Annual Report (1924),* 116.

18 *EPHD Annual Report (1928),* 78; *(1929),* 76; *(1930),* 78; *SBH, Ninth Annual Report (1927), op. cit.* (note 16), 110.

19 Lack of 'respectable' clothing for visiting the clinic was often a deterrent to women; see *Glasgow MOH Annual Report (1926),* 162.

20 *EPHD Annual Report (1928),* 77; *(1929),* 75; *(1932),* 69; *(1936),* 87; *Glasgow MOH Annual Report (1925),* 155.

21 For the significance of default in this campaign, see below, ch. 8.

22 For the broader implications of this process of taxonomy and control in the creation of 'technologies of power' over sexuality, see especially, M. Foucault, *The History of Sexuality, Vol. 1: An Introduction* (London: Random House, 1979).

23 See, e.g., *EPHD Annual Report (1920),* xxii, 54; *(1921),* xvii; *(1924),* 59; *(1931),* 76; *Glasgow MOH Annual Report (1929),* 157.

24 *SBH/DHS, Annual Reports.*

25 *Glasgow MOH Annual Report (1923),* 20; *(1925),* 138; *(1929),* 157–8; *Dundee MOH Annual Report (1935),* 109.

26 A. K. Chalmers, 'The Notification and Control of Venereal Diseases', *Public Health,* 42 (1928–9), 105. On the application of evolutionary notions of atavism to contemporary explanations of sexuality, see L. Bland and F. Mort, 'Look Out For The "Good Time" Girl: Dangerous Sexualities as a Threat to National Health', in *Formations of Nation and People* (London: Routledge and Kegan Paul, 1984), 138.

27 See, e.g., J. Brown, 'Social Control and the Modernisation of Social Policy, 1890–1929', in P. Thane (ed.), *The Origins of British Social Policy* (London: Croom Helm, 1978), 126–9.

28 *Glasgow MOH Annual Report (1923),* 20.

29 *Glasgow MOH Annual Report (1927),* 157; A. S. M. Macgregor, 'The Powers and Responsibilities of Local Authorities in the Venereal Diseases Campaign', *Proceedings of the Imperial Social Hygiene Congress* (London: BSHC, 1927), 228.

30   See, e.g., *EPHD Annual Report (1920)*, xxiii; *(1921)*, xvi; *(1923)*, 20;
     Glasgow MOH Annual Report (1927), 157; A. K. Chalmers, 'The
     Need for a Policy', *Proceedings of the Imperial Social Hygiene Congress*
     (London: BSHC, 1924), 118.

31   L. Bland, 'Marriage Laid Bare: Middle-Class Women and Marital
     Sex 1880s–1914', in J. Lewis (ed.), *Labour and Love: Women's
     Experience of Home and Family 1850–1940* (Oxford: Basil Blackwell,
     1986), 136.

32   L. A. Hall, *Hidden Anxieties: Male Sexuality, 1900–1950* (London:
     Polity Press, 1991), 36.

33   It was estimated that in the period 1925–9, the proportion of new
     female cases in Dundee ceasing to attend VD clinics before
     completing a course of treatment was *c.* 43% while for men the
     default rate was *c.* 26%. In contrast, in Glasgow, the respective
     default rates were *c.* 10% and ca. 50%. For Scotland as a whole,
     male default rates for the same period were in the order of 28%,
     twice the level for female patients. See *Annual Reports of the SBH and
     the MOH for Dundee and Glasgow.*

34   In some quarters of Scottish medical opinion, there was a firm belief
     that men possessed a 'more recently acquired, and in consequence,
     less stabilised standard of sex morality'. See, e.g., Chalmers, *op. cit.*
     (note 26), 108.

35   See, e.g., *SBH, Ninth Annual Report (1927)*, *op. cit.* (note 16), 118;
     Glasgow MOH Annual Report (1927), 150.

36   L. W. Harrison, 'Local Authorities and Notification: Discussion',
     Proceedings of the Imperial Social Hygiene Congress, op. cit. (note 30),
     126; *Report of Committee of Inquiry on Venereal Disease* (London:
     HMSO, 1923), para. 19.

37   Thus, although recorded default rates rose by *c.* 40% in Glasgow for
     the period 1923–9, the average number of attendances per patient
     nearly doubled from 24.3 to 40 (*Glasgow MOH Annual Report
     (1929)*, 153).

38   Chalmers, *op. cit.* (note 26), 108.

39   See, e.g., *Glasgow MOH Annual Report (1926)*, 162; *EPHD Annual
     Report (1938)*, 134: 'the patient's own statement of the reason why
     she does not attend well is that the cost of coming into the central
     clinic even once a week is "the price of a loaf of bread"'.

40   See, e.g., *Glasgow MOH Annual Report (1929)*, 153–62; *Aberdeen
     MOH Annual Report (1937)*, iii–v.

41   *Glasgow MOH Annual Report (1929)*, 153–62; NAS, HH
     64/122/37, Memorandum on 'Defaulting' by I. N. Sutherland,
     Senior Medical Officer, 21 Nov. 1944.

42 On recidivism, see especially, L. Radzinowicz and R. Hood, *The Emergence of Penal Policy in Victorian and Edwardian England*, Vol. 5 of L. Radzinowicz, *A History of English Criminal Law and its Administration from 1750* (London: Stevens, 1986), 306–10; V. A. C. Gatrell, 'Crime, Authority and the Policeman-State', in F. M. L. Thomson (ed.), *Cambridge Social History of Britain 1750–1950, Vol. 3: Social Agencies and Institutions* (Cambridge: Cambridge University Press, 1990), 306–10.

43 Gatrell, *op. cit.* (note 42), 310.

44 See, e.g., *EPHD Annual Report (1920)*, 54; *(1931)*, 76; *(1936)*, 83. Scottish public health officials habitually employed the term 'girl' to denote 'young woman' when discussing the incidence and control of VD. This served to reinforce their presentation of sexually active, single women as regressive and in need of special protection and restraint. On the association between the 'degenerate sexuality' of the woman and child, see S. L. Gilman, 'Sexology, Psychoanalysis, and Degeneration: From a Theory of Race to a Race to Theory', in J. E. Chamberlin and S. L. Gilman (eds), *Degeneration: The Dark Side of Progress* (New York: Columbia University Press, 1985), 87. On the development of 'problem girl' strategies elsewhere, see especially, A. Mooij, *Out of Otherness: Characters and Narrators in the Dutch Venereal Disease Debates, 1850–1990* (Amsterdam/Atlanta: Rodopi, 1998), ch. 3; J. Sangster, 'Incarcerating "Bad Girls": The Regulation of Sexuality through the Female Refuges Act in Ontario, 1920–1945', *Journal of the History of Sexuality*, 7 (1996), 239–75; C. Strange, *Toronto's Girl Problem: The Perils and Pleasures of the City 1880–1930* (Toronto: University of Toronto Press, 1995), ch. 5; R. M. Alexander, *The 'Girl Problem': Female Sexual Delinquency in New York, 1900–1930* (Ithaca and London: Cornell University Press, 1995), ch. 2.

45 *SBH/DHS Annual Reports; Census of Scotland 1931, Preliminary Report* (Edinburgh: HMSO, 1931).

46 *EPHD Annual Report (1920)*, 54. See also NAS, ED15/256, Evidence to Young Offenders (Scotland) Committee, 6 May 1926, q. 9565.

47 *EPHD Annual Report (1924)*, 59; *(1932)*, 70; *(1933)*, 83; *(1936)*, 83; *Glasgow MOH Annual Report (1923)*, 19.

48 *EPHD Annual Report (1921)*, 41–2.

49 See, e.g., *ibid.*, *(1928)*, 77; *(1931)*, 76; *(1934)*, 75; *(1938)*, 13; *Glasgow MOH Annual Report (1925)*, 153.

50 See especially the evidence of social workers before the Scottish Committee on Young Offenders (1926), NAS, ED 15/256.

51 *EPHD Annual Report (1931)*, 76; *(1934)*, 75. For a contemporary review of institutional responses to the problem of sexually promiscuous girls, see especially C. Neville Rolfe, 'Sex-Delinquency', in H. Llewellyn Smith (ed.), *The New Survey of London Life and Labour, Vol. IX: Life and Leisure* (London: P. S. King, 1935), ch. 11.

52 ECA, EPHD Papers, Box 34, file 15/1. The Conference was jointly sponsored by the Scottish Committee of the NCCVD and Edinburgh PHC.

53 *EPHD Annual Report (1931)*, 76; *Glasgow MOH Annual Report (1926)*, 162.

54 Lees, e.g., criticized existing homes as 'in many cases ... little better than prison life' (*EPHD Annual Report (1921)*, 41).

55 See, e.g., *Edinburgh Council of Social Service Annual Report (1926)*, 10–12. For contemporary concern over the correlation between domestic work and VD and its implications for the job placement strategies of 'rescue' institutions, see *Aberdeen MOH Annual Report (1924)*, 126–7; ECA, EPHD Papers, Box 34, file 15/1.

56 For the ideology of such homes, see, L. Mahood, *The Magdalenes: Prostitution in the Nineteenth Century* (London: Routledge, 1990), 3, 78–9, 81; L. Mahood, 'The Wages of Sin: Women, Work and Sexuality in the Nineteenth Century', in E. Gordon and E. Breitenbach (eds), *The World is Ill Divided: Women's Work in Scotland in the Nineteenth and Early Twentieth Centuries* (Edinburgh: Edinburgh University Press, 1990), 30–7; see also, Edinburgh Central Library, *Annual Reports of Edinburgh Magdalene Asylum (1920–39)*.

57 Edinburgh Central Library, Edinburgh Magdalene Asylum, Sub-Committee Minute Book, 12 April 1920.

58 *Edinburgh Council of Social Service, Annual Report (1926)*, 10–12, *(1927)*, 19; *(1928)*, 16. The Committee's objectives and rhetoric in part reflected the Council's origins as the local branch of the Charity Organisation Society.

59 Edinburgh Central Library, *Annual Reports of Edinburgh Rescue Shelter; EPHD Annual Report, (1929)*, 75; *(1936)*, 88; *Glasgow MOH Annual Report (1926)*, 162. For similar liaison between rescue and medical agencies in England, see Neville Rolfe, *op. cit.* (note 51), 313–14, 329. Continuing research on the asylums may also reveal welfare, police and medical authorities to have colluded in the use of the Mental Deficiency and Lunacy (Scotland) Act of 1913 to institutionalize infected girls as 'moral imbeciles'. In England, although VD 'was never deemed to be evidence of mental defect, the continuation of behaviour which placed one in danger of contracting

or spreading the disease could encourage such a diagnosis'. See, M. Thompson, *The Problem of Mental Deficiency: Eugenics, Democracy, and Social Policy in Britain c. 1870–1959* (Oxford: Clarendon Press, 1998), 251.

60   L. Bland, '"Cleansing the Portals of Life": The Venereal Disease Campaign in the Early Twentieth Century', in M. Langan and B. Schwarz (eds), *Crises in the British State 1880–1930* (London: Hutchison, 1985), 201.

61   See L. Bland, '"Guardians of the Race" or "Vampires upon the Nation's Health"? : Female Sexuality and its Regulation in Early Twentieth-Century Britain', in E. Whitelegg *et al.*, *The Changing Experience of Women* (Oxford: Martin Robertson, 1982), 375–88.

62   W. Robertson, 'Treatment and Control of Venereal Diseases', *EMJ*, 19 (1917), 368; *Glasgow MOH Annual Report (1921)*, 8; *(1922)*, 10. It was symptomatic of this attitude that, in the reports of VD Medical Officers, young infected women were often referred to as 'infective material'.

63   See, e.g., *Glasgow MOH Annual Report (1922)*, 10; *(1923)*, 19, 21.

64   Public Record Office [PRO], MH 55/198, Draft memo. by David Lees for the Medical Advisory Committee of the BSHC, Dec. 1930, 2.

65   On this view, see Bland, *op. cit.* (note 60) 202. For the local distinction between the two groups as vectors, see *Glasgow MOH Annual Report (1922)*, 10; *(1923)*, 19; D. Lees, 'Methods of Securing the Maximum Efficiency of a Venereal Diseases Clinic', *Proceedings of the Imperial Social Hygiene Congress, op. cit.* (note 30), 141–2.

66   Bland, *op. cit.* (note 61), 377–8; *op. cit.* (note 60), 200–1; L. Bland, 'In the Name of Protection: The Policing of Women in the First World War', in J. Brophy and C. Smart (eds), *Women-In-Law: Explorations in Law, Family and Sexuality* (London: Routledge and Kegan Paul, 1985), 42.

67   See especially, Bland, *ibid.*, 23–49; Bland and Mort, *op. cit.* (note 26), 131–51; NAS, HH 31/16, Papers relating to Scottish Women Patrols.

68   L. Mahood and B. Littlewood, 'The "Vicious" Girl and the "Street-Corner" Boy: Sexuality and the Gendered Delinquent in the Scottish Child-Saving Movement, 1850–1940', *Journal of the History of Sexuality*, 4 (1994), 549–78; L. Mahood, *Policing Gender, Class and Family: Britain 1850–1940* (London: UCL Press, 1995), ch. 6.

69   ECA, Edinburgh Town Council Minutes, 1 May 1924; *EPHD Annual Report (1926)*, 56; *Glasgow MOH Annual Report (1925)*, 141.

70   *EPHD Annual Report (1935)*, 82; *Glasgow MOH Annual Report*

(1925), 141.

71   *EPHD Annual Report (1930)*, 76–7; *(1933)*, 83; *(1934)*, 35; *Glasgow MOH Annual Report (1926)*, 162; *(1933)*, 118; *(1934)*, 143; *(1935)*, 134. For similar developments in VD social work overseas and its function within a similar tradition of middle-class moral philanthropy, see A. Mooij, *op. cit.* (note 44), ch. 3.

72   *Edinburgh MOH Annual Report (1937)*, 100–1.

73   ECA, Edinburgh Town Council Minutes, 1 April 1924.

74   Thus, in Edinburgh in 1928, it was claimed that some 80% of women and child defaulters returned for further observation, treatment and advice as a result of domiciliary visits. By 1932, the success rate was estimated at 90% (*EPHD Annual Report (1928)*, 77; *(1932)*, 69).

75   See, e.g., *EPHD Annual Report (1928)*, 77–8; *(1929)*, 75; *(1930)*, 77.

76   For a copy of the standard letter issued to male defaulters, see *Glasgow MOH Annual Report (1920)*, 86.

77   This was commonly attributed to the fact that the typical male defaulter belonged to 'a hardened, incorrigible section who furnished false particulars' (*Dundee MOH Annual Report (1935)*, 109).

78   *EPHD Annual Report (1929)*, 74.

79   *Ibid. (1930)*, 76; *(1932)*, 70.

80   *Ibid. (1932)*, 70.

81   *Dundee MOH Annual Report (1936)*, 109.

82   NAS, HH 65/121/81; HH 65/122/39, discussion papers on DORA Regulation 33B, 1942; *EPHD Annual Report (1943)*, 24. Leading clinicians at the Royal Infirmary of Edinburgh were strongly in favour of more aggressive contact tracing in dealing with infectious diseases. Sir Robert Philip, Professor of Tuberculosis, urged that dispensary staffs 'should be a mobile force, ready to hunt down the enemy in a systematic search for all cases in their area' (*British Medical Journal [BMJ]*, 2 July 1932, 3).

83   NAS, HH 65/117/65, W. A. Horne [Senior Deputy MOH, Glasgow], 'Incidence of Venereal Diseases in Glasgow', 3 Dec. 1943. Due to the threat of assault, male nurses were in fact rarely used for contact tracing (communication from retired consultant venereologist, 21 June 1995).

84   NAS, HH 65/116/85, Department of Health for Scotland to MOH Kirkwall, 18 Nov. 1939.

85   See, e.g., *Glasgow MOH Report (1930)*, 192.

86   *Glasgow MOH Annual Report (1920)*, 9; Chalmers, *op. cit.* (note 3), 404. For a similar reluctance to advocate chemical prophylaxis overseas, see A. Brandt, *No Magic Bullet: A Social History of Venereal*

Sin and Suffering

Disease in the United States since 1830 (Oxford: Oxford University Press, 1987), 158; P. J. Fleming, 'Fighting the "Red Plague": Observations on the Response to Venereal Disease in New Zealand 1910–45', *New Zealand Journal of History*, 22 (1988), 63.

87   See, e.g., D. Lees, *Practical Methods in the Diagnosis and Treatment of VD* (Edinburgh: Livingstone, 1927), 176–7, 325–6, 381, 390, 419, 553; *SBH, Instructions to Patients Suffering from Syphilis* (Edinburgh: HMSO, July 1919). A 'mental diet' often formed part of the pharmacopoeia, designed to divert the patient from 'pictures ... and literature of a sexually stimulating variety' and from the 'melancholy joys' of 'the continuous contemplation of his genitals' (L. W. Harrison, Special Adviser on VD, Ministry of Health), *Modern Diagnosis and Treatment of Syphilis, Chancroid and Gonorrhoea* (London: Constable, 1924), 285–6, 321).

88   ECA, EPHD Papers, file 15/11, Minutes of the Scottish Executive Committee of the BSHC, 20 Oct. 1933.

89   See especially, *Dundee MOH Annual Report (1938)*, 122; *EPHD Annual Report (1938)*, 131–3.

90   Lees, *op. cit.* (note 87), 299, 536; Harrison, *op. cit.* (note 87), 10–11, 403. Debate focused in particular on the significance of the Wassermann Test in determining the mix and duration of treatment with arsenobenzol compounds and mercury.

91   *SBH, Seventh Annual Report (1925)*, *op. cit.* (note 6), 68.

92   D. Lees, *op. cit.* (note 65), 138; *EPHD Annual Report (1925)*, 57; Harrison, *op. cit.* (note 87), 181–3.

93   *Dundee MOH Report (1937)*, 119–20; *EPHD Annual Report (1937)*, 99.

94   See F. J. T. Bowie *et al.*, 'Treatment of Gonorrhoea by M. and B. 693', *BMJ*, I (1939), 712–24; Brandt, *op. cit.* (note 86), 173.

95   This symmetry is well captured in David Lees' obituary in *The Scotsman*, 28 March 1934: 'While he was healing their bodies, he was influencing their minds. Many a poor stray has through his quiet talks decided to have another try at life again.'

96   Lees, *op. cit.* (note 87), 537–8.

97   *Ibid.*, 171; *EPHD Annual Report (1925)*, 55; Harrison, *op. cit.* (note 87), 410; L. Findlay [Venereologist to Royal Hospital for Sick Children, Glasgow], *Syphilis in Childhood* (London: Hodder and Stoughton, 1919), 121–2.

98   J. Weeks, *Sex, Politics and Society: The Regulation of Sexuality since 1800* (London and New York: Longman, 1989), 228.

99   See especially, Brandt, *op. cit.* (note 86), 137–8; F. Mort, *Dangerous Sexualities: Medico-Moral Politics in England since 1830* (London:

132

Sin and Suffering

Routledge and Kegan Paul, 1987), 208–9; J. Cassel, *The Secret Plague: Venereal Disease in Canada, 1838–1939* (Toronto: University of Toronto Press, 1987), ch. 9. As in the United States, this legitimation was reinforced by the impact of new technologies for the diagnosis and treatment of VD on the authority of the medical profession in sexual matters; see Brandt, *op. cit.* (note 86), 120.

100 Foucault, *op. cit.* (note 22), 26, 36, 41–2, 145.

101 Armstrong, *op. cit.* (note 14).

102 *Ibid.*, 12.

103 Mort, *op. cit.* (note 99), 199.

104 D. Evans, 'Tackling the "Hideous Scourge": The Creation of the Venereal Disease Treatment Centres in Early Twentieth-Century Britain', *Social History of Medicine,* 5 (1992), 431.

105 The view that 'amateur' prostitutes were predominantly working class and that they demonstrated the 'wayward sexual mores of the labouring classes' underpinned Australian VD procedures in the interwar period, and similar assumptions shaped social hygiene ideology in France, Canada, and the USA. See D. R. Tibbits, 'The Medical, Social and Political Response to Venereal Diseases in Victoria 1860–1980', Monash University, Ph.D. thesis (1994), 181; Brandt, *op. cit.* (note 86), 22, 157; C. Quétel, *History of Syphilis* (Oxford: Polity Press, 1990), 181, 204; J. Sangster, *op. cit.* (note 44), 246–8, 265, 274; R. M. Alexander, *op. cit.* (note 44), 33–4, 39–40.

106 Armstrong, *op. cit.* (note 14), 103–6.

107 P. J. Fleming, 'Shadow over New Zealand: The Response to Venereal Disease in New Zealand 1910–45', Massey University, Ph.D. thesis (1989), 9, 72, 175; Tibbits, *op. cit.* (note 105), 182; Sangster, *op. cit.* (note 44), 252, 264–6; Alexander, *op. cit.* (note 44), 41; C. Strange, *op. cit.* (note 44), 128–9.

108 It is significant that, while Reformatory and Industrial Schools could refuse admission on grounds of 'moral considerations', this was rarely applied to boys. In contrast, 'girls who were suspected prostitutes, found living in brothels, victims of assault and incest, or suffering from venereal disease were frequently rejected' and referred to Magdalene homes. See Mahood, *op. cit.* (note 68), 53.

6

Images of Social Hygiene:
VD Propaganda in Interwar Scotland

The Organization of Propaganda

The moral agenda underlying VD administration in Scotland was perhaps most clearly reflected in the propaganda work undertaken. The Royal Commission on Venereal Diseases had concluded that 'the evils which [led] to the spread of venereal diseases [were], in great part, due to want of control, ignorance and inexperience' and that to combat the 'great scourge', medical strategies would have to be complemented by an upgrading of public awareness and of 'the moral standards and practice of the community'.[1] Accordingly, as the main strategy of prevention, the VD Regulations of 1916 empowered Scottish health authorities to liaise with the police, with medical and educational authorities, and with social hygiene agencies, in the provision of 'instructional lectures' and 'the diffusion of information' on questions relating to VD. The regulations laid particular stress on the need to highlight their 'far-reaching and disastrous effects on the social efficiency of the family'.[2]

Scottish health officials fully endorsed the views of the Royal Commission and continued to regard moral hygiene and education as a fundamental aim of VD policy and a precondition of any effective medical advance against the 'social evil'.[3] A major constraint upon the success of the new VD services was perceived to be ignorance; ignorance of the prevalence of VD, of its 'incalculable ravages' upon family and racial health, of the medical facilities available and the vital importance of early and professional treatment, and, above all, of the moral and sexual conduct conducive to its transmission and elimination. Accordingly, administrators and clinicians welcomed the efforts of social hygiene agencies to 'educate for chastity' and to preach the importance of sexual continence for physical and racial health. For David Lees, 'propaganda' was a vital adjunct to medical science in furthering the cause of public health and optimizing the use of the clinics, while for Medical Officers of Health such as A. K. Chalmers and W. L. Burgess, who perceived the First World War as having fractured sexual norms, education in sexual hygiene was imperative to counter 'the lower moral code sapping the vigour of our youth' and to alert the young of 'the moral and physical dangers which imperilled them'.[4]

The organization and content of propaganda was shaped by a variety of social forces and ideologies and could often be contentious. As recommended by the Royal Commission on Venereal Diseases, the prime responsibility for the preparation and dissemination of materials rested with local health authorities in collaboration with local branches of the National Council for Combating Venereal Diseases [NCCVD] (subsequently the British Social Hygiene Council [BSHC]), which enjoyed accredited status with the Scottish Board of Health [SBH] for funding out of the Venereal Diseases Grant.[5] During the period of post-war demobilization, the National Council in London played an extremely pro-active role in trying to pump-prime and co-ordinate the educational work of Scottish local authorities, but after the establishment of a Scottish Committee in 1921, responsibility for propaganda was formally devolved upon its local branches.[6]

Within each branch, the Medical Officer of Health and VD Medical Officer were decisive in determining policy with respect to the content and targeting of information, often on the basis of the pattern of attendance at the clinics.[7] Nonetheless, other medics, educationalists, social workers, church leaders, and social hygiene and purity activists making up the NCCVD/BSHC local executive committees also shaped VD propaganda, as did members of local Public Health and National Health Insurance Committees.[8] Purity organizations, such as the purity department of the British Women's Temperance Association, which supplemented the NCCVD's literature with their own tracts, were particularly vocal on the issue.[9] In Scotland, the Alliance of Honour was especially concerned to ensure that VD literature and lectures addressed ethical aspects of the question. Founded in 1903 as an inter-denominational youth purity organization devoted to the inculcation of a high and single standard of chastity, the Alliance was strongly represented in the East of Scotland, where it launched a series of educational campaigns in liaison with the NCCVD, with whom it often shared the patronage of local civic leaders.[10]

On issues of social hygiene education, the new-found social authority of the public health professions had also to be shared with the older authority exercised by the Scottish clergy. The Scottish churches viewed VD propaganda as part of a broader campaign for moral reform to counter the spiritual debilitation of war and post-war shifts in social mores, and were highly influential in validating the content and format of local educational initiatives.

EAST LOTHIAN COUNTY AND BURGHS PUBLIC HEALTH.

VENEREAL DISEASES.

Although these diseases occur as the result of immoral conduct,
they may be spread in other ways.

THE EFFECTS OF THESE DISEASES
upon the individual and upon the race are:
GRAVE AND FAR REACHING.

It has been demonstrated that

PROMPT RECOGNITION AND SYSTEMATIC TREATMENT
of these diseases will enable the patient to avoid these
grave after-consequences.

Arrangements have been made for

FREE TREATMENT FOR ALL.

Persons suffering from these diseases can have treatment

UNDER CONDITIONS OF SECRECY.

Patients may attend for treatment and consultation at the
EDINBURGH ROYAL INFIRMARY.

Male Patients attend on:—			Female Patients attend on:—		
MONDAYS. WEDNESDAYS FRIDAYS SATURDAYS	}	At 10 A.M.	MONDAYS THURSDAYS	}	At 10 A.M.
TUESDAYS FRIDAYS:	}	At 5 P.M.	THURSDAYS -		At 3 P.M.

Further information as to these facilities, and copies of a special leaflet on the dangers
of Venereal Diseases, can be obtained from the

COUNTY MEDICAL OFFICER OF HEALTH.

ADDRESS YOUR LETTER IN THIS WAY—

Private.

County Medical Officer of Health,
County Public Health Office,
Haddington.

Plate 6.1
Local authority VD propaganda, 1922
(*Haddington Courier and East Lothian Advertiser*, 3 March 1922)

According to the SBH, by 1925, a comprehensive programme of 'propaganda work' was under way. This included 'meetings, lectures, and exhibitions of films, both for laymen and for the medical profession; conferences with local health authorities, education authorities, and other public bodies; lectures at large public works and to social organisations; exhibition of suitable posters; advertisements and articles in newspapers, trade union journals and women's periodicals, and distribution of appropriate literature, including leaflets for foreign seamen printed in most continental languages'.[11] Despite the best efforts of the NCCVD/BSHC to standardize procedures, the mix and format and targeting of propaganda varied widely across the country, with considerable deference to local sentiment. Thus, some local health authorities preferred to issue their own VD posters rather than the more explicit posters of the Council *(see Plate 6.1)*, fearing that the latter might offend public opinion and purity activists.[12] For similar reasons, the issue of where VD posters might appropriately be displayed was often contentious. Glasgow Corporation's Sub-Committee on VD agonized over the issue for years, and was extremely reluctant to sanction their display other than in the men's toilets at railway stations.[13] Indeed, even this limited distribution of posters encountered opposition.[14]

The format of public meetings and lectures was also shaped by a mix of medico-moral and professional agendas, with particular regard to the need to control the access and response of working-class audiences to information on VD, and to ensure that sexual propriety was observed and that individual issues of sexual hygiene were firmly located within broader obligations to public morality and racial health.

Overarching the propaganda work of the NCCVD/BSHC in the 1920s was a series of public meetings held in collaboration with the major health authorities. These were a means of raising Scottish public consciousness of the incidence and effects of venereal infection and of networking the voluntary and governmental agencies dealing with the disease.[15] The meetings were carefully orchestrated to manufacture civic consensus on the issue and to represent both the medical and moral strands of social hygiene discourse. Typically, meetings would be chaired by a local civic or church dignitary with contributions from the Medical Officer of Health, a leading clinician, a representative of the executive committee of the NCCVD, a local minister, and a social purity activist.

Lecture programmes were similarly arranged so as to ensure that information on VD was appropriately disseminated and contextualized. In the early years, there was concern to focus lectures on 'responsible people'; on the moral gatekeepers in local society such as teachers, purity activists, social workers, and community nurses.[16] Thus, in 1919, lectures in Edinburgh were reserved for groups such as the local branches of the National Vigilance and Women Citizens' Association, the Matron's Association, voluntary health visitors, and dispensary and poorhouse nurses.[17] A professional monopoly on the dissemination of medical knowledge was strictly adhered to, and specialist lectures were normally delivered by either a venereologist or infectious diseases officer. Where medical slides were used to illustrate talks, they had to be approved by the Medical Officer of Health.[18] Lectures on the medical aspects of VD were differentiated according to the sex of the audience, partly for reasons of propriety but also in recognition of prevailing gendered perceptions of health.[19]

Lectures and slide-shows to wider public audiences, which in the West of Scotland frequently numbered in excess of 800, were also often gender-specific, especially in the early part of the interwar period, and normally subject to an age restriction. Talks to male and female adolescent groups were always conducted separately. It was customary for lectures to be chaired by either a local minister or Medical Officer of Health, reflecting the professional power structure within the social hygiene movement, and for the lectures to provide a focal point for the supervised and 'appropriate' distribution of literature, whose promiscuous distribution amongst uninformed members of the public was viewed as an incitement to prurience.[20] As the dissemination of medical information was perceived as part of a broader process of social and moral regeneration, typically, a series of lectures was grouped so as to provide an ethical and biological framework for the discussion of VD. Precedence was given to the evolutionary aspects of sex in animals and plants and to the health 'responsibility of citizenship' and its implications for national efficiency.[21]

From the start, Scottish local health authorities were alive to the potential of the cinema as a medium for VD propaganda. As early as 1917, Dundee Public Health Committee arranged with the proprietors of its cinema theatres to screen public announcements relating to its VD campaign *(see Plate 6.2)*. Subsequently, both documentary films and fictional propaganda films such as *The End of the Road, Flaw, Damaged Goods*, and *John Smith and Son* were widely used as a means of popular education in social hygiene.[22] In the 1920s, attendances at cinema performances at times exceeded 3000,[23] and this level of public interest was sustained into the 1930s. For example, an estimated 26,000 people attended VD propaganda films in Scotland in the four months ending 30 January 1932, with

THE HIDDEN PLAGUE

—————————————

By order of the Government the Town Council is starting a campaign against Venereal Diseases.

This is in the interests of

PERSONAL HEALTH
and
NATIONAL EFFICIENCY

It is up to you to **HELP** where and when you can.
A Royal Commission has declared that Venereal Diseases are sapping the vitality of the Nation.
They say that not less than one-tenth of the population in large cities are infected with Syphilis, acquired or congenital, while those infected with Gonorrhoea greatly exceeds this.

THINK OF IT

These two diseases are the chief causes of-

BLINDNESS
DEAFNESS
MENTAL
ENFEEBLEMENT

Plate 6.2
Transcript of cinema announcement, Dundee 1917
(courtesy of Dundee City Archives)

an average attendance of 665.[24] Even in the more remote areas, VD films were widely exhibited with the aid of mobile 'cinemotors' *(see Plate 6.3)*.[25]

However, significant constraints were imposed by the authorities on the exhibition of VD propaganda films in Scotland. Some SBH officials shared the reservations of several Medical Officers of Health about the value and appropriateness of the message being projected in some of the dramatized documentary films. For example, the Board's medical member, Sir Leslie Mackenzie, feared their 'confusion of two orders of ethical values – the treatment of a person for disease as disease, and the treatment of a person for moral delinquency as moral delinquency'.[26] In general, the Board favoured instructional films that focused upon 'the natural history of the infective micro-organisms ... and upon the demonstrated facility of destroying those germs so long as they remain[ed] on the surface'.[27]

In addition, as in England, the social purity movement in Scotland had reservations about the content and venue of the propaganda films exhibited. As Kuhn has revealed, a crucial problem for social purity organizations, such as the National Vigilance Association and National Council for Public Morals, was 'the instability of propaganda films as bearers of meaning' and of ensuring that the films would be read for their 'social hygiene' content and not be of 'pornographic interest to their audiences'. Additional concerns related to the conditions in which such films were viewed, with the darkness and intimate seating of the cinema being viewed as a risk to public morality.[28] In many instances, social hygiene organizations negotiated with the commercial distributors over the conditions under which VD propaganda films would be shown. Even when this was not the case, Scottish local

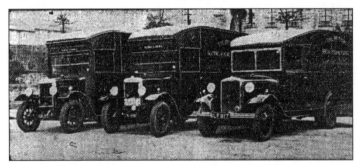

Plate 6.3

Three of the cinemotors used by the British Social Hygiene Council in rural areas in interwar Scotland (*Scotsman*, 2 April 1935)

authorities strictly regulated performances in terms of the age, gender, and social composition of the audience, according to the perceived suitability of each film.[29] Normally, films were screened as part of a longer meeting organized by social hygiene and purity agencies and were customarily introduced by Medical Officers of Health or local VD Medical Officers.[30]

Social Hygiene Education in Schools

The Royal Commission on Venereal Diseases had considered specific instruction on sex hygiene to be 'undesirable' for the elementary school curriculum. However, it had strongly recommended that such instruction be introduced in evening continuation schools, in public and secondary schools, and in all teachers' training colleges,[31] and these proposals attracted substantial support in post-war Scotland. The Scottish Committee of the NCCVD campaigned widely for instruction on 'hygiene' to be accorded 'an adequate place in all permanent educational arrangements' and lobbied the Scottish Education Department accordingly. It established local committees to liaise with educational leaders and pressure groups and concentrated much of its early lecture programmes on schoolteachers.[32] Various purity organizations were also active in promoting the cause of sex education as a means of combating VD. The East of Scotland Branch of the National Vigilance Association mounted a hard-fought campaign to introduce moral hygiene instruction into secondary and continuation schools, as did the Dundee and Glasgow Branches of the Alliance of Honour.[33] Meanwhile, in Aberdeenshire, the Scottish Band of Hope secured permission to lecture on hygiene and temperance in the local authority schools.[34]

Health officials and clinicians, often inspired by eugenics, were also extremely active in canvassing the need for sexual issues to be addressed in schools as part of more general education on personal hygiene and racial health.[35] Similarly, while reserving specific instruction on VD for infectious diseases courses for adolescents over 16, the Scottish Association of Medical Women advocated systematic training in biology and physiology including reproduction 'and their moral and racial significance, for all young people of all classes by specially qualified teachers'.[36]

At the same time, as Mort has indicated, the issue of sex education, especially in elementary schools, became the 'sharp focus for disagreement' within the medico-moral alliances of the social hygiene movement.[37] A considerable body of Scottish public opinion,

142

including many teachers and some leading educationalists, was fearful of a policy of 'sexual enlightenment in youth'. In the view of Sir Henry Keith, President of the Scottish Education Authorities' Association, addressing a conference on 'The Social Evil' in Glasgow in 1921, 'it was a moot point whether they did not do more harm by giving information at an early age which otherwise would not occur to the young mind'.[38] Similarly, receiving evidence in 1925, a Scottish Office Committee encountered a commonly held opinion that, in the absence of properly trained teachers, sex education would lead 'to the very precocity and malpractice which it [was] designed to prevent', and that 'a second-hand familiarity with the facts of sexual vice [could not] fail to be injurious to youth'.[39]

At a local level, there was often tension between medics and purity groups over the control and content of hygiene instruction. In particular, purity groups, along with church leaders, were concerned that in conveying information on VD, moral issues and ideals should remain to the fore and that the 'whole subject' should be lifted 'to a higher sphere by purifying the thoughts of the rising generation'.[40] For their part, many teachers and education authorities in working-class areas of Scotland feared that such instruction might prove disruptive with pupils and raise sectarian issues.[41] Thus, Glasgow's Local Education Authority decided to discontinue the teaching of sex hygiene in its schools in 1920 and subsequently resisted all attempts by the Public Health Committee to reverse the decision.[42]

The Departmental Committee on Sexual Offences Against Children and Young Persons in Scotland did recommend in 1926 that parental guidance on sexual hygiene should be subsequently followed up by instruction by doctors and teachers in the schools as part of more general physical training.[43] In addition, a number of Joint VD Committees continued to lobby the educational and medical establishment, but given a continuing lack of professional and public consensus on the issue, and the reluctance of English authorities to introduce new provisions, the Scottish Education Department [SED] was forced in 1929 to leave the matter 'to the discretion of individual authorities'.[44]

In the 1930s, the Scottish Committee of the BSHC collaborated with the Salvation Army and the Church of Scotland in providing illustrated lectures to juveniles in residential schools and children's homes.[45] It also sought to upgrade the provision of biology in schools as a basis for dispelling ignorance on matters of social hygiene, and initiated discussions between venereologists, public health officers, the SED, the Educational Institute for Scotland and the teachers' training colleges. Evidence was submitted to the Committee on the Scottish Health Services stressing the medical benefits to be gained from health education initiatives but evidence would suggest that, as in England, the school curriculum in Scotland remained largely impervious to the propaganda of the Social Hygiene Movement.[46]

The Message of VD Propaganda

The language of VD propaganda in interwar Scotland was clearly shaped by eugenics and the politics of national efficiency with its demonology of racial poisons and degeneration. As Kuhn has observed, such propaganda was not merely an effect of the moral panic produced by the Report of the Royal Commission on Venereal Diseases. It actively participated in it by 'constructing, reconstructing and circulating discourses' in which the moral and spiritual state of the nation was conflated with its physical health, with VD the focus of and metaphor for broader fears surrounding the degenerative effects of atavistic, 'uncontained sexuality', allegedly induced by the impact of war and post-war social change upon conventional moral controls.[47] VD propaganda commonly highlighted the impact of 'The Deadly Peril' on industrial and racial efficiency and the disgenic

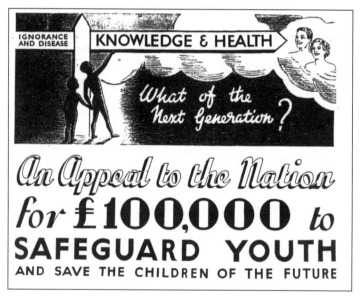

Plate 6.4
British Social Hygiene Council Appeal, 1935
(*Scotsman*, 2 April 1935)

144

effects of immoral (i.e. extra-marital) intercourse upon infant mortality and disablement.[48] Private sexual practices were defined as an issue of public and racial health to be regulated by the sexual health 'responsibilities of citizenship'.[49]

A prime responsibility was 'enlightenment'. According to the materials distributed and exhibited by the Scottish Committee of the NCCVD/BSHC, the high incidence of VD was primarily a function of 'ignorance rather than barbarity'. Central to the iconography of its posters and literature was the identification of 'ignorance' with moral corruptibility and 'disease', in juxtaposition to 'knowledge and health' *(see Plates 6.4 and 6.5)*. 'Ignorance the Great Enemy' featured prominently in the social epidemiology of VD articulated in pamphlets and films, and public awareness of the salient facts about VD was identified as pivotal to its control.[50] There was, therefore, a 'Duty of Knowledge' and 'it was a matter of honour for all who [had] at heart the welfare of the human race and of their kith and kin ... to familiarise themselves with the facts', so that 'the dark menace of

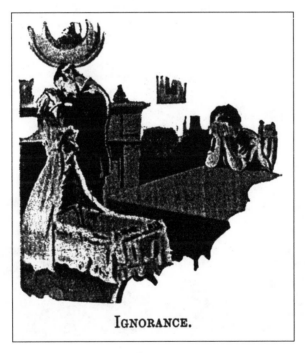

IGNORANCE.

Plate 6.5
The role of 'Ignorance' in the iconography of VD
(*The Seafarer's Chart of Healthy Manhood* (BSHC, 1925))

145

venereal diseases [might] be dispelled before the sunshine of enlightenment'.[51] Above all, in order 'to stamp out the scourge', and to protect future generations, it was imperative that information on social hygiene should be disseminated to the youth of the nation.

It was equally imperative that such knowledge should be 'correct knowledge'; authoritative knowledge enunciated, on the one hand, by properly qualified medical practitioners, and on the other, by professionals whose brief was public morality. In VD literature, documentary films and allegorical cartoons, such as *The Road to Health*, it was medical expertise that formed the bridge from the gloomy depths of depravity and disease to the enlightened paths of racial health and national efficiency *(see Plate 6.6)*. In all types of VD propaganda, the practitioner was allocated a pivotal role in articulating the medico-moral prescriptions of the Social Hygiene Movement. In films such as *Damaged Goods*, the doctor was either depicted 'as part of a setting (surgery, laboratory) connoting status and specialised knowledge', or positioned in relation to other characters as the dispenser of wisdom. As Kuhn observes: 'Everything about this man's appearance and expression convey[ed] rectitude, sternness, strictness and rigorously unbending correctness. From this elevated position, his enunciation of information – "the facts" about VD –

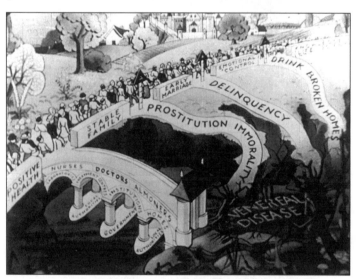

Plate 6.6
Imagery in *The Road to Health*
(courtesy of National Film and Television Archive)

acquire[d] a peculiarly authoritative quality, as [did] his instructions and injunctions to other characters'.[52] Significantly, medication was never illustrated independently of the physician, as it was his personal authority which symbolized the power of modern healing. This presentation of professional expertise and authority was heavily gendered. The power of medical science was personified by male doctors, and nurses and midwives never figured alone.

Within VD propaganda materials, there was a vigorous representation of the penalties of non-compliance with professional advice and of recourse to herbalists and other quacks.[53] Such penalties, central to the narrative of films such as *Deferred Payment*, *The Gift of Life* and *John Smith and Son*, and to many of the NCCVD/BSHC's leaflets, were most commonly illustrated by a caricature of the archetypal 'syphilitic runt' destined for either premature death or degeneration *(see Plate 6.7)* or of the sightless victim of gonorrhoeal ophthalmia. In such images, the sins of self-indulgent parents who failed to defer to the new 'heroic' therapies of medical science were visibly visited upon the next generation.

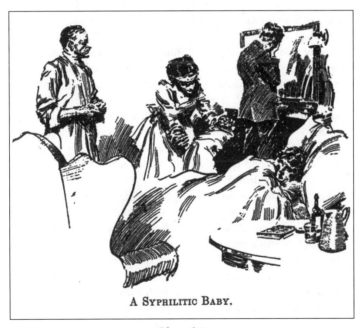

A SYPHILITIC BABY.

Plate 6.7
Depiction of the archetypal syphilitic runt
(*The Seafarer's Chart of Healthy Manhood* (BSHC, 1925))

147

Similarly, defaulters from treatment were depicted as 'condemning themselves to live under the shadow of a great peril, a peril as ominous as the menace of Vesuvius – liable to burst at any moment into terrible activity'. Their only salvation was 'to continue treatment *until given a clean bill of health by the doctor, and to dismiss all thoughts of marriage until a cure [had] been definitely pronounced*'.[54]

Although educational in content, VD propaganda materials were expressly circulated as a form of 'moral inspiration' towards a 'higher moral standard'. As with the public health reports of the period, pamphlets, posters, and film and lecture scripts subscribed to an aetiology and epidemiology of VD that recognized an explicit taxonomy of guilt and blame. VD was represented not just as a physical disease but as the penalty for moral turpitude and sexual intemperance. It was as much the immorality as the infectivity of 'impure sexual intercourse' that threatened racial health and the integrity of the family in society and which in films such as *Trial for Marriage* stood to be condemned. Social hygiene propagandists did avoid the more negative proscriptions on sexuality of the purity movement, but they continued to identify social health and evolution with moral self-restraint and 'a noble sex life' within the confines of responsible parenthood. Similarly, curative regimes of treatment and follow-up were commonly presented as involving a moral as well as physical process of rehabilitation with the rewards of medical science and adherence to qualified treatment predicated upon compliance with a moral regime of sexual abstention and reform. There was a clear ideological conflation of moral redemption ('salvation' was the metaphor commonly employed in propaganda material) with submission to professional treatment, in which 'the power of Science and the rewards of moral virtue [were] constituted as mutually dependent'.[55]

The moral dimension of VD propaganda was, however, firmly shaped by a male-produced discourse and both echoed and reinforced prevailing double standards of sexual morality. As in other countries,[56] Scottish propaganda materials were acutely gendered in their representation of the causes and spread of venereal infection. They commonly represented sexually active women as the major source and vector of infection, albeit with a strong shift in focus from professional prostitutes to so-called 'amateurs'; young women who had casual sex on a non-pecuniary basis and whose alleged indifference to health precautions rendered them the more virulently infectious.[57]

In contrast, men were typically represented as the recipients of disease. Sometimes, in leaflets such as *The Seafarer's Chart of Healthy Manhood*, or films such as *Deferred Payment*, men's sexual indiscretions were clearly identified as a threat to family and racial health, but even where male culpability *was* emphasized, the prostitute or casual good-time girl remained the constant point of reference as the root source of VD. Men were rarely depicted as wilfully evil vectors of infection. More usually, propaganda portrayed the contraction of VD by men as a function of ignorance and misguided susceptibility to the attentions of predatory women, especially when their moral inhibitions were loosened by alcohol. Even where the demoralization of a woman had been caused by male exploitation, it was the loss of female chastity that was held to be central to the spread of disease.[58]

Within this presentation of the causes and diffusion of VD, social hygiene propaganda both reflected and reaffirmed powerful assumptions about the nature and socially desirable boundaries of female sexuality. Women were accorded a strictly limited set of sexual roles. They could either opt for the passive sexuality of the wife and mother, or, as sexual initiator, be stigmatized as a prostitute and the reservoir of disease. There was no acceptable sphere for non-marital female sexual activity, which was clearly defined by social hygienists as diseased and pathological. Healthy female sexuality was identified with reproduction and, within VD propaganda, positive depictions of women as sexual participants were always accompanied by images of children and motherhood.

Similarly, it was conformity by women to the ideals of chastity and maternity that, according to the Social Hygiene Movement, was critical in the containment of VD and the preservation of racial health, and it was upon women that the responsibility for maintaining the moral integrity of society was primarily devolved. Typical was the injunction of Mary Scharlieb, in her lectures for the NCCVD and Alliance of Honour, that:

> The men are what the women make them and unless the wives and mothers of the country do their duty, and uphold the standard of purity, the nation ... and our magnificent empire must follow the empires of olden days into utter ruin.[59]

Such sentiments, perpetuating the assumption that male self-control was problematic, and that their moral behaviour was ultimately the responsibility of their female partners, were frequently aired in social hygiene leaflets such as *How Girls Can Help*, and films such as *The End of the Road*. Significantly, NCCVD/BSHC lecturers were recommended to close with a slide of the Madonna and 'a few words on the power of womanhood to save the next generation through the purity and good of woman's life'.[60]

The experience of VD was also expressed in gender-specific terms. While male sickness was often represented in the context of manpower needs and racial efficiency, it was also portrayed as an individual disaster on its own terms. In contrast, women's venereal illnesses were always linked to maternity, by reference either to sterility or to the presence of congenitally ill children. The emotional appeal of the propaganda was directed not at the disabilities of the mother but at the sickness of the child and especially the degeneration of the family.[61] The sexual health of the single woman was only accorded a separate identity as a source and carrier of venereal disease, or as a function of 'moral imbecility'.[62] Similarly, while information leaflets for men stressed their responsibility for their own 'physical and mental efficiency' and for the health of their families (including their faithfully chaste future brides), no reference was made to the health of their sexually active girlfriends or consorts. Moreover, while men might rehabilitate themselves by compliance with professional treatment, single women remained permanently tainted by their sexual initiation, notwithstanding their medical cure.

Notes

1 *Final Report of the Royal Commission on Venereal Diseases [RCVD], PP 1916 (Cmd. 8189) XVI*, 60.

2 *Local Government Board for Scotland, Public Health (Venereal Diseases) Regulations and Memorandum on Schemes for the Diagnosis, Treatment and Prevention of Venereal Diseases* (Edinburgh: HMSO, 1916), 4, 7, 10.

3 *SBH, Sixth Annual Report, PP 1924–5 (Cmd. 2416) XIII*, 63.

4 D. Lees, 'VD in City Life', *Journal of State Medicine*, 40 (1932), 92–3; *Glasgow MOH Annual Report (1921)*, 8; *Dundee MOH Annual Report (1920)*, 46.

5 On the social politics of the NCCVD's propaganda work, see especially B. Towers, 'Health Education Policy 1916–26: Venereal Disease and the Prophylaxis Dilemma', *Medical History*, 24 (1980), 70–87. Some £600 was sanctioned by the SBH for 'propaganda' work in Scotland for the year 1921–2, rising to £1000 in 1929–30.

6 Edinburgh City Archives [ECA], File 15, Box 34, DRT 14, Edinburgh Corporation Town Clerk's Department, VD General File.

7 ECA, File 15/11, Box 36, DRT 14, Minutes of Scottish Committee of the British Social Hygiene Council [SCBSHC], 20 Oct. 1933; *Royal Commission on National Health Insurance, Minutes of Evidence*

(London: HMSO, 1926), q. 20847.

8 See, e.g., ECA, File 15, Box 34, DRT 14; Files 15(1) and 15(2), Box 8, DRT 14; Glasgow City Archives [GCA], Public Health Department Newscuttings; Dundee City Archives [DCA], Town Clerk's Papers, File 344, NCCVD 1918 and 1919. The fact that, in Scotland, the government grant for propaganda work was paid to social hygiene and purity agencies by the local authorities and not directly by the SBH, also produced a more varied pattern of provision.

9 GCA, Glasgow Public Health Department Newscuttings, 1921–2.

10 See, e.g., *Dundee MOH Annual Report (1920)*, 45; ECA, File 15, Box 34, DRT 14, Edinburgh Branch, Alliance of Honour to Edinburgh Branch, NCCVD, 2 Feb. 1918; Northern Health Services Archives [NHSA], Aberdeen PHC Minutes, 15 Dec. 1919.

11 *SBH, Seventh Annual Report, PP 1926 (Cmd. 2674) XI*, 84.

12 See, e.g., GCA, Glasgow Corporation Minutes, Sub-Committee on VD, 21 Oct. 1929; Fife County Archives, Glenrothes, Fife and Kinross Joint VD Committee, Minutes, 2 May 1927.

13 GCA, Glasgow Corporation Minutes, Sub-Committee on VD, 17 Sept. 1919, 16 June 1921, 21 March 1923, 18 Feb. 1925.

14 J. Weeks, *Sex, Politics and Society: the Regulation of Sexuality since 1800* (London: Longmans, 1981), 216. In part, this stemmed from a concern that posters might be just a first step towards the introduction of prophylactic ablution centres in men's toilets.

15 During the period 1921–9, the Scottish Committee of the NCCVD/BSHC organized 400 public meetings, with an attendance of over 175,000 people. See *Glasgow Herald*, 19 Oct. 1929.

16 See, e.g., DCA, Dundee PHC Minutes, 28 Aug. 1917.

17 ECA, File 15/1, Box 34, DRT 14, Report of Edinburgh Branch of NCCVD to Local Government Board for Scotland, Oct. 1919.

18 See, DCA, Town Clerk's Correspondence, File 344, NCCVD 1919.

19 Recent research suggests that VD propaganda was also an area of expertise in which medical women were able to find an important role for themselves, 'both in the practice of medicine and in the dissemination of moral advice' (E. Thomson, 'Women in Medicine in Late-Nineteenth and Early Twentieth-Century Edinburgh: A Case Study', University of Edinburgh, Ph.D. thesis (1998), 246, 261–9).

20 For accounts of typical meetings, see, e.g., *Glasgow Herald*, 13 March 1917, 3 Dec. 1921.

21 See, e.g., GCA, Glasgow Public Health Department Newscuttings; *Dundee MOH Annual Report (1920)*, 456; *(1921)*, 367. Broader lecture titles such as 'Sex and Heredity' were also found to avoid the

stigma that many people attached to attending advertised talks on
VD. See ECA, File 15/2, Box 8, DRT 14, A. Chalmers Watson to
Town Clerk, 4 July 1919.

22 See, e.g., *Glasgow MOH Annual Report (1926)*, 154; ECA, EPHD
Files 15/5, 15/11, Box 36, DRT 14. On the social politics
surrounding the emergence of a new cinematic genre of propaganda
films, see especially, A. Kuhn, *Cinema, Censorship and Sexuality
1909–25* (London: Routledge, 1988).

23 Contemporary Medical Archives Centre [CMAC], SA/BSH, A2/7,
Extract from Minutes of the Scottish Committee of the NCCVD,
22 Jan. 1923.

24 *Glasgow MOH Annual Report (1925)*, 141; Editorial, 'The Social
Evil', *Glasgow Herald*, 24 Nov. 1922; ECA, EPHD, 15/11, Box 36,
DRT 14, SCBSHC Minutes.

25 Thus, in the autumn of 1925, the cinemotors travelled extensively in
the rural areas of Lanarkshire and Wigtownshire, with an average
attendance of 125. CMAC, SA/BSH, A2/9, Extract from Minutes of
Executive Committee of SCBSHC, 2 Dec. 1925.

26 *Glasgow Herald*, 3 Dec. 1921; W. E. Whyte, 'Place of the Local
Authority in the VD Campaign (Scotland)', *Proceedings of the
Imperial Social Hygiene Congress* (London: NCCVD, 1924), 103.

27 *SBH, Ninth Annual Report, PP 1928 (Cmd. 3112) X*, 109. The
Ministry of Health also censored VD propaganda films. For
example, it refused to sanction *Social Hygiene for Women* for
exhibition other than to select audiences of nurses, midwives, health
visitors and teachers. Similarly, it refused permission for *Whatsoever a
Man Soweth* to be on general release for mixed audiences. Limited
exhibition to single-sex audiences was permitted as long as this was
approved by the Medical Officer of Health and 'the bedroom scene
omitted'. (CMAC, SA/BSH, C1/5, Minutes of NCCVD
Propaganda Committee, 17 Nov. 1924, 15 Dec. 1924).

28 A. Kuhn, *The Power of the Image: Essays on Representation and
Sexuality* (London: Routledge and Kegan Paul, 1985), 123–7; Kuhn,
op. cit. (note 22), 42, 112–13, 120. The more general efforts of the
social purity movement to censor film material and to regulate access
to cinemas in Scotland are discussed in V. E. Cree, *From Public
Streets to Private Life. The Changing Task of Social Work* (Aldershot:
Avebury, 1995), 26.

29 DCA, Town Clerk's Papers, File 344, A. C. Gotto to Secretary,
Dundee Branch NCCVD, 11 June 1920. In the mid-1930s,
Damaged Lives was initially shown to separate audiences of men and
women, with mixed showings for married couples at the weekends

(*Public Health*, 46, No. 12 (Sept. 1933), 384). For additional constraints on distribution imposed by the British Board of Film Censors, see Kuhn, *op. cit.* (note 22), 67–8, 132.

30 See, e.g., ECA, File 15/11, Box 36, DRT 14, SCBSHC minutes; *Royal Commission on National Health Insurance, Mins of Ev.* (London: HMSO, 1926), q. 20847.

31 *Final Report of the RCVD, op. cit.* (note 1), 60.

32 See, e.g., ECA, File 15(2), Box 8, DRT 14, EPHD, VD.

33 Cree, *op. cit.* (note 28), 29; DCA, Town Clerk's Papers, File 344, NCCVD 1918, Minutes of Meeting between Dundee Educational Authorities and Joint Committee of NCCVD and Alliance of Honour, 1 Nov. 1918; ECA, 15/1, Box 34, DRT 14, Conference of NCCVD Propaganda Committee, 7 Dec. 1918, 9. The Alliance of Honour claimed the support of the Scottish Education Department in introducing hygiene lectures under the existing education code.

34 NHSA, E2/6/1, E2/6/5, E2/6/10, Education Authority for County of Aberdeen, Minutes of Proceedings (1919–20), 194; (1923–4), 77; (1928–9), 76.

35 See, e.g., the views of Edinburgh's MOH, ECA, File 15/1, Box 34, DRT 14, Conference Minutes, 9.

36 CMAC, SA/MWF Uncat. 56, Scottish Association of Medical Women, Memorandum 1919.

37 F. Mort, *Dangerous Sexualities: Medico-Moral Politics in England since 1830* (London: Routledge and Kegan Paul, 1987), 196–7.

38 *Glasgow Herald*, 3 Dec. 1921, 10.

39 *Report of Departmental Committee on Sexual Offences against Children and Young Persons in Scotland, PP 1926 (Cmd. 2592) XV*, 36.

40 See, e.g., *GMJ*, 90 (1918), 44–6.

41 For similar fears elsewhere, see Mort, *op. cit.* (note 37), 197; J. Cassel, *The Secret Plague: Venereal Disease in Canada 1838–1939* (Toronto: University of Toronto Press, 1987), 244.

42 GCA, Glasgow Corporation Public Health Sub-Committee on VD, Minutes, 21 Jan. 1920, 19 May 1926. On the contest between various discourses over the appropriate source of "'proper' knowledge about the body and its sexuality' in interwar Britain, see Kuhn, *op. cit.* (note 22), 110–13.

43 *Departmental Committee on Sexual Offences, op. cit.* (note 39), 36.

44 CMAC, SA/BSH, A2/9, A2/10, Extracts from Minutes of SCBSHC, 2 Dec. 1925, 4 July 1927, 6 Dec. 1928; NAS, HH 60/278, *Scottish Education Department Circular No. 79*, 16 Jan. 1929.

45 CMAC, SA/BSH, A2/12, A2/14, Extracts from Minutes of SCBSHC, 2 March 1931, 7 Dec. 1933.

46 ECA, 15/11, Box 36, DRT 14, SCBSHC Minutes, 10 June 1932, 23 Feb. 1933; CMAC, SA/BSH, F8, Minutes of BSHC Educational Advisory Board, 20 June 1934; BSH A2/15, Extracts from Minutes of SCBSHC, 5 March 1934, 5 Nov. 1934; *Training for Citizenship: A Report of the Advisory Council on Education in Scotland, PP 1943–44 (Cmd. 6495) III*, 12. On England, see Mort, *op. cit.* (note 37), 196–8; Steve Humphries, *A Secret World of Sex: Forbidden Fruit: The British Experience 1900–50* (London: Sidgwick and Jackson, 1988), ch. 2.

47 A. Kuhn, *op. cit.* (note 28), 129–30.

48 These were frequently juxtaposed in slide-shows with the beauty and sanctity of procreative reproduction in nature.

49 For similar discourses in Continental VD propaganda, see A. Mooij, *Out of Otherness: Characters and Narrators in the Dutch Venereal Disease Debates 1850–1990* (Amsterdam/Atlanta: Rodopi, 1998), ch. 2; F. L. Bernstein, 'Envisioning Health in Revolutionary Russia: The Politics of Gender in Sexual-Enlightenment Posters of the 1920s', *Russian Review*, 57 (1998), 191–217.

50 *The Tragedy of Ignorance* was one of the most widely exhibited films in Scotland in the late 1920s (CMAC, SA/BSH/C1/7, BSHC Propaganda Committee Film Report for 1929). On the broader significance of 'ignorance' in the narrative interpretation of VD propaganda films, see Kuhn, *op. cit.* (note 28), 105.

51 ECA, File 15, Box 34, DRT 14, EPHD Files, *The Deadly Peril of Venereal Diseases*, 3; GCA, Glasgow Public Health Department Newscuttings; Kuhn, *op. cit.* (note 22), 106, 109.

52 Kuhn, *op. cit.* (note 28), 109–10.

53 See, e.g., DCA, Town Clerk's Papers, File 344, NCCVD 1918, NCCVD Warning Leaflet, 'Some Perils of Venereal Disease: No. 3, The Folly of Self-Drugging'; File 344, NCCVD 1919, NCCVD Leaflet, 'Quackery and Venereal Disease'.

54 DCA, Town Clerk's Papers, NCCVD 1919, NCCVD Warning Leaflet, 'Living Beneath Vesuvius'.

55 Kuhn, *op. cit.* (note 28), 111–12; Kuhn, *op. cit.* (note 22), 104. It was precisely this need for a moral as well as medical response to the threat of VD that persuaded Scottish public health authorities to reject the propaganda literature of the Society for the Prevention of VD whose leaflets, while advocating abstention from 'irregular sexual intercourse', focused primarily on the use of medical prophylaxis in the form of packets of potassium permanganate and calomel ointment (GCA, Glasgow PHC Minutes, 20 April 1920; Sub-Committee on Clinical Services, 21 Nov. 1930, 7 Aug. 1931, 19

May 1933; DCA, Dundee PHC Minutes, 15 May 1933; ECA, Edinburgh PHC Minutes, 16 May 1933, 15 Dec. 1936). For the broader implications of the venereal prophylaxis debate in Britain, which in fact centred primarily in the south of England, see S. M. Tomkins, 'Palmitate or Permanganate: The Venereal Prophylaxis Debate in Britain 1916–26', *Medical History*, 37 (1993), 382–98; Towers, *op. cit.* (note 5), 70–87; R. Davenport-Hines, *Sex, Death and Punishment: Attitudes to Sex and Sexuality in Britain since the Renaissance* (London: William Collins, 1990), ch. 6.

56   See, e.g., F. L. Bernstein, *op. cit.* (note 49); P. J. Fleming, '"Shadow over New Zealand": The Response to Venereal Disease in New Zealand 1910–1945', Massey University, Ph.D. thesis (1989), ch. 3.

57   See, e.g., the role of Hermani in *Trial for Marriage* and Doris, the Bridesmaid, in *John Smith and Son*. This shift is well captured in the NCCVD warning leaflet No. 4, *Some Perils of Venereal Disease: How Great is the Risk of Infection* (1918): 'Can Venereal Disease be caught from a professional prostitute only? No ... The payment of money makes no difference. "Amateurs" are even more dangerous than "Professionals".' (DCA, Town Clerk's Papers, File 344, NCCVD, 1918).

58   Thus, in the film *Damaged Goods*, it is the girl who has resorted to prostitution who according to the Doctor sums up 'the whole problem' of VD, rather than the employer who has sexually assaulted her, or her male clients.

59   M. Scharlieb, 'Purity and the Nation's Welfare', in *Facing the Problem: A Call to Womanhood* (London: Alliance of Honour, 1925), 8. See also DCA, Town Clerk's Papers, File 334, NCCVD, 1920, NCCVD, *Hints to Lecturers.*

60   ECA, EPHD File 15/1, Box 34, DRT 14, Text for Slide Show, 'Love-Marriage-Parenthood'.

61   See, e.g., the plots of *John Smith and Son* and *Deferred Payment*, National Film and Television Archive, shotlists and viewing copies.

62   See, e.g., DCA, Town Clerk's Papers, File 344, NCCVD, 1918, A. F. Tredgold, *Mental Deficiency in Relation to Venereal Disease* (NCCVD Pamphlet).

7

Outcomes:
The Impact of Public Health Provisions 1918–39

The Incidence of VD in Interwar Scotland

The celebrated conclusion of the Royal Commission on Venereal Diseases in 1916 that 'the number of persons ... infected with syphilis, acquired or congenital, cannot fall below 10 per cent of the whole population in the large cities, and the percentage affected by gonorrhoea must greatly exceed this proportion'[1] continued to inform the social politics surrounding the administration of sexually transmitted diseases in Scotland for much of the interwar period. It fuelled contemporary crisis perceptions of the incidence of the 'social evil' and of its implications for the health, efficiency, and social morality of the nation, and continued to be quoted by Scottish public health administrators well into the 1920s.[2]

Yet, after 1923, there was little effort on the part of social commentators and medical officials in Scotland to test this dramatic claim. For the most part, a defeatist attitude to quantifying the problem prevailed. Thus, in the early 1920s, the Scottish Board of Health were at pains to stress that 'no reliable measure existed of the level of venereal diseases within the community' and that estimates of their incidence in Scotland had 'to be founded largely upon conjecture'.[3] Similarly, as late as 1934, the Department of Health for Scotland endorsed the consensus view of Scottish venereologists that, in the absence of any system of compulsory notification, the level of infection in the country remained 'unknown'.[4] Very occasionally, Medical Officers of Health were prepared to speculate tentatively about trends in the incidence and severity of syphilis or gonorrhoea at the local level, but they were either unwilling or unable to quantify their impressions.

There were three main sources of information upon which estimates of the incidence of VD might have been based: the Registrar-General's mortality reports, the results of Wassermann and other testing for syphilis, and the case records of the local authority VD treatment centres.

Mortality Data

Several contemporary studies sought to use mortality statistics as a means of establishing the incidence of VD, and specifically syphilis, within the Scottish community.[5] The problems of using such data were legion. Death certification grossly understated the prevalence of syphilis. Difficulties of diagnosis, such as the tendency of secondary diseases (for example, cerebral haemorrhage) to mask the underlying syphilitic cause of death, and the widespread and natural reluctance of practitioners to certify private patients in a family practice as dying from VD, rendered the returns 'worthless as an absolute statement of the number of deaths'.[6]

However, mortality figures from locomotor ataxia (tabes dorsalis) and general paralysis of the insane [GPI] were regarded as a useful, albeit crude index of its 'progress or regress'.[7] As these diseases were invariably caused by syphilis and were more accurately certified, trends over time could be interpreted with more confidence. As *Figure 7.1* reveals, statistics of interwar recorded deaths from locomotor ataxia and GPI in Scotland did not entirely justify crisis perceptions. After 1920, there was a clear and sustained downturn in

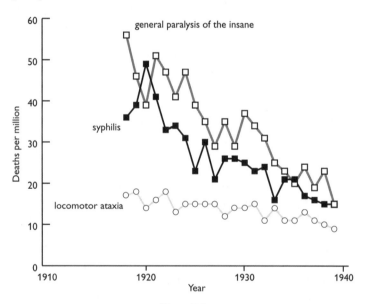

Figure 7.1
Scottish Deaths per Million of Population from
Syphilis and Parasyphilitic Diseases 1918–39
(*Source:* Registrar General for Scotland Annual Reports)

158

the incidence of mortality from GPI, with the annual level of deaths averaged for the period 1935–9 some 61 per cent down on deaths for the period 1915–19. Mortality figures for tabes were more stable but they also declined on trend after the mid-1920s, with the five-yearly averages recording a downturn of some 28 per cent for the interwar period.[8]

The task of estimating the relationship between mortality data and the incidence of VD was highly problematic, especially at a time when new forms of treatment such as the use of arsphenamines were transforming the relationship between the morbidity and mortality rates of syphilis. However, inspired by contemporary debate over the issue and by a concern to counter complacency from the smaller local authorities, medical experts within the Scottish Board of Health sought in the early 1920s to provide crude estimates.

Thus, Frederick Dittmar, Medical Inspector of the Board, attempted to establish the approximate extent of syphilitic infection within the community by aggregating along with syphilis a proportion of the mortality for a range of associated diseases.[9] He argued that the percentage represented by such deaths to total annual deaths would be 'at least about the same, and possibly greater' than 'the proportion of the population affected by syphilis'. On this basis, he posited an incidence of syphilis within the Scottish community of *circa* 6 per cent for 1911–15. Similar calculations for selected interwar years indicate a steady fall to 3 per cent by the late 1930s.[10]

Meanwhile, his colleague, T. F. Dewar, sought to gain traction on the issue by exploiting medical evidence that between 2 to 3 per cent of syphilitic cases died of locomotor ataxia and GPI, and that mortality rates from syphilis calculated upon this ratio would reflect the proportion of the living population infected at a previous date.[11] On the basis of assumptions about the average age at infection and expectation of life, Dewar's methodology yields a prevalence of syphilitic disease of *circa* 4.7 per cent for 1920 falling to *circa* 3.7 per cent of the population by 1925.

While such estimates were markedly lower than those of the Royal Commission on Venereal Diseases, they still indicated an alarming level of infection within the interwar Scottish community; especially at a time when public health experts widely agreed that gonorrhoea was at least three to four times as prevalent as syphilis.[12]

Evidence from Wassermann and Other Testing

More confident estimates of the incidence of syphilis in interwar Scotland might have been based upon the results of Wassermann and other forms of blood testing. However, prevalence testing for epidemiological purposes was notably absent from contemporary health practice in Scotland. One major constraint was the lack of consensus within the medical profession over the reliability of the Wassermann Test and over its interpretation for the purposes of venereology. Knowledge of the 'physical basis of the reactions' was still rudimentary and lack of standardization in the application of the Wassermann Test rendered comparative analysis of findings hazardous. In particular, the value of Wassermann reactions in infants as an indicator of congenital syphilis was increasingly questioned.[13] In addition, there were logistical and medico-legal problems involved in obtaining a random sample of blood donors.[14] At best, an unselected sample of public hospital patients might be obtained, which inevitably reduced the validity of reaction findings for estimating the incidence of VD in the general population.

Nonetheless, a scatter of studies *was* undertaken in the 1920s, based primarily upon samples of maternal, placental and infantile

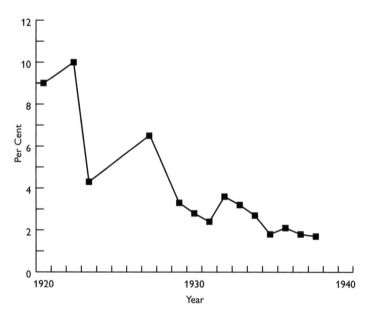

Figure 7.2
Incidence of Syphilis in Interwar Scotland
based on Wassermann and Kahn Tests
(*Source:* see note 20)

160

blood taken at maternity hospitals and ante-natal clinics in Glasgow and Edinburgh from 'the hospital class'.[15] Wassermann reaction tests yielded adult syphilis incidence figures varying from 3.3 per cent to 10 per cent and averaging 6.3 per cent.[16] Dewar's attempt to investigate a genuinely random sample from a 'moderately sized and centrally situated' Scottish garrison town yielded a finding of 4.3 per cent.[17] Such samples again indicate a significant decline in the incidence of syphilis in Scotland during the 1920s.

Due to the growing practice within Scottish maternity hospitals of routinely testing all expectant mothers for syphilis, coupled with the increasing adoption of the more reliable Kahn precipitation test to supplement the Wassermann reaction test, the historian has available much firmer evidence for the 1930s.[18] For example, statistics of testing undertaken at the Elsie Inglis Memorial Hospital and the Royal Maternity Hospital in Edinburgh reveal that during the period 1934–8, some 1.99 per cent of patients were positive. For the same period, Glasgow ante-natal clinics yielded a positive rate of 1.85 per cent.[19] In spite of the class and sex specificity of the data, figures for Glasgow also facilitate a longer-run perspective of trends in Scottish syphilis, especially when integrated with previous case studies involving Wassermann testing in the 1920s *(see Figure 7.2)*.[20] The interwar trend is seen to have been sharply downwards with the fall being concentrated in the 1920s. Thereafter, despite a temporary upswing in the incidence of syphilis in the early 1930s, the falling trend was sustained at a more modest rate. Over the whole period 1920–39, Scottish syphilis levels within these socio-economic groups is seen to have dropped by 80 per cent and by some 70 per cent by 1930.

Evidence from Scottish VD Clinics

The activity reports of the local authority VD clinics established after 1916 represent another important source of information on the incidence and distribution of VD in interwar Scotland. As a data base, such information does have significant limitations. The numbers attending clinics were not merely a reflection of shifts in the incidence of VD. They often varied, both over time and between health authorities, according to the quality of the medical staff and the facilities provided, particularly in the early years of the service.[21] They were also sensitive to shifts in public awareness of the seriousness of specific venereal infections, as in the upswing in gonorrhoea cases after 1927.[22] Likewise, the introduction of new diagnostic techniques could create the illusion of an upswing in the prevalence of disease, as with the impact in the 1930s of routine ante-natal screening upon the numbers of females with syphilis.[23] The use of 'new cases' as an index of the incidence of sexually transmitted diseases was also complicated by the difficulty of distinguishing new infections from re-infections or from secondary manifestations of old infections previously untreated, and by the tendency of many patients to migrate 'between several different clinics'.[24] Above all, it was widely agreed by medical authorities that the numbers attending the clinics were only a proportion of those infected within the community.

Nonetheless, despite these limitations, the data collated by the VD clinics furnish some useful indicators of medium- and long-term trends in the temporal, sexual, and geographical incidence of VD in interwar Scotland. An index of the volume of new cases diagnosed as having VD *(see Figure 7.3)* reveals a fairly level profile of activity for total numbers, except for an upswing in the late 1920s. In contrast, the specific indices for syphilis and gonorrhoea cases are widely divergent. Both display upswings in the late 1920s followed by sharp downturns in the early 1930s, but whereas gonorrhoea is on a rising trend, the trend for syphilis is sharply downwards.

This divergence was clearly reflected in changes in the relative

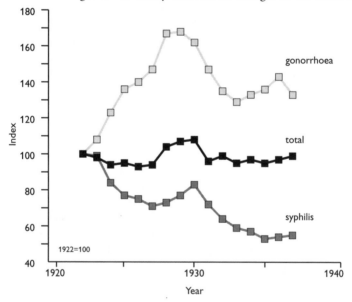

Figure 7.3
Scottish VD Clinics: Index of New Cases 1922–37
(*Source:* SBH/DHS Annual Reports)

incidence of the two infections in patients attending the clinics. At the start of the 1920s, syphilis was the dominant disease, representing some 48 per cent of infected patients, but by 1924, gonorrhoea already exceeded syphilis as a proportion of Scottish cases. By 1930, the proportion of patients diagnosed as suffering from syphilis had dropped to 36 per cent, and continued to fall to 26 per cent in 1938. Meanwhile, the proportion of cases diagnosed with gonorrhoea had risen from 38 per cent in 1922 to 56 per cent in 1930, before declining to 50 per cent in the late 1930s.[25] Comparative analysis of Scottish and English clinic data reveals a very similar configuration in the interwar indices for all new cases. There is also a close symmetry between the time series for new syphilitic cases in the two countries. For gonorrhoea, the marked rise in numbers in the 1920s is a common feature but is more pronounced in Scotland (a rise of some 68 per cent as compared with 36 per cent).

A breakdown by sex of Scottish VD cases attending clinics *(see Figure 7.4)* reveals a rising trend in the numbers of both male and female patients in the 1920s. However, female numbers diverged sharply downwards after 1932. The long-term downtrend in syphilis cases was shared by both sexes but their short-term upswing in the late 1920s was primarily a male phenomenon. The volume of male and female gonorrhoea cases displayed a similar profile over time

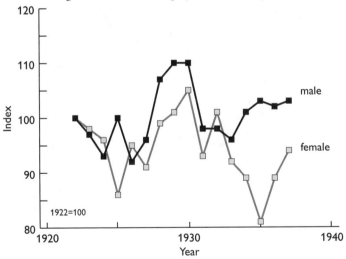

Figure 7.4
Index of New VD Cases by Sex at Scottish Clinics 1922–37
(*Source:* SBH/DHS Annual Reports)

163

with a substantial and sustained rise to *circa* 1930, then a downturn to the mid-1930s before levelling out on a par with the mid-1920s. However, the index of female gonorrhoea cases is markedly more volatile than that for male patients.[26]

How far a comparison between clinic data for specific cities can illuminate real variations in the regional incidence of interwar VD in Scotland is problematic. Diagnostic and recording practices were rarely standardized. Local shifts in the organization or quality of provisions often produced significant fluctuations in both the volume and gender of new cases, with institutional considerations clearly outweighing epidemiological factors.[27] Nonetheless, comparative data for Edinburgh, Glasgow, Aberdeen and Dundee *(see Figure 7.5)* do furnish some indication of how far VD Schemes diverged in the pattern of cases encountered.[28]

Indexed time series of all new venereal cases at clinics in Glasgow and Edinburgh display very similar profiles, fluctuating modestly around a shallow downtrend. In contrast, activity levels at Dundee and Aberdeen clinics exhibit for the bulk of the interwar period wider variations around a sharply rising trend. The data would suggest that this divergence was primarily a function of proportionately sharper

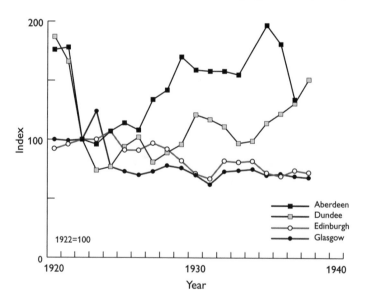

Figure 7.5
Index of New VD Cases at Scottish City Clinics: 1920–38
(*Source:* SBH/DHS Annual Reports)

164

rises in gonorrhoea north of the Forth. All the cities conform to the national trend in the changing proportion of VD attributable to syphilis, although Edinburgh's short-term upswing during 1927–31 is markedly more pronounced. Similar series for gonorrhoea also broadly follow the Scottish pattern, but with significant variations in their range. However, a good deal of this variation had less to do with the relative incidence of the disease than with differing practices of classifying non-specific venereal infections.

The use of data from the VD clinics to measure the actual proportion of Scottish interwar society suffering from sexually transmitted diseases is highly problematic. On the assumption held by contemporary venereologists that those seeking private treatment from practitioners for syphilis represented some one-third of the numbers attending public clinics, and that the ratio of gonorrhoea to syphilis was in the order of 3–4:1, a very crude lower estimate of the extent of new infection within the population can be obtained *(see Tables 7.1 and 7.2)*. Marked regional variations in levels of infection are revealed, with Glasgow two to three times the national incidence. Their significant decline over the interwar period is equally apparent, with levels of infection in the major urban centres in the 1930s only half those prevailing in the 1920s.

Table 7.1
Estimated proportion of the Scottish population newly
infected with syphilis and gonorrhoea 1922–37:
Assuming ratio of gonorrhoea to syphilis of 3:1

	1922–37 annual %	1922–29 annual %	1930–37 annual %
Scotland	0.41	0.47	0.35
Glasgow	0.79	1.05	0.57
Edinburgh	0.67	0.90	0.44

Table 7.2
Assuming ratio of gonorrhoea to syphilis of 4:1

	1922–37 annual %	1922–29 annual %	1930–37 annual %
Scotland	0.51	0.58	0.44
Glasgow	0.98	1.30	0.71
Edinburgh	0.84	1.12	0.53

By the standards of the later twentieth century, the levels of venereal infection in interwar Scotland were relatively high. Data from clinics would suggest that the incidence of syphilis and gonorrhoea in the later 1920s and 1930s was some four to six times greater than that for the period 1950–80.[29] Historical comparisons of ante-natal Wassermann Test results are far from reliable, but evidence from the Edinburgh Royal Infirmary points to a similar ratio between interwar and post-war infection rates.[30]

Nonetheless, for all its deficiencies, the evidence does indicate a dramatic improvement in the health and quality of life for a significant minority of the Scottish community after the First World War. In particular, all the indicators suggest that there was a dramatic fall in the incidence of syphilis as a killing and disabling disease as compared with levels prevailing both before and during the First World War. Certainly, interwar medical authorities and politicians who continued to cite the estimates of the Royal Commission on Venereal Diseases were grossly exaggerating the extent of syphilitic infection within the community, and the intuition of Glasgow's Medical Officer of Health in 1934 that the prevalence figure of 10 per cent quoted by the Commission 'might now be put at from three to four per cent' appears more consistent with the available facts.[31] The social implications of the rising trend in new cases of gonorrhoea are more difficult to interpret, as this was clearly a function not only of its prevalence in Scottish society but of improved medical facilities and the growing public awareness of the seriousness of the disease.

The Impact of Public Health Measures

It is impossible to measure with any precision the impact of public health measures upon the incidence and social repercussions of VD in interwar Scotland. As the Scottish Board of Health observed in its annual report for 1927: 'From a statistical point of view, no confident inference can be made' and 'it is difficult to prove that the work of the centres, enormous in aggregate as it has been, has had any considerable result in eliminating syphilis and gonorrhoea'.[32] In particular, it was difficult to assess how far shifts in the virulence and incidence of VD were a function of the application of new chemotherapies as distinct from longer-term biological changes in the micro-organisms and the susceptibility of the host population.[33]

Interwar clinicians and social hygiene activists were, however, disposed to place more emphasis on the power of their expertise to affect change. Thus, David Lees was adamant as to the cost-effectiveness of VD Schemes 'alike in the prevention of disease, in the cure of existing infectious disease, and in the alleviation of suffering to many individuals', while his successor, R. C. Batchelor, regarded the interwar medical advances in Scottish venereology as 'phenomenal' and as furnishing 'the happiest of auguries for the future attainment of the highest possible measure of health and longevity for all the community'.[34] Similarly, the Scottish Committee of the British Social Hygiene Council [BSHC] claimed that its activities had played a vital role in the success of the VD Schemes and significantly reduced the social havoc wreaked by the 'Great Scourge'.[35]

While it was impossible to obtain any convincing measure of the impact of VD provisions upon the pool of venereal infection within the community, these claims were arguably not without foundation. Given the continuing variation between clinics in methods of diagnosis and treatment, official returns as to levels of 'cure' must be treated with a good deal of caution. Nonetheless, according to the Annual Reports of the Scottish Board of Health/Department of Health for Scotland, some 22 per cent of syphilis cases and 49 per cent of gonorrhoea cases attending Scottish VD centres during the interwar period were discharged as 'cured'.[36] Moreover, while lacking 'final tests as to cure', an additional 28 per cent of syphilis cases and 15 per cent of gonorrhoea cases completed at least one course of treatment and were often non-infectious. They thus presented a greatly reduced risk to public health.[37]

By the late 1920s, there was increasing evidence that the clinics had substantially reduced the mortality and disablement formerly associated with untreated or partially treated VD. The Scottish Board of Health was in no doubt but that 'many who in former years would have passed into the chronic stages of either syphilis or gonorrhoea, with resulting aneurism, heart disease, paralysis or tabes, on the one hand, or stricture, or in the case of women, pelvic inflammation, on the other, are now either restored to health, or at least have their conditions so much ameliorated that disability is averted and life prolonged'.[38] It was believed that intensive treatment of early syphilis by the dual therapy of '914' and bismuth had dramatically reduced the incidence of syphilis of the central nervous system and had led, along with the administration of induced malarial therapy to hospital patients in the early stages of general paralysis, to the 20 per cent fall in the GPI cases admitted to Scottish asylums over the period 1922–31. Malarial therapy had also significantly reduced mortality from GPI in the asylums and appeared to have arrested the disease in many patients.[39] As David Henderson, Physician-Superintendent to the Royal Edinburgh Hospital, reported in 1935:

It is not too much to say that the introduction of malarial therapy in the treatment of general paralysis has marked an epoch in psychiatric treatment. Prior to its introduction, cases of general paralysis might form from 10 to 20 per cent of our admission rate, and death within the space of five years was the usual result. Since the use of malarial therapy was started, the admission rate of general paralysis has decreased by two-thirds or thereabouts, and a large number of those admitted can be successfully treated and discharged fit and able to resume their former occupations. Furthermore, many such cases can be treated successfully in general hospitals or nursing homes, thereby obviating the necessity of mental hospital treatment.[40]

The impact of the VD Schemes was perhaps most visible in the declining incidence of congenital syphilis and reduced levels of infant mortality and disablement due to venereal infection. Recorded cases of congenital syphilis in Scotland fell steadily from 1500 in 1921 to 540 in 1935. Clinicians and health administrators largely attributed the fall to the collaborative work of the VD and ante-natal clinics and the school medical services whose combined efforts also achieved a dramatic reduction in the level of child blindness associated with gonococcal ophthalmia.[41]

Moreover, there were indications that VD propaganda was securing a higher and earlier take-up of qualified medical advice and treatment. In particular, both the rising proportion of new cases found to be non-infectious, rising from 11 per cent in 1922 to 28 per cent in 1932, and the rising ratio of gonorrhoea to syphilis cases at the clinics, were widely regarded as indicators of an increasing public awareness of the gravity of venereal infections and their sequelae.[42]

From the standpoint of VD clinicians, perhaps the most valuable effect of propaganda was to encourage a growing proportion of patients to report in the early stages of their disease when the condition was more readily amenable to treatment, the duration of treatment lessened and the period of likely infectivity within the family and community minimized.[43] Systematic evidence for this is lacking. Nonetheless, scattered data do suggest that the critical importance of early treatment was gradually appreciated by those at risk, although significant variance is evident in the behaviour of male and female patients *(see Table 7.3)*. Evidence of increases in the number of average attendances per case was also viewed as reflecting the impact of propaganda on patient compliance, although this could equally have reflected shifts in the pattern of therapy and the availability of resources.[44]

Table 7.3:
New Cases of Acquired VD at Glasgow VD Centres:
Stage of Infection [%]

Year	% acute syph*		acute gon.		chronic gon.	
	m	f	m	f	m	f
1925	45	38	80	67	20	33
1934	54	24	89	65	11	35
1937	65	42	92	90	8	10

*primary, secondary and latent in the first year of infection.
Sources: *Glasgow MOH Annual Report* (1925), 149; (1934), 138; (1937), 131.

Yet, despite the best efforts of clinicians and social hygiene activists, there remained serious gaps in the public health provisions for VD in interwar Scotland. While the number of cases recorded at the clinics represented only a fraction of 1 per cent of the population, even the most conservative estimates of the incidence of VD placed it substantially higher. As the Scottish Board of Health admitted, even allowing for private treatment, it was 'likely that a fair number of infected persons [were] receiving no treatment at all'.[45]

This shortfall was especially marked in the case of female sufferers. Clinicians encountered a vast amount of ignorance at the female clinics about the nature of VD and of its medium- and long-term effects. As the Board recorded in 1928:

> There is often revealed an almost incredible ignorance with regard to the manifestations of one or other of the maladies in question, or even as to the nature and significance of general indications of ill-health; many of the women who suffer from these ailments or their sequelae apparently regarding the pain, weakness or discharge or other local indications of derangement as not so much signs of illness as natural evils, the general portion of their sex.[46]

As a result, as Table 7.3 indicates, a significantly lower proportion of women attended the clinics in the earliest and most curable stages of VD. In Dundee, in 1933, only 4.7 per cent of female syphilitic patients reported in the primary stages of the disease as compared with 25.6 per cent of male patients.[47] Similarly, as late as 1938, the ratio of male to female syphilis patients at Edinburgh clinics attending for treatment in the sero-negative primary stage of the

169

disease was more than 9:1.[48] In Glasgow, it was estimated that syphilitic women receiving inadequate or no treatment outnumbered those receiving proper medical care by at least 3:1 and by possibly as high as 8:1.[49]

Ignorance, coupled with the asymptomatic course of gonococcal infection in many women, ensured a similar asymmetry in the timing of admissions for gonorrhoea. While physiological and sociological factors were also relevant, this delay in treatment may well explain the fact that, although the number of female out-patients at the VD centres was substantially less, female cases accounted for as much as 67 per cent of in-patient days for syphilis and 70 per cent of in-patient days for gonorrhoea during the interwar period.[50] This was almost certainly also a legacy from the lack of medical provision for women sufferers during and immediately after the First World War.

Perhaps the most depressing feature of the Scottish data was the continuing preponderance of male patients receiving treatment for gonorrhoea at the clinics, varying between 75 and 80 per cent of new cases throughout the interwar period, despite the view of public health officials and general practitioners that its actual prevalence within the community was more even between the sexes.[51] While the estimated ratio of gonorrhoea to syphilis in the population was 3 or 4:1, the ratio for female out-patients, though rising on trend, only averaged 0.9:1 for the interwar period. While health standards for the mass of the population were steadily improving, this 'dark figure' of unreported and untreated infection represented a lasting and significant threat to the health and fertility of Scottish women.

The propaganda work of the Scottish Committee of the BSHC and local Public Health Committees was clearly only partially successful in raising public awareness of the nature of VD. As the Medical Officer of Health for Aberdeen lamented in 1935, 'ignorance' was still 'amongst the greatest factors that one has to contend with in dealing with venereal diseases'.[52] Well into the late 1920s, much of the public was oblivious of the existence of the VD clinics.[53] Venereal infection was often trivialized. In particular, gonorrhoea was frequently dismissed 'as a cold in the pipe' and, in some districts of Scotland, the discharge was 'considered a good thing for the patient, "running off" in some mysterious way, disordered or unhealthy blood'.[54] Popular myths and stereotypes surrounding the origins and transmission of the disease survived until after the Second World War, including the fear that it could be readily caught from toilet seats and eating utensils, and 'the appalling and unwarranted belief' that it could be cured by intercourse with a virgin.[55] According to medical and police authorities, this notion inspired many sexual offences against children and the communication of VD continued to feature as an aggravating offence in many High Court indictments for sexual assault on young girls.[56]

Nor was the Social Hygiene Movement successful in reducing the moral stigma surrounding VD in Scotland. By emphasizing the role of individual conduct and perpetuating its association with infidelity, immorality and promiscuity, it failed to eradicate the 'popular stigma which consign[ed] all venereally infected individuals ... to the same social category of moral outcasts'.[57] Public opinion continued to view those afflicted with VD as 'moral lepers' rather than as cases of infectious disease with the inevitable avoidance of professional treatment and recourse to quacks. Jessie Kesson's autobiographical novel, *The White Bird Passes,* vividly captures contemporary prejudice surrounding venereal infection, with the Matron of Skene children's home in Aberdeenshire refusing to release her to attend to her dying syphilitic mother.[58]

However, the primary concern of venereologists and local health authorities in interwar Scotland was the apparent failure of VD propaganda to change the sexual behaviour of patients and to secure their compliance with treatment regimes. Clinicians reported a disturbingly high incidence of re-infection. For example, in 1927, it was reported that at the Broomielaw Municipal Clinic in Glasgow 'more than half the total number of cases treated (both syphilis and gonorrhoea) had formerly undergone a course of treatment, followed by cessation of symptoms, and had returned, after an interval, for treatment of fresh symptoms, which they attributed to re-exposure to infection'.[59] In the opinion of Glasgow's Medical Officer of Health, such evidence of venereal recidivism clearly indicated the cynical exploitation of the clinics by 'libertines'.[60] Unfortunately, the detailed case notes for patients at the Edinburgh clinics have been destroyed, but the surviving summary registers for the period convey a very similar story.

The continuingly high level of default from treatment, despite the best efforts of social hygiene propaganda, was also perceived by the Scottish medical establishment as severely compromising the efficiency of the VD services and as the major factor determining the 'stubborn' level of infection within the community.[61] Around one-third of patients attending Scottish VD clinics during the 1920s failed to complete their course of treatment, while another quarter withdrew before 'final tests for cure' had been conducted. Levels of default varied markedly, with Glasgow clinics having the highest default rate, averaging some 65 per cent for the period 1921–9 as compared with the national average of 56 per cent.[62] Even in Edinburgh, which was recognized as having the best compliance record, a default rate for the 1920s of 34 per cent was recorded. As a result of more developed 'follow-up' procedures, levels of default did decline in the 1930s but the national annual average for the period 1930–7 was still 46 per cent.

Although the repercussions of such default levels cannot be quantified, they clearly had serious implications for the spread of VD within the family and wider community. Moreover, they raised fundamental questions in Scottish public health debate as to the adequacy of voluntary strategies for containing the 'Great Scourge', and the need for additional controls.

Notes

1 *Final Report of the Royal Commission on Venereal Diseases [RCVD]*, PP 1916 (Cd. 8189) XVI, 23.

2 See, e.g., *Glasgow Medical Officer of Health [MOH] Annual Reports (1914–1919)*, 93; *Aberdeen MOH Annual Report (1924)*, 26.

3 T. F. Dewar, 'On the Incidence of Venereal Disease in Scotland', *Edinburgh Medical Journal [EMJ]*, 30 (1923), 314.

4 *Department of Health for Scotland [DHS], Sixth Annual Report*, PP 1934–5 (Cmd. 4837) IX, 86.

5 F. Dittmar, 'The Prevalence of Venereal Diseases in Scotland', *Transactions of the Incorporated Sanitary Association of Scotland* (1919), 45–55; T. F. Dewar, *op. cit.* (note 3), 316–21; D. White, 'Thoughts on the Prevalence of Syphilis', *British Journal of Venereal Diseases [BJVD]*, I (1925), 136–45.

6 *RCVD, PP 1916 (Cd. 8189) XVI*, 6; Minutes of evidence of Dr J. C. Dunlop, Superintendent of Statistics, Office of Registrar General for Scotland, *PP 1914 (Cd. 7475) XLIX*, qq. 1325–1592. As one medical correspondent admitted: 'The general practitioner whose honesty was such as to compel him to insert the word "syphilitic" in front of "cerebral haemorrhage" ... would very soon find himself minus a practice' (*BMJ*, ii (1920), 257).

7 White, *op. cit.* (note 5), 139; Dewar, *op. cit.* (note 3), 319.

8 *Annual Reports of Registrar General for Scotland;* see especially, 1947, 28, Table J (2). Data on mortality from congenital syphilis strongly reinforces this picture. The mortality rate for syphilis in children under the age of one fell by 67% in the period 1920–5 and by 90% in the period 1920–38.

9 Dittmar, *op. cit.* (note 5), 45–55.

10 For details, see R. Davidson, 'Measuring "The Social Evil": The Incidence of Venereal Disease in Interwar Scotland', *Medical History*, 37 (1993), 171–2.

11 Dewar, *op. cit.* (note 3), 316–21.

12 Dittmar, *op. cit.* (note 5), 53; *Edinburgh Public Health Department [EPHD] Annual Report (1930)*, 74.

13 *Medical Research Committee, Special Report No. 14: The Wassermann Test* (London: HMSO, 1918), 3–5; *Medical Research Council, Special Report No. 78: The Serum Diagnosis of Syphilis: the Wassermann and Sigma Reactions Compared* (London: HMSO, 1923), 3; *Special Report No. 82:* J. N. Cruikshank, *Maternal Syphilis as a Cause of Death of the Foetus and of the New-Born Child* (London: HMSO, 1924), 5, 23.

14 Dewar, *op. cit.* (note 3), 329.

15 For details, see Davidson, *op. cit.* (note 10), 172–4.

16 Interestingly, these findings are broadly consistent with the incidence of syphilis found in serological tests on geriatric patients in Glasgow undertaken in the 1960s. See J. G. Pritchard *et al.*, 'The Old Morality: A Study of Serological Tests for Venereal Infection in Elderly People', *BJVD*, 43 (1967), 18–24.

17 Dewar, *op. cit.* (note 3), 321–9.

18 According to the recollections of one doctor who undertook clinical training in the VD Department of Edinburgh Royal Infirmary at the end of the 1930s, '[P]ermission was not asked for these tests; it was routine.' (R. P. Cookson, *A Doctor's Life* (Sussex: Book Guild Ltd, 1991), 59).

19 *EPHD Annual Report (1933)*, 40–1; *(1936)*, 52; *(1937)*, 97; *Glasgow MOH Annual Report (1934)*, 206; *(1935)*, 210; *(1936)*, 189; *(1937)*, 202; *(1938)*, 186.

20 Sources: *Glasgow MOH Annual Reports;* Dewar, *op. cit.* (note 3), Cruikshank, *op. cit.* (note 13).

21 Dewar, *op. cit.* (note 3), 339; *SBH, Third Annual Report, PP 1922 (Cmd. 1697) VIII*, 25; *Ninth Annual Report, PP 1928 (Cmd. 3112) X*, 107; *Aberdeen MOH Annual Report (1922)*, 85; *(1935)*, 49–50; *(1936)*, iv; *Dundee MOH Annual Report (1929)*, 24.

22 *SBH, Ninth Annual Report, op. cit.* (note 21), 121; *Tenth Annual Report, PP 1928–29 (Cmd. 3304) VII*, 219; *Aberdeen MOH Annual Report (1935)*, 49–50.   ·

23 *EPHD Annual Report (1933)*, 79; *Dundee MOH Annual Report (1937)*, 21.

24 C. N. Rolfe, 'The Prevention of Venereal Disease', *Journal of State Medicine*, XXXIV (1926), 356.

25 Davidson, *op. cit.* (note 10), 177, Graph 8.

26 *Ibid.*, 179–80, Graphs 10–11.

27 See, e.g., *Dundee MOH Annual Report (1922)*, 38; *Aberdeen MOH Annual Report (1922)*, 85.

28 See also above, ch. 4.

29 *SBH/DHS, Annual Reports; Department of Health, Communicable Diseases (Scotland) Unit: Annual Summaries of Sexually Transmitted Diseases.*

30 *EPHD Annual Reports.*

31 *Glasgow MOH Annual Report (1934)*, 10.

32 *SBH, Ninth Annual Report, op. cit.* (note 21), 121.

33 R. J. Peters [Assistant MOH, Glasgow Corporation], 'The Mass Experiment in the Treatment of Syphilis', *Glasgow Medical Journal [GMJ]*, 116 (1931), 101–2. Despite contemporary panic surrounding the effects of 'racial poisons' upon national efficiency, evidence to the Royal Commission on VD from some Scottish clinicians had suggested that, at least for syphilis, there were indications of a trend decline in the virulence of the disease in Scotland from the last quarter of the nineteenth century. See especially the evidence of Dr J. C. Dunlop, Office of Registrar-General for Scotland, *PP 1914 (Cd. 7475) XLIX*, q. 1407; Dr John Barlow, President of RCPS Glasgow, *PP* 1916 (Cd. 8190) *XVI*, q. 19, 261.

34 *EPHD Annual Report (1937)*, 96; D. Lees, 'Venereal Diseases in City Life – Observations on their Effect on the Community', *Journal of State Medicine*, 40 (1932), 92.

35 *Scotsman*, 2 April 1935.

36 The Scottish Board of Health specified a rigorous standard of cure for VD. For syphilis, a patient's blood had to give a negative response to Wassermann tests for a period of two years. For gonorrhoea, a range of conditions had to be met. These included the absence of all clinical symptoms of disease for one month after the cessation of treatment, the absence of all evidence of disease on bacteriological and cultural examination of the discharges from the urethra, cervix etc., the absence of lesions under urethroscopic examination, a negative result from the administration of a vaccine designed to provoke any latent disease, and a negative result from a complement fixation test (*SBH, Seventh Annual Report, PP 1926 (Cmd. 2674) XI*, 70, 76). However, how far these criteria were in practice adhered to in the clinics, is debateable.

37 *SBH/DHS, Annual Reports.*

38 *SBH, Ninth Annual Report, op. cit.* (note 21), 121.

39   *Annual Reports of General Board of Control for Scotland (1931), PP 1931–2 (Cmd. 4163) XI,* xxiii; *(1935), PP 1935–6 (Cmd. 5124), XIII,* xxvi; *(1937), PP 1937–8 (Cmd. 5715) XIII,* xxii.

40   Lothian Health Services Archives [LHSA], LHB 7/7/15, *Royal Edinburgh Hospital, Annual Report for 1935,* 11.

41   *DHS, Eighth Annual Report, PP 1936–7 (Cmd. 5407) XI,* 85; *EPHD Annual Report (1931),* 75; *(1934),* 70; *(1936),* 86; Peters, *op. cit.* (note 33), 99–100.

42   *SBH, Ninth Annual Report, op. cit.* (note 21), 121; *Tenth Annual Report, op. cit.* (note 22), 219; *Dundee MOH Annual Report (1928),* 133; *Glasgow MOH Annual Report (1925),* 144; *(1926),* 154.

43   See, e.g., *Dundee MOH Annual Report (1936),* 109; *EPHD Annual Report (1925),* 54; *(1935),* 74; *Glasgow MOH Annual Report (1928),* 110–11.

44   Average attendances at Glasgow clinics increased from 24.8 in 1924 to 34.32 in 1933 (*Glasgow MOH Annual Reports*).

45   *DHS, Sixth Annual Report, op. cit.* (note 4), 87.

46   *SBH, Ninth Annual Report, op. cit.* (note 21), 108. See also *EPHD Annual Report (1935),* 77.

47   *Dundee MOH Annual Report (1933),* 104.

48   *EPHD Annual Report (1938),* 132.

49   *Glasgow MOH Annual Report (1929),* 147.

50   *SBH, Annual Reports,* Statistical Appendices.

51   *Glasgow MOH Annual Report (1923),* 116; *(1932),* 134; *EPHD Annual Report (1934),* 71; *(1936),* 83.

52   *Aberdeen MOH Annual Report (1935),* 51.

53   *SBH, Ninth Annual Report, op. cit.* (note 21), 108.

54   M. Archibald [Assistant Surgeon, Glasgow Lock Hospital], 'The Position of the General Practitioner in Anti-Venereal Disease Schemes', *Proceedings of the Imperial Social Hygiene Congress* (London: NCCVD, 1924), 188.

55   *Glasgow MOH Annual Report (1922),* 86; Mass Observation Archives, University of Sussex, Box DR 59, File 478, Glasgow Respondent 2554, Nov. 1942.

56   *Report of Departmental Committee on Sexual Offences against Children and Young Persons in Scotland, PP 1926 (Cmd. 2592) XV,* 15; NAS, AD 15, High Court Precognitions.

57   See, e.g., *Aberdeen MOH Annual Report (1935),* 51.

58   J. Kesson, *The White Bird Passes* (Edinburgh: B&W Publishing, 1996 edition), 124.

59   *Glasgow MOH Annual Report (1927),* 155.

60   *Ibid., (1925),* 150.

61   *EPHD Annual Report (1926),* vi–vii; *Glasgow MOH Annual Report (1922),* 10; *(1923),* 20–1; *(1928),* 155.

62   *SBH/DHS, Annual Reports; Glasgow MOH Annual Report (1929),* 151.

8

'A Scourge to be Firmly Gripped': The Campaign for VD Controls in Interwar Scotland

The Context

By the early 1920s, a great deal of public and professional opinion in Scotland was in favour of more stringent controls; sentiments that were to be formalized in three separate bills over the course of the decade. Drafted 'for the better protection of young children', the Venereal Disease (Children) (Scotland) Bill of 1923 proposed that all cases of congenital syphilis and gonorrhoeal ophthalmia in children under the age of five should be notifiable and that Medical Officers of Health should be empowered to examine and test parents of infected children with a view to ensuring their adequate treatment in the interests of the family and public health.[1] Although more local in its application, the Edinburgh Corporation (Venereal Disease) Bill of 1928 was more far-ranging in its provisions for the compulsory treatment of VD. The Medical Officer of Health was empowered to compel anyone believed to be infectious, and who refused to seek and to sustain treatment, to undergo treatment by a qualified private practitioner or clinic and to continue it until certified cured or non-infective. Similarly, parents of children suffering from disease of syphilitic or gonorrhoeal origin could be required to submit to medical examination and a complete course of treatment. Initially, the Bill also provided for the committal to hospital by warrant of any infected persons believed to be a threat to public health (such as those defaulting from treatment at the clinics) and their detention for treatment.[2] Finally, drafted along similar lines, the Glasgow-sponsored Venereal Disease (Scotland) Bill of 1928 sought to make it a legal duty of infected persons (and parents of a syphilitic child) to place themselves under treatment by a medical practitioner until certified as non-infective. The Bill proposed a system of 'conditional' notification (i.e. notification of defaulters) with ultimate power for a Medical Officer of Health to prosecute and detain.[3]

These proposals aroused fierce public debate both at Westminster and in the counsels of Scottish local government, and became the focus for extensive pressure-group activity. They raised a range of fundamental and contentious issues relating to the liberty of the individual, to the role of the medical profession and the local state in the control of sexually transmitted diseases, to the medico-legal implications of compulsory treatment, and to the right of Scottish health legislation to deviate from the diktat of Whitehall. This chapter examines the impulses and constraints operating upon the Scottish campaign for VD controls and the social politics surrounding its evolution and eventual defeat.

The Impulses

The Scottish campaign for VD controls could point to solid precedent. Under the 1889 Infectious Diseases Notification Act and the 1897 Public Health (Scotland) Act, Medical Officers of Health possessed powers to examine and to isolate infected persons and to prosecute those endangering public health in cases of infectious disease. Even with diseases such as TB and ophthalmia neonatorum, which attracted social stigma and presented problems of defining infectivity and treatment, controls including notification had been introduced.[4] More specifically, Scottish proposals were consistent with the interventionist thrust of much previous public debate over the spread of VD. The Royal Commission on the Poor Laws had recommended that public assistance authorities should have 'power to detain cases of venereal disease when medically certified to be dangerous to others'.[5] While subscribing to a broadly voluntarist strategy, the Royal Commission on Venereal Diseases had advocated compulsory treatment for infected Poor Law patients and prisoners. It had also anticipated that improvements in medical facilities and a heightened public awareness of the social costs of VD might lead to an acceptance of more coercive measures.[6] Indeed, the Commissioners had admitted that 'the application of compulsion to cases in which there is no sense of responsibility, where no restraint is thought of, and where contagion is in its most active and virulent form, can be defended on strong public grounds'.[7]

Subsequently, wartime concern over military efficiency and the reconstruction debates surrounding civilian health produced a range of emergency regulations and longer-term proposals designed to penalize the spread of VD.[8] Moreover, while the Trevethin Committee, the major post-war public inquiry into the prevention of venereal infection, favoured the retention of a voluntary system of public clinics, it *was* prepared to endorse local, experimental measures of compulsion against those evading or defaulting from

178

treatment as a means of building up 'a body of experience of great value in determining future policy'.[9]

At the forefront of the Scottish campaign for such measures were many of the surgeons and clinicians most closely involved in the diagnosis and treatment of VD. As we have seen in Chapter 2, some of the more interventionist views aired before the Royal Commission on VD had come from Scottish venereologists. Subsequently, the leading activist for controls and draftsman of the Edinburgh Venereal Disease Bill was David Lees, Clinical Medical Officer in charge of the Edinburgh Corporation VD Scheme. As early as 1920, Lees pressed the Public Health Committee for sanctions against the 'irresponsible class' who ignored or defaulted from full treatment. 'It is', he wrote, 'an anomaly in Public Health Administration that known sources of venereal infection ... should be allowed with impunity to go about, a source of danger not only to themselves but to the community at large.'[10] Thereafter, in his official reports and in the counsels of the British Medical Association [BMA] and the British Social Hygiene Council [BSHC], he fought unremittingly for the extension of notification to VD, and for compulsory treatment. To combat congenital syphilis and ophthalmia neonatorum, he was prepared on explicitly 'eugenic principles' to contemplate controls on marriage and conception and the enforced treatment of pregnant women known to be infected.[11] For Lees, 'what was needed was not a discontinuance of the voluntary system, but a strengthening of it; not an infringement of the liberty of any subject who deserved liberty, but definitely and avowedly an infringement of the liberty of the libertine'.[12] Such views were typical of a generation of social hygienists operating in the field of public health in the 1920s, whose outlook towards VD had been shaped by service in the medical corps during the First World War, and who were concerned to establish the professional status of their expertise as venereologists.[13]

Also playing a strategic role within the Scottish campaign for VD controls were the Medical Officers of Health.[14] The medico-moral politics of war and reconstruction had endorsed their concern to contain the threat of 'the social evil'. They not only represented a powerful pressure group. They also articulated the views of clinicians to local politicians and the community. To A. Maxwell Williamson, Medical Officer of Health for Edinburgh, 'the continuation of a treatment centre without any accompanying compulsion represent[ed] simply the revolution of an endless chain'. Leaving active sources of possible infection 'to roam at large' merely negated any preventive role of the clinics. In view of the stringent controls over 'innocent sufferers' from other infectious diseases, he questioned why 'such undue delicacy and leniency should be shown towards those wilfully contracting and disseminating venereal disease' and advocated legal powers to compel them to submit to and sustain treatment until certified as cured.[15] His successor, William Robertson, subscribed to similar views. According to Robertson, VD was 'a menace to the manhood and future generation of this country' and a 'scourge to be firmly gripped'. Armed with the rhetoric of social hygiene, he protested that:

> The clean must be protected from the unclean and the unclean must be made clean .... If we have power to segregate contacts in the case of smallpox, typhus, or any other infectious disease, we should have analogous powers when dealing with venereal diseases. If we have power to take specimens of blood, swabs, and smears in one class of infectious diseases, we should have that power for all infections .... The need is for immediate and vigorous repressive action.[16]

Robertson concurred with Lees that permissive schemes, 'coupled with moralising and the offering of advice', were inadequate as medical strategies.[17] As he concluded in his annual report for 1927, 'we may as well cry for the moon to come down to earth as we need expect to get the better of venereal diseases by voluntary methods'.[18]

Other Medical Officers of Health in Scotland were more ambivalent towards the introduction of compulsory powers. Nonetheless, there were specific aspects of the problem, such as congenital disease and the continuing high incidence of 'defaulting', where there was a growing consensus in support of legislation. For example, the Medical Officer of Health for Dundee was persuaded by the level of default in local clinics to advocate compulsory notification and treatment for 'persistently neglectful patients'.[19] Similarly, A. K. Chalmers, Medical Officer of Health for Glasgow, while opposing general measures of compulsion, was prepared to advocate State intervention to reduce the incidence of congenital syphilis and gonorrhoeal ophthalmia. In his view, 'in the presence of positive evidence that a following generation is suffering from transmitted disease, controversy should cease and action begin ... as no one ... would question the right of the State to take action for the protection of the oncoming generation from causes of race-deterioration which are so well established'.[20] Accordingly, he campaigned for an amendment to the Public Health Acts to compel parents of venereally infected children to seek treatment, and took responsibility for drafting the Venereal Disease (Children) (Scotland)

Bill in 1923.[21]

Critical to the impact of clinicians and Medical Officers of Health upon public policy towards VD was their success in shaping the views of Scottish local government. There was strong precedent for local authorities in Scotland pioneering health legislation. For example, the Edinburgh Local Act of 1879 imposing compulsory notification for infectious diseases predated general legislation by a decade.[22] Throughout the 1920s, all the major authorities repeatedly lobbied the Scottish Board of Health for additional powers.[23] In March 1923, a conference of Scottish local authorities resolved that the existing law was 'inadequate to secure the proper control and treatment of venereal disease' and that the Board should initiate a system of notification and legal compulsion upon all infected persons to undergo and sustain professional treatment. In 1924, Glasgow Corporation approved a similar motion incorporating a specific 'compulsitor' upon parents of congenitally infected children to seek treatment. Thereafter, this motion became the template for a score of representations to the Board of Health from smaller local authorities throughout Scotland. After a succession of resolutions and deputations during the years 1925–7 urging the Board to broaden the application of infectious disease regulations to VD, West of Scotland authorities drafted the Venereal Disease (Scotland) Bill. Meanwhile, in the course of its campaign for compulsory legislation, Edinburgh Corporation organized a series of meetings in 1927 and the early months of 1928 designed to secure the backing of all Scottish local authorities for its own Venereal Disease Bill.

The Convention of Scottish Royal Burghs also played an active role, reviving its long-standing interest in the regulation and containment of 'pestilential infections' dating back to the eighteenth century. On grounds of public economy, the Convention regularly urged the need for the compulsory notification of VD 'accompanied by legislation of an inhibitory nature' to ensure the proper completion of treatment.[24]

The social and economic effects of default from treatment and its associated venereal recidivism remained a central concern of all protagonists in the Scottish campaign.[25] The incidence of default was regarded as undermining the cost-efficiency of the clinics. At all levels of Scottish health administration during the 1920s, the issue of 'wasted expenditure' and 'the interest of the taxpayer and ratepayer' were repeatedly cited in support of greater controls over those infected with VD. The free provision of treatment without associated powers to regulate sexual behaviour was widely condemned in a period of draconian public expenditure cuts, especially as VD was perceived to be primarily the self-inflicted outcome of promiscuity.[26] Thus, Mary Liston regularly warned her defaulting patients that she was 'not going to waste public money on them' and threatened to charge them '10/- for treatment if attendance is not regular or orders carried out'. However, as she lamented to Lady Astor, 'I cannot carry out this threat in practice. I have to waste public money over and over again merely to relieve symptoms not to affect a cure.'[27]

Moreover, the existence of a substantial body of defaulters endangering their own health and transmitting infection to others was viewed as fundamentally inconsistent with the aims of preventive medicine and the moral objectives of the Social Hygiene Movement with its stress on self-control in the interests of racial progress. Scottish public health reports in the 1920s identified the defaulters as sexually 'atavistic' recidivists requiring coercive measures. It was both a medical and moral imperative that this 'most offensive portion of the population be identified and circumscribed'.[28] Such views were reinforced by growing evidence of the devastating impact of male default upon family health, and the protection of women and children against the sexual indulgence of infected menfolk became a recurrent theme in public health debate over the introduction of VD controls.[29]

Sharing these concerns was the Scottish Committee of the National Council for Combating Venereal Diseases/British Social Hygiene Council. As in England, the Council played a vital part in raising Scottish public consciousness of the incidence and effects of venereal infection and in networking the voluntary and governmental agencies dealing with the disease. However, the roles of the Council in England and Scotland increasingly diverged. Between 1918 and 1922, the National Executive Committee in London submitted a series of proposals to the Local Government Board and Ministry of Health in favour of measures to secure the 'continuous treatment of infective persons' and to penalize defaulters, but the Ministry of Health warned it that any public commitment to compulsion would be contrary to government policy and would jeopardize its subsidy for propaganda work. Thereafter, the English Council rapidly revised its strategy, refocused on educational issues and moral propaganda, and adopted either an agnostic or broadly voluntarist approach to interwar debate over VD.[30] In contrast, the Scottish Committee adhered to a compulsionist stance and gave increasing priority to co-ordinating a campaign for controls. In so doing, it was able to draw not only upon its special relationship with central government, but also upon a membership that included many of the strategic personnel in Scottish venereal medicine and public health.

From the early 1920s, the Scottish Committee pressed the Board of Health for statutory powers to compel those infected with VD to submit to a full course of treatment. It was particularly concerned to regulate defaulters who offended against both the moral and hygienic aims of the Council. The apparent use of the clinics as a prophylactic by such 'sexual libertines' was considered to be as morally indefensible as the issue of 'prophylactic packets' or the provision of self-disinfection ablution centres.[31] The Committee organized the conference of Scottish local authorities in March 1923, drafted its resolutions on compulsory notification and treatment, and co-ordinated subsequent lobbying of the Board of Health.[32] For the remainder of the 1920s, it continued to service and support the campaign for controls conducted by the local authorities. The Committee exerted increasing pressure on the Board to 'give a lead' while encouraging the major cities to experiment with local schemes of compulsion;[33] a level of involvement in marked contrast to the position of 'interested observer' claimed by the Council in England.[34]

The response of women's organizations to VD controls also varied geographically. While Scottish legislation such as the Edinburgh Corporation Bill encountered fierce opposition from a range of feminist pressure groups, local branches of the Women Citizens' Association, Co-operative Women's Guild, and the National Council of Women *were* often prepared to give their conditional support. They shared the view of the Public Health Departments that greater powers were necessary to reduce the wilful or negligent spread of VD and to protect the welfare of women and children. In addition, they saw the opportunity in local legislation to regulate male sexual behaviour as part of the contemporary struggle for women's rights. They did not view additional sanctions as undermining the principle of 'equal citizenship' but as reinforcing it by denying the right of infected men to 'pollute the springs of life' through marital intercourse. Female proponents of controls dismissed the agitation of other feminist groups such as the Women's Freedom League and the Association for Moral and Social Hygiene as unrepresentative of informed opinion in Scotland and as reflecting only the dogmatic and outdated 'abolitionist' views of upper-middle-class suffragists from London and Plymouth.[35] It is difficult to explain this divergence within the women's movement. Some members of the London executive of the Association for Moral and Social Hygiene argued that the absence of anti-regulationist sentiment north of the border might be attributed to the absence of

Contagious Disease legislation in nineteenth-century Scotland.[36] However, Scottish women's groups *had* participated in the campaign against Contagious Diseases legislation, and women's organizations had also opposed the use of the Burgh Police Acts to regulate prostitution in the Scottish cities.[37]

The Scottish Board of Health

The response of the Scottish Board of Health to the campaign for VD controls was ambivalent. During the immediate post-war years, it was concerned to promote a voluntary strategy that encouraged patients to seek treatment in the early and most infectious stages of the disease. It feared that compulsory notification would alienate public opinion from the clinics and be valueless without a comprehensive system of compulsory treatment which would in turn raise intractable issues of civil liberty.[38] However, by 1921, faced with growing evidence of evasion and default from treatment, the Board adopted a more interventionist stance, questioning 'whether in the interests of the community it should not be made a matter of compulsion that persons contracting these diseases shall have recourse to treatment, and shall continue in attendance for a period sufficient to ensure full result therefrom'.[39]

The Board agreed with clinicians and Medical Officers of Health that it was unacceptable for defaulters, suffering 'in the main from self-inflicted infections', to endanger public health and waste public money. It also agreed that the parents of children suffering from congenital syphilis or gonorrhoeal ophthalmia were prime and legitimate targets for compulsion, and in 1923 commissioned Thomas Dewar, head of the Board's Infectious Diseases Section, and A. K. Chalmers, Medical Officer of Health for Glasgow, to draft a bill sanctioning the notification and compulsory treatment of infected parents in the interests of 'child welfare'. This was subsequently forwarded to the Ministry of Health as the Venereal Disease (Children) (Scotland) Bill in August 1923.[40]

However, despite intensive lobbying from Scottish local authorities, from the British Social Hygiene Council and from many of its own Medical Inspectors, the Board remained reluctant to grasp the nettle of more general controls by the introduction of a Public Health Amendment Act or a more liberal interpretation of its powers pertaining to the control of 'epidemic, endemic or infectious disease' under the Public Health (Scotland) Act of 1897. Senior officials viewed compulsion as raising not only contentious issues of freedom and social equity (in terms of both class and gender) but also serious

184

medico-legal issues, given the dangers associated with treatment involving arsenobenzol compounds.[41] In their opinion, 'it [was] better to make it a statutory offence not to resort to treatment rather than to force the individual to submit to treatment'.[42] Torn between sympathy for the objectives of the Scottish campaign and doubts as to the political and administrative expediency of controls, the Board of Health preferred to shift the onus of responsibility back onto the local authorities. Thus, reviewing policy options in April 1924, H. L. Fraser, Principal Assistant Secretary, concluded that:

> If ... a responsible local authority, who have all the facts before them, come to the Board with a definite resolution to extend the Infectious Diseases Notification Schedule to VD, I have no doubt the Board would give their approval. It is one thing to advise caution and quite another to refuse consent to a definite proposal put forward by a responsible local authority who desire to try the experiment.[43]

However, although such experiments were consistent with the recommendations of the Trevethin Committee, efforts by the Board in 1924–5 to encourage local initiatives were firmly rejected by the Ministry of Health. In the view of the Ministry, public policy towards VD should focus on education rather than compulsory regulations and any 'special measures' contemplated by Scottish local authorities would have to be subjected to full parliamentary scrutiny.[44]

Thereafter, to the frustration of Thomas Dewar and many of the medical inspectorate, the Board of Health retreated to a somewhat more reactive but no less ambivalent stance on VD issues.[45] Publicly, it continued to endorse the demand of local authorities, clinicians and social workers for sanctions against defaulters, especially as a means of reducing conjugal and congenital infection.[46] It was also prepared to encourage the major Scottish local authorities to test the issue of controls in Parliament by means of Private Bill procedure.[47] However, when faced with specific proposals, as in the Edinburgh Corporation Bill, it proved unsupportive. In particular, it criticized the powers of detention and compulsory treatment in the Bill for shifting the focus of reform away from prevention and 'import[ing] into public health administration a new and contentious principle of compulsory cure'.[48] The dormancy of existing measures for the compulsory removal for treatment of TB patients was regarded as a significant indicator of public resistance to such powers.[49]

The Board proposed instead more modest powers enabling the Medical Officer of Health to require a person believed to be suffering

185

from VD to seek treatment and to take proper precautions to avert the spread of infection, under penalty of a fine. Yet, senior officials admitted that their primary concern was less the nature of the provisions *per se* than their propensity to alienate public opinion and that the distinction between the two strategies was largely academic. As they conceded, apart from segregation and 'complete continence coupled with rigid aseptic practice in personal and family hygiene', there was not 'in practice any effective precaution against the spread of infection except treatment'.[50] The vacillation of the Scottish Board of Health over the issue of VD controls in the 1920s reflected in part its lack of a coherent operational philosophy and the differing views of its medical experts and generalist administrators. It also reflected the sheer complexity of legislating for sexually transmitted diseases. Particularly significant were the socio-legal and political problems of reconciling the coercive sentiments of the Scottish campaign with the more libertarian strands of British public and professional opinion.

The Constraints

A decisive factor inhibiting Scottish legislation was the attitude of the Ministry of Health as shaped by its Principal Medical Officers, Sir Arthur Newsholme and Sir George Newman, and by its Advisor on Venereal Diseases, Colonel L. W. Harrison.[51] Throughout the interwar period, the Ministry adhered to a policy of voluntary treatment underpinned by a State-subsidized programme of social hygiene education. It was opposed to the compulsory notification and treatment of VD, 'medically, administratively, and socially'. In the Ministry's view, existing notification procedures were inappropriate for VD with its acute social stigma and its often protracted and poorly defined infectivity. It anticipated considerable public resistance to notification, with patients deterred from seeking medical treatment in the early, most infective stages of VD and an increasing recourse to quacks. Particular concern was expressed at the possible deterrent effect of notification for pregnant women and infants upon attendance at ante-natal and child welfare centres. Moreover, given the uneven access of practitioners to the technology of bacteriological and other tests, the Ministry of Health predicted that any system of compulsory notification for VD would only be partial and 'turn out to be a class measure, affecting only the poorer section of the community' attending public treatment centres. Proposals for the compulsory treatment of infected persons were similarly dismissed as 'a fundamental threat to the liberty of the subject under English law' and to the established principles of public health policy. The Ministry considered that they would encourage the concealment of infection and delay in seeking medical advice. The issues of who should be compelled to submit to treatment, and at what stage of infection, were regarded as highly problematical and would, in the view of Whitehall, tend to resolve in inequitable controls which targeted public rather than private patients and which alienated 'poorer class families' from the medical services.

A powerful argument deployed by the Ministry of Health and shared by other opponents of compulsory legislation was the difficulty of implementing VD controls given the absence of generally accepted standards of non-infectivity, treatment, and cure.[52] As in the USA, this lack of consensus surfaced in all the major interwar debates on the State regulation of sexually transmitted diseases in Britain. In the early 1920s, it figured prominently in the rejection of public self-disinfection schemes by Whitehall and by leading pressure groups such as the National Council for Combating Venereal Diseases.[53] It was a decisive factor in the decision of the Trevethin Committee to recommend the continuation of voluntary provisions,[54] and was a central thrust of the opposition to Scottish proposals for compulsory treatment. As Dr Graham Little, MP and Consultant Dermatologist, observed in moving the rejection of the Edinburgh Corporation Bill:

> In a disorder in which neither methods of treatment nor tests of cure are stabilised by present knowledge, such a requirement is a medical absurdity as well as a monstrous infringement of individual liberty.[55]

The inability of many medical practitioners, through lack of expertise or facilities, or through sheer apathy, to apply modern and consistent methods of diagnosis and cure to venereal cases (especially to gonorrhoea) was also regarded by many public health officials as a major obstacle to any scheme of compulsory notification or treatment.[56] As late as 1927, Sir George Newman echoed the views of many venereologists in complaining of 'the technical inefficiency, the slip-shod methods, the antiquated notions, the degree of ignorance and indifference that mark[ed] the reactions of too large a proportion of medical men towards venereal problems'.[57]

Another important criticism levelled at the Scottish campaign for controls was that its use of default statistics exaggerated the threat of VD to public health. The view of the Ministry of Health, endorsed by the Trevethin Committee, was that many patients who discontinued treatment early were non-infectious. Whitehall argued that many cases of syphilis attending clinics were already past the infectious stage, that the standard of cure was so high that many cases of gonorrhoea were non-infective well before the completion of treatment, and that many so-called 'defaulters' moved to other treatment centres or opted to continue treatment under private practitioners.[58] Thus, despite the fact that performance indicators for VD clinics in England and Wales were markedly worse than for those in Scotland,[59] the Ministry of Health was disposed to focus instead upon the overall trend decline in default and its legitimation of a voluntary strategy for confronting 'the social evil'.[60] Meanwhile, the high default rates in overseas countries which *had* adopted compulsory measures, such as Australia, were regularly cited by opponents of Scottish legislation.[61]

Disagreement amongst Scottish Medical Officers of Health and local authorities over the extent and type of compulsion to be adopted also significantly weakened the case for controls. There was broad agreement amongst Scottish medical officers that congenital infection and defaulting should be legislated against, but they differed markedly over more generic measures. In particular, the commitment of medical officers in Edinburgh to compulsory treatment was not always shared by their counterparts in Glasgow. A. K. Chalmers, whose views were regularly sought by the Board of Health, rejected such proposals 'as an invasion of individual liberty'. In his view:

> To penalise ... in some way for spreading infection [was] logical enough, but to compel ... to undergo a particular form of treatment [was] to suggest an analogy with crime, and [was] opposed to every principle which has hitherto guided the evolution of medical and surgical methods for the relief of disease.

He feared that such regulation would 'alter the whole relation of the public to Public Health Administration' and provide a dangerous precedent for the 'sterilisation of the "unfit" and the extinction of all recessive types'.[62] Representations from local authorities to the Scottish Board of Health displayed a similar polarity between those favouring compulsory notification as a means of tracing and penalizing the wilful transmission of VD and those opting for 'conditional notification' [i.e. notification restricted to defaulters] as the basis of compulsory treatment.[63] Moreover, Scottish venereologists were often equally divided as to the precise nature of the VD controls that should be introduced and the extent to which they should be contingent upon improved medical facilities.[64]

Underpinning all health policy-making in interwar Britain was the need to secure the co-operation of the medical profession. Its generally negative reaction to proposals for more stringent VD regulations was therefore viewed in government circles as a major obstacle to legislation. BMA branch support for local measures might occasionally be elicited, as in Liverpool in 1920 and Edinburgh in 1928,[65] but general legislation received limited support from the profession. From the outset, although in favour of the detention of Poor Law patients, the BMA was firmly opposed to the compulsory notification of VD and this was confirmed by a canvass of BMA opinion in 1923.[66] Proposals for the compulsory treatment of VD received an equally hostile response when debated at BMA meetings.[67]

Many factors, ranging from empirical uncertainties, through medico-legal concerns, to professional self-interest, motivated this reaction. Despite advances in venereology, the medical profession still differed over the extent of VD in the community. Therapy for syphilis and gonorrhoea remained the subject of heated debate, and correct dosages, length of treatment, and definitions of cure continued to be contested in the medical journals.[68] Doctors therefore lacked a stable 'scientific' consensus upon which interventionist strategies might securely be based.

In addition, doctors were very concerned at the legal implications of VD controls. A number of high court judgments in the early 1920s had already threatened the confidentiality of proceedings at VD clinics. Quite apart from specific liability for slander in cases of wrongful notification and for damages arising from the compulsory use of arsenobenzol compounds, it was feared that the involvement of practitioners in the systematic disclosure of information and the imposition of regimented treatment would further undermine the concept of medical privilege and the confidence of patients in qualified medical practice. The extent of unqualified 'quackery' still existing in the treatment of VD in interwar Britain, despite the 1917 Venereal Disease Act, and to which patients might be diverted, added substance to this fear.[69]

Medical opposition to VD controls in interwar Britain also reflected ongoing struggles for power and status within the medical profession itself.[70] Friction between general practitioners and Medical Officers of Health had attended the introduction of infectious disease legislation in the late nineteenth century. In particular, notification procedures involving secondary (bacteriological) diagnosis 'often undermined the general practitioner's authority'.[71] After 1900, as scientific advances opened the way for State medicine to take a more interventionist stand in the fight against VD, and the technology of diagnosis and treatment became more sophisticated, these tensions increased. Within this context, municipal proposals for compulsory notification and/or treatment were viewed as yet a further threat to private practice and resisted accordingly.[72]

A wide range of women's organizations with roots in the suffrage movement also vigorously resisted Scottish demands for VD controls. Experience of wartime controls, pre-eminently the notorious DORA 40D, had provided damning evidence of the degree to which, under a patriarchal legal and enforcement system, punitive purity legislation, designed to contain VD, discriminated against women.[73] Organizations such as the influential National Union of Societies for Equal Citizenship [NUSEC] were therefore hostile towards further attempts to criminalize the transmission of VD. The Union predicted that compulsory notification and treatment would in practice target prostitutes and female patients of public clinics, that such measures would revive some of the more detestable features of the Contagious Diseases Acts and degenerate into ill-disguised sexual harassment. Instead, it advocated a preventive strategy of moral education and social hygiene.[74]

The Association for Moral and Social Hygiene [AMSH] articulated similar views. Having spearheaded the campaign against DORA 40D, it then co-ordinated much of post-war feminist resistance to local authority controls.[75] The AMSH deployed a range of familiar arguments: the deterrent effect of compulsion on patients seeking early treatment, its violation of professional confidentiality, the lack of any convincing comparative evidence from overseas that compulsion enhanced the efficiency of clinics, and the medical, ethical and legal dangers of imposing controls on a medical profession that was ill-trained in new diagnostic and curative techniques. The neglect of individual 'moral reclamation' arising out of a health policy centred on physical treatment was also criticized. However, the AMSH's strongest concern was the bias with which Medical Officers of Health would exercise their powers. On past evidence, it argued that private patients 'of good social position' would be exempt from coercion while sanctions would be focused on working-class offenders attending the public clinics. Gender discrimination would also be systemic, with prostitutes and 'denounced women' being treated as scapegoats for promiscuity within the community as a whole.

The Medical Women's Federation [MWF] provided a further important strand of opposition to Scottish proposals for VD controls. As with the NUSEC and the AMSH, the Federation articulated the medico-moral strategy of the Social Hygiene Movement, with the concept of 'promiscuity' central to its causal and curative ideologies. It opposed notification for VD on the grounds that there was no legally accepted criterion of infectivity and that, if associated with compulsory treatment, it would 'lead to concealment of early cases and delay in treatment during the curable stage'. The practical and medico-legal difficulties of penalizing the transmission of sexually transmitted diseases were regarded as insurmountable. Instead of coercive measures, the MWF recommended a series of 'constructive' social reforms designed to promote sexual continence in *both* sexes, including 'facilities for early marriage', improved housing conditions, and improved provisions for sex education and 'mixed-sex rational recreation'.[76] Significantly, several of the more influential female venereologists in Scotland also subscribed to a voluntarist viewpoint. Thus, Nora Wattie of Glasgow Corporation Public Health Department 'pronounced against both notification and compulsory attendance' and advocated better staff resourcing of clinics and the development of more systematic contact-tracing procedures. Likewise, Helen Murrell, Assistant Venereologist at the Royal Infirmary of Edinburgh, opposed legal sanctions and recommended improved accommodation for infectious prostitutes and hostels for girls, these to be linked with existing social organizations and supplemented by separate homes for cases of congenital syphilis and vulvo vaginitis.[77]

The Outcome

In the event, the Scottish campaign for the more rigorous State regulation of VD proved abortive. The Venereal Disease (Children) (Scotland) Bill was firmly rejected by the Ministry of Health in 1923–4 on medical, social and administrative grounds, and subsequently pigeon-holed by the Scottish Board of Health.[78] However, the critical set-back to the campaign came in April 1928, when the Edinburgh Corporation (Venereal Disease) Bill was opposed by the Government on its second reading in the House of Commons and defeated in division by 156 votes to 93.[79]

In 1927, events leading up to this defeat focused in Edinburgh. By April 1927, a Provisional Order Bill incorporating VD controls had been drafted on the advice of the Public Health Committee and local opposition from women's organizations had already emerged. However, in June, the Parliamentary Chairman of Committees ruled that the VD clause raised sufficiently broad and contentious issues as to justify a separate private bill procedure. This was duly activated by the Corporation in late December. By January 1928, local debate had begun to formalize into rival organizations with a developing repertoire of pressure-group tactics. While Edinburgh Corporation mobilized the support of other Scottish local authorities, a vocal Protest Committee had been formed, co-ordinated by the AMSH and NUSEC and channelling feminist opposition to the Bill.

The first reading of the Bill on 10 February 1928 elevated the debate to a national level. Thereafter, it figured prominently in the correspondence of *The Times* and periodical press, and in the editorials of professional organs such as the *British Medical Journal*. The national executives of interest groups such as the British Social Hygiene Council, the BMA, and the Society of Medical Officers of Health began to canvass and to co-ordinate responses to the Bill. Meanwhile, both supporters and opponents of VD controls shifted the thrust of their lobbying to central government, circularizing MPs, targeting influential groups such as the Parliamentary Medical Committee and lobbying the Scottish Office.

The first reading of the Edinburgh Corporation (Venereal Disease) Bill had also activated a vigorous debate in Whitehall. While objecting to the emphasis of the Bill upon the compulsory treatment of VD rather than the penalization of its transmission, the Scottish Board of Health urged the Government to permit a free debate on second reading. It stressed the strength of feeling within the Scottish local authorities and the encouragement that the Board had given them to introduce private legislation as a means of advancing public debate on the issue. Initially, the Scottish Office were in broad agreement. Sir John Gilmour, Secretary of State for Scotland, and Walter Elliot, Vice-President of the Board and Parliamentary Under-Secretary of State, concurred that a preventive strategy in line with existing infectious disease controls would have been preferable. They were also of the view that *some* form of legislation was needed. They viewed local experimentation in health legislation as an appropriate means of government growth and considered that a second reading would be a valuable means both of raising public awareness of the continuing problem of VD and of obtaining a thorough and informed investigation of policy options in Committee.

However, by the 15 March, the Scottish Office had revised its position and declared its intention of opposing the Bill on second reading. To some extent, this *volte-face* reflected the reservations of Sir James Leishman and Sir Leslie Mackenzie, Permanent Members of the Scottish Board of Health, who had, since the early 1920s, consistently voiced a preference for the modification of existing regulations rather than for innovatory controls. The criticisms levelled at the Bill by A. K. Chalmers, former Medical Officer of Health for Glasgow, were also influential. However, despite protestations to the contrary by Gilmour, the decisive factor was clearly the attitude of the Ministry of Health. On the advice of Sir George Newman and Colonel Harrison, Neville Chamberlain opposed the Bill's second reading on the grounds that it constituted a radical and undesirable departure from existing principles of public health administration which would pose a serious threat to civil liberty without significant benefit to community health. He refused to permit Scottish experimentation in VD controls that might impact upon English public health procedures and persuaded the Cabinet to oppose the measure.

As it became known that the Cabinet were proposing to put on a Government three-line whip against the Bill, an unprecedented step for private legislation, the specific issue of VD regulations became increasingly subsumed within a broader constitutional debate over Scottish legislative autonomy. A major cultural renaissance and new political alignments in Scotland in the 1920s had produced a resurgence of Scottish Nationalism, fuelled by a range of Whitehall proposals designed to reduce the autonomy of Scottish central and local government.[80] Given this backdrop, news of the Bill's obstruction elicited a predictably hostile response from Scottish civic leaders. Typical was the reaction of Edinburgh's Lord Provost who vehemently protested at the treatment of a national capital as if it were 'a fourth-rate mushroom English city'.[81] Many Scottish politicians, including Conservative Unionist MPs, predicted that such tactics would be electorally damaging and play into the hands of the Scottish Home Rule campaign.[82] The presence of a large contingent of English feminists, led by Lady Astor, at Edinburgh protest meetings only served to exacerbate the situation.

In a lively, four-hour, second reading debate on 19 April 1928 all the major arguments for and against compulsion in the administration of VD were rehearsed, from broad constitutional issues, through issues of social equity, morality and medico-legal ethics, to the practicalities involved. Conflicting interpretations were predictably placed upon the recommendations of the Royal Commission on Venereal Diseases and the Trevethin Committee and on the lessons to be drawn from domestic precedent and overseas example. The debate reflected the range of interest groups and ideologies involved, with considerations of medical science in juxtaposition with conventional feminist arguments and a promiscuous appeal to the needs of economy, eugenics, professional integrity and 'equal citizenship'.

Both sides of the debate attracted cross-party support in the division. The ayes included an unholy alliance of committed Labour MPs such as Emmanuel Shinwell along with ex-service Tories such as Rear-Admiral Tufton Percy Hamilton Beamish, Conservative member for Lewes. The noes were equally varied: Labour members for urban constituencies such as David Kirkwood and Arthur Greenwood voting alongside highland Liberals such as Sir Murdoch Macdonald and Tory feminists such as Lady Astor. Nevertheless, a breakdown of votes by party reveals that on the issue of VD controls, Labour members were the most supportive of innovation and Liberal members the least. Some 35 per cent of the Conservative members attending voted for the Bill as compared with 45 per cent of the Labour members and only 13 per cent of the Liberals. Significantly, while Scottish MPs represented only 13 per cent of those opposing the Bill, they constituted 23 per cent of its supporters, while MPs from London and the Home Counties were overwhelmingly against the measure.[83]

The defeat of the Edinburgh Corporation Bill inevitably slowed the momentum of the Scottish campaign for VD controls. In the light of events and the evident reluctance of the Scottish Office to support any compulsory measure explicitly involving treatment, the Venereal Disease (Scotland) Bill sponsored by Glasgow Corporation was dropped.[84] However, throughout the remainder of the interwar period, local authorities and public health committees continued to lobby the Scottish Board of Health (as of 1928, the Department of Health for Scotland) for additional powers with which to regulate those who ignored or discontinued treatment.[85] The Department, mindful of the continuing opposition to controls in the Ministry of Health, remained reluctant to encourage new initiatives. It did provide fresh data on the incidence of default in its annual reports as a basis for 'legitimate debate', but its view in the mid-1930s was that public and parliamentary opinion had not shifted sufficiently to make legislation politically viable.[86] Representations to the Ministry of Health from the Convention of Scottish Royal Burghs received a similar response.[87]

However, in 1936, the Report of the Committee on the Scottish Health Services gave fresh impetus to the campaign for controls. Persuaded by the weight of local authority and medical opinion, the majority of the Committee recommended that 'because of the serious effects of syphilis on the race', compulsory notification should be introduced along with powers 'to require infected persons to undergo treatment until they [were] no longer a danger to others'. With a view to the recent history of such proposals, it pointedly added that, if it was deemed 'inexpedient to apply a system of compulsory treatment over the whole country, powers should be given to the larger local authorities ... to adopt compulsory measures on an experimental basis'.[88] Further momentum was added by the widely publicized findings of a New York inquiry comparing unfavourably the performance of British voluntary procedures with the compulsory measures operating in Scandinavia.[89] In 1937, renewed pressure from Scottish members of the BSHC Executive led to the appointment of an inter-departmental committee to investigate these claims.[90] Meanwhile, evidence from opinion polls indicated that public opinion was shifting in favour of more rigorous VD controls.[91] Predictably, these findings became the focus of renewed pressure on the Department of Health for Scotland and Ministry of Health for action, but in the event, they were soon to be subsumed within the more general debate over VD regulations occasioned by the outbreak of the Second World War.

The Implications

The defeat of this first phase of the Scottish campaign for VD controls serves to illuminate the socio-medical politics of interwar Britain. Underlying the various strands of opposition to compulsion was a broader societal resistance to State intervention. Compulsory notification and treatment posed fundamental issues of personal liberty and the inquisitorial rights of Government. Such measures ran counter to the traditional values of liberal individualism and voluntarism that had so tenaciously survived into the interwar period, despite the collectivism of war and reconstruction.[92] These values permeated the reports and recommendations of the Royal Commission on Venereal Diseases and the Trevethin Committee and continued to resonate in health policy-making circles. They were further reinforced by the growing association of VD controls in Europe with totalitarian regimes.

To some extent, this resistance to compulsory regulations incorporated a growing critique of the role and power of the expert in democratic society. The heroes of Victorian government growth, such as the Medical Officers of Health, were increasingly viewed by social commentators as a potential threat. In the cause of social advancement and the discharge of ostensibly neutral, civil duties, it was feared that professional groups would collude with the State in the erection of authoritarian controls.[93] These concerns were frequently aired in the debate over Scottish VD proposals. Thus, at a major protest meeting against the Edinburgh Corporation Bill in March 1928, Lady Astor declared that 'they had not come to Edinburgh to praise Caesar but to bury him. The more they looked at this bill ... the more it smacked of Caesar'.[94] As the Scottish Board of Health observed, there was an overriding fear in some quarters that 'any legislation, however moderate and however wisely safeguarded, might prove a harsh and even tyrannous weapon in the hands of unwise officials, even though their unwisdom were based upon mistaken zeal'.[95] More specifically, there was a strong residue of Shavian distrust of medical science and officialdom surviving into the interwar period. Opposition to VD controls in part re-enacted the libertarian campaigns of the 1890s and 1900s against compulsory notification of infectious diseases and compulsory vaccination, with a similar fear of a 'professional despotism' based upon the social claims of an uncertain medical technology.[96]

Notes

1 Public Records Office [PRO], Ministry of Health Papers, MH 55/183, Bill papers.
2 National Archives of Scotland [NAS], HH 33/595/1–16, Bill papers.
3 NAS, HH 33/595/16a, 18, Bill papers.
4 *52 & 53 Vict. (1889), ch. 72; 60 & 61 Vict. (1897), ch. 38.*
5 *Royal Commission on the Poor Laws and Relief of Distress [RCPLRD], PP 1909 (Cd. 4499) XXXVII,* 276.
6 *Royal Commission on Venereal Diseases [RCVD], PP 1916 (Cd. 8189) XVI,* 50–1, 53.
7 *Ibid.,* 51.
8 L. Bland, '"Cleansing the Portals of Life": The Venereal Disease Campaign in the Early Twentieth Century', in M. Langan and B. Schwarz (eds), *Crises in the British State 1880–1930* (London: Hutchinson, 1985), 203; F. Honigsbaum, *The Struggle for the Ministry of Health 1914–1919* (London: G. Bell & Sons, 1970), 45.
9 *Report of Committee of Inquiry on Venereal Disease* (London: HMSO, 1923), 10.
10 *Edinburgh Public Health Department [EPHD] Annual Report (1920),* 54.
11 *Ibid. (1921),* 41; *(1923),* 48; *(1925),* 55; *(1927),* 61; *Proceedings of the Imperial Social Hygiene Congress* (London: NCCVD, 1924), 135–47.

12 *British Medical Journal [BMJ]*, ii (1928), 64–5. For biographical
    details, see *British Journal of Venereal Diseases [BJVD]*, 10 (1934),
    79–81; Medical Society for the Study of Venereal Diseases, Scottish
    Branch [MSSVDSB], Minutes, 19 Dec. 1928. Similar views were
    expressed by Mary Liston, Assistant Medical Officer, Edinburgh VD
    Scheme. See University of Reading Library, MS/1/1/229, Nancy
    Astor Papers, Liston to Lady Astor, 20 Jan. 1928, 12 Feb. 1928. I
    am indebted to Dr R. L. Wolfe for alerting me to this
    correspondence.

13 A. S. Wigfield, 'The Emergence of the Consultant Venereologist',
    BJVD, 48 (1972), 549–52.

14 There was also widespread support from Medical Officers of Health
    [MOH] elsewhere in the United Kingdom. Of the MOH in the
    leading 'provincial centres' surveyed in 1922, 69% considered that
    public opinion was 'ripe for demanding legislative protection for
    VD', and 86% favoured some form of 'modified notification and
    compulsory continuous treatment' (British Medical Association
    [BMA] Archives, B/322/1/1, Papers of Special Committee on the
    Notification of VD 1922–3).

15 *EPHD Annual Report (1919)*, xx–xxi; *(1920)*, xxi–xxiii; *(1921)*,
    xvi–xvii.

16 W. M. Robertson, 'The Administrative Control of Venereal Disease',
    Transactions of the Incorporated Sanitary Association of Scotland
    (1919), 63–4.

17 *EPHD Annual Report (1923)*, vii; *(1926)*, vi–vii.

18 *Ibid.*, vii.

19 *Dundee MOH Annual Report (1923)*, 49; *(1925)*, 33–5; *(1926)*, 42.

20 A. K. Chalmers, 'The Notification and Control of Venereal
    Diseases', *Public Health*, 42 (1928–9), 104–9.

21 *Glasgow MOH Annual Report (1920)*, 10; *(1923)*, 22; PRO, MH
    55/183, Bill papers.

22 *42 & 43 Vict., ch. 132*, clause 208.

23 For the following account, see especially, NAS, HH 33/595/10,
    Chronological Note of Representations to Scottish Board of Health
    in favour of Venereal Disease Legislation (1921–28); HH 65/116,
    items 1–2, 5–9, 33, 45–6.

24 Edinburgh City Archives [ECA], Minutes of Convention of Scottish
    Royal Burghs, 4 May 1922, 7 June 1922, 3 April 1928.

25 On the incidence of default and its central role within contemporary
    discourse surrounding VD, see above, chs 5 and 7.

26 See, e.g., *EPHD Annual Report (1926)*, vi–vii; NAS, HH 65/115/4,
    Resolution from Convention of Scottish Royal Burghs, 9 June 1922;

NAS, HH 65/116/2, Minutes of Deputation from Glasgow Corporation, 23 May 1924.

27 University of Reading Library, MS/1/1/229, Nancy Astor Papers, M. Liston to Lady Astor, 12 Feb. 1928.

28 *Glasgow MOH Annual Report (1928)*, 155; *(1929)*, 157.

29 See, e.g., A. K. Chalmers, *op. cit.* (note 20), 107–8; NAS, HH 33/595/18, Memorandum by Dr A. S. Macgregor, 14 April 1928. In 1926, the male default rate at Glasgow clinics for syphilis was twice the female rate and for gonorrhoea, 4.5 times as high (NAS, HH 33/595/18).

30 Contemporary Medical Archives Centre [CMAC], SA/BSH, A1/7, National Council for Combating Venereal Diseases [NCCVD], Resolutions, 1918–22; A2/7, Minutes of NCCVD Executive Committee, 11 April 1923; *Health and Empire*, Vol. 1, no. 3 (Jan.–Feb. 1922), Editorial, 17–18; Vol. 1, no. 12 (May 1923), 96–7.

31 NAS, HH 65/115/5, Memorandum on 'Venereal Disease: The Need for Further Legislative Powers', by W. E. Whyte (Secretary, Scottish Committee), 1 July 1922. The Scottish Committee Chairman, Dr McGregor Robertson, believed that libertarian sentiments had to yield to 'the interests of public welfare and to the necessity of a national danger' (*Health and Empire*, Vol. 1, no. 6 (May 1922), 46–7).

32 NAS, HH 65/116/3. In response to concern from the NCCVD Executive Committee that such campaigning contravened government policy, the Scottish Committee retorted that it was only representing Scottish local authority opinion and that, as it was financed by the Scottish Board of Health, 'the wishes of the Ministry of Health did not apply to their country' (CMAC, SA/BSH, A2/7, Minutes of National Executive Committee, 11 April 1923).

33 NAS, HH 65/116/2, 27, 37; HH 33/595/8.

34 *Health and Empire*, Vol. 13, no. 1 (1928), 4.

35 NAS, HH 33/595/13, Edinburgh Corporation Bill: Representations in favour; GD/333/3, 6, 9–10, Papers of the Edinburgh Women Citizens' Association [EWCA]. However, local branches varied widely in their response. Thus, the Falkirk Branch of the WCA remained committed to 'moral and non-coercive measures' (Falkirk District Museums History Research Centre, Falkirk WCA, Minutes, 13 Feb. 1923, 22 Jan. 1928).

36 Fawcett Library, AMS/43, Minutes of Association for Moral and Social Hygiene [AMSH], Executive Committee, 8 Nov. 1927.

37 National Library of Scotland, Minto Papers, MS 12357, ff.162–91, Letters concerning the Contagious Disease Act; L. Mahood, *The Magdalenes: Prostitution in the Nineteenth Century* (London:

Routledge, 1990), 146–8.

38   NAS, HH 65/113, Papers relating to the 1918 Sexual Offences Bill; *Annual Report of the Local Government Board for Scotland, PP 1919 (Cmd. 230) XXV*, xii–xiv.

39   *Scottish Board of Health [SBH], Second Annual Report, PP 1921 (Cmd. 1319) XIII*, 43.

40   PRO, MH 55/183, Bill papers; A. K. Chalmers, *op. cit.* (note 20), 109.

41   NAS, HH 65/116/27, Memorandum on 'Notification' by H. L. Fraser, 6 Aug. 1924; *Medical Research Council, Special Report No. 66, Report of Salvarsan Committee, Toxic Effects Following the Employment of Arsenobenzol Preparations* (London: HMSO, 1922).

42   NAS, HH 65/116/20, Notes by H. L. Fraser, Aug. 1924.

43   *Ibid.*

44   NAS, HH 65/116/32, Ministry of Health to SBH, 22 Oct. 1924.

45   Dewar's irritation was long-standing. As early as August 1922, he had minuted his superiors: 'Shades of Bruce and Burns – that we should always be abjectly waiting for a lead from England!' (NAS, HH 65/115/6). Thereafter, his views increasingly diverged from those of Sir Leslie Mackenzie, Medical Member of the Board, who advocated a cautious policy of 'education and social propaganda' with only a marginal adjustment to the isolation clauses of existing public health legislation to restrain habitual defaulters. Mackenzie had long held that, while compulsory controls were in principle entirely consistent with the protection of public health, 'measures of direct repression' were unlikely to succeed with a civilian population (*RCPLRD, PP 1910 (Cd. 4978) XLVI*, 185; Sir L. Mackenzie, 'The Administrative Control of Venereal Disease in Scotland', *Proceedings of the Imperial Social Hygiene Congress* (London: NCCVD, 1924), 23–8; 'In Memory of Dr Thomas F. Dewar', *Health and Empire*, 4, no. 4 (1929), 298–30; T. F. Dewar, 'Problems in the Administrative Control of Venereal Disease from the Departmental Point of View', *Health and Empire*, Vol. 1, no. 10 (1922–3), 81).

46   *SBH, Eighth Annual Report, PP 1927 (Cmd. 2881) X*, 107–8; *Ninth Annual Report, PP 1928 (Cmd. 3112) X*, 118.

47   NAS, HH 65/116/33, 38.

48   NAS, HH 33/595/8, Venereal Disease Legislation: Memorandum for the President's Information.

49   NAS, HH 33/595/10, Further notes on Edinburgh Corporation Bill. For a comparative perspective, see especially, L. Bryder, *Below the Magic Mountain: A Social History of Tuberculosis in 20th Century Britain* (Oxford: Clarendon Press, 1988), 103–9.

50 NAS, HH 33/595/10, Further notes on Edinburgh Corporation
   Bill.
51 The following synopsis is based upon A. Newsholme, *The Last
   Thirty Years in Public Health: Recollections and Reflections on my
   Official and Post-Official Life* (London: Allen and Unwin, 1936),
   164; J. M. Eyler, *Sir Arthur Newsholme and State Medicine
   1885–1935* (Cambridge: Cambridge University Press, 1997),
   277–94; G. Newman, 'The Administrative Control of the Venereal
   Diseases in England', *Proceedings of the Imperial Social Hygiene
   Congress* (London: NCCVD, 1924), 18–23; *idem, The Building of a
   Nation's Health* (London: Macmillan, 1939), 134; A. King, 'The Life
   and Times of Colonel Harrison', *BJVD*, 50 (1974), 391–403; NAS,
   HH 33/595/5, Observations by Ministry of Health on Bradford and
   Liverpool Corporation Acts; PRO, MH 55/183, Venereal Disease
   (Children) (Scotland) Bill, Bill papers.
52 Despite dramatic advances in the science of venereology, the precise
   impact of Salvarsan on syphilitic infectivity remained a contentious
   issue as did the reliability of the Wassermann Test as a diagnostic
   tool. See, e.g., *Medical Research Council, Special Report no. 78: The
   Serum Diagnosis of Syphilis: The Wassermann and Sigma Reactions
   Compared* (London: HMSO, 1923), 3.
53 PRO, MH 55/191, Minute by F. J. Coutts, 30 April 1925.
54 *Report of the Committee of Inquiry on Venereal Disease* (London:
   HMSO, 1923), para. 22.
55 *Hansard [HC]*, 216, col. 456, 19 April 1928.
56 *SBH, Seventh Annual Report, PP 1926 (Cmd. 2674) XI*, 81; PRO,
   MH 55/191, Memorandum by Sir G. Newman on the
   recommendations of the Trevethin Committee, 6 June 1923.
57 *Proceedings of the Imperial Social Hygiene Congress* (London: British
   Social Hygiene Council [BSHC], 1927), 238. See also above, ch. 4.
58 L. W. Harrison, 'Local Authorities and Notification: Discussion',
   Proceedings of the Imperial Social Hygiene Congress (London:
   NCCVD, 1924), 126; *Report of the Committee of Inquiry on Venereal
   Disease, op. cit.* (note 54), para. 19.
59 The respective percentages of cases discharged after completion of
   treatment were 43/30 for 1924 and 43/39 for 1929.
60 *Annual Report of the Ministry of Health, PP 1924 (Cmd. 2218) IX*, 8;
   PP 1927 (Cmd. 2938) IX, 45.
61 *The Shield*, 5 (Nov. 1927), 147; *Hansard [HC]*, 216, Col. 450, 19
   April 1928.
62 *Glasgow MOH Annual Report (1920)*, 9–10; *(1923)*, 21; NAS, HH
   333/595/16, Memorandum by A. K. Chalmers on Edinburgh

A Scourge to be Firmly Gripped

Corporation Bill. See also MSSVDSB Minutes, 19 Dec. 1928.
63 NAS, HH 65/116/27, Memorandum by H. L. Fraser, 6 Aug. 1924.
64 See, e.g., MSSVDSB Minutes, 20 Jan. 1937.
65 E. W. Hope, 'The Prevention of Venereal Disease', *Journal of State Medicine*, XXIX (1921), 336; NAS, HH 33/595/10, Edinburgh Corporation Bill papers.
66 Northern Health Services Archives [NHSA], 1/15/6, BMA, Memorandum as to the Organization of Measures for Prevention and Treatment of Venereal Disease, Feb. 1917; *BMJ Supplement*, 4 Aug. 1923, 152. 'Conditional' notification was rejected by 46 divisions to 14, general notification by 60 to 4.
67 See especially the rejection of David Lees' motion at the 1928 Annual Conference, *BMJ*, 4 Aug. 1928, 64–6.
68 See especially *BMJ*, 8 Aug. 1914, 280–7; L. W. Harrison, 'The Value of a Scientific Outlook to the Worker in Venereal Disease', *BJVD*, 1 (1925), 81–5; *Lancet*, 18 Jan. 1930, 159. For variance on these issues amongst Scottish venereologists, see MSSVDSB, Minutes, 19 Dec. 1928, 25 March 1931, 18 March 1932, 29 March 1933.
69 BMA Archive, B/322/1/1, Minutes of Special Committee on the Notification of VD, 1922–3; *BMJ*, 10 Feb. 1923, 250; *Lancet*, 3 March 1928, 454; F. G. Crookshank and A. W. Ewart Wort, 'Medico-Legal Problems in Relation to Venereal Disease', *BJVD*, 2 (1926), 36–58; W. D. Thompson, 'The Medico-Legal Aspects of Venereal Disease', *ibid.*, 12 (1936), 88–108.
70 See above, ch. 4.
71 D. Porter and R. Porter, 'The Enforcement of Health: The British Debate', in E. Fee and D. Fox (eds), *Aids: The Burdens of History* (Berkeley/London: University of California Press, 1988), 108.
72 *Ibid.*, 114. For similar intra-professional conflict in the USA, see A. M. Brandt, *No Magic Bullet: A Social History of Venereal Disease in the United States since 1880* (Oxford: Oxford University Press, 1985), 40–6.
73 Bland, *op. cit.* (note 8), 203–4.
74 Fawcett Library, A1/5–6, Minutes of National Union of Societies for Equal Citizenship [NUSEC], Executive Committee; NAS, HH 33/595/9, Edinburgh Corporation Bill papers, NUSEC to SBH, 17 April 1928.
75 See especially, Bland, *op. cit.* (note 8), 203; Fawcett Library, AMS/43, Minutes of the AMSH Executive Committee, 1924–9; 'Treatment of Venereal Disease: The Movement Towards Compulsion', *The Shield*, Vol. 5 (Nov. 1927), 117–24.
76 CMAC, SA/MWF/A11, Minutes of Medical Women's Federation

[MWF], Standing Committee on Venereal Diseases; PRO, MH 55/203, MWF, 'Some Suggestions as to the Duty of the State in the Control of Venereal Disease'; NAS, HH 33/595/9, MWF to SBH, 21 March 1928.

77 MSSVDSB, Minutes, 20 Jan. 1937.

78 PRO, MH 55/183, Venereal Disease (Children) (Scotland) Bill 1923–4, Bill papers.

79 The following account is primarily based upon: NAS, HH 33/595, Edinburgh Corporation Bill papers; HH 81/22–3, Private Legislation Procedure, Counsel Notebooks; GD/333, Records of the EWCA; ECA, Minutes of the Public Health Committee, Lord Provost's Committee, and Edinburgh Town Council; *EPHD Annual Reports*; Fawcett Library, AMS/43, Minutes of the AMSH Executive Committee; A1/5, Minutes of the NUSEC Executive Committee; *Hansard [HC]* 216, cols 446–510, 19 April 1928; University of Reading Library, MS/1/1/229, Nancy Astor Papers, Correspondence relating to the Edinburgh Corporation Bill.

80 H. J. Hanham, *Scottish Nationalism* (London: Faber, 1969), 107, 117–18; C. Harvie, *No Gods and Precious Few Heroes: Scotland 1914–1980* (London: Edward Arnold, 1981), 129–35; I. Levitt, *The Scottish Office: Depression and Reconstruction 1919–59* (Edinburgh: Scottish History Society, 1992), 11–14.

81 *Scotsman*, 21 March 1928.

82 NAS, HH 33/595/12, Correspondence of Sir John Gilmour, March and April 1928.

83 *Hansard [HC]* 216, Cols 508–10; M. Stenton and S. Lees, *Who's Who of British Members of Parliament*, Vols 3 & 4 (Sussex: Harvester Press, 1979, 1981). 67% of Labour MPs attended the debate. Participation rates for Conservative and Liberal MPs were 31% and 34% respectively.

84 NAS, HH 33/595/16a, Bill papers.

85 NAS, HH 65/116/50, 52, 56, Representations from Local Authorities. See also representations from the Royal Sanitary Association of Scotland (CMAC, SA/BSH, A2/14, Extract from Minutes of BSHC Scottish Committee, 7 Dec. 1933).

86 *DHS, First Annual Report, PP 1929–30 (Cmd. 3529) XIV*, 103; NAS, HH 65/116/61, Minute, 22 Nov. 1934.

87 PRO, MH 55/1326, Convention of Scottish Royal Burghs to Ministry of Health, 9 May 1935.

88 *Report of the Committee on Scottish Health Services, PP 1935–6 (Cmd. 5204) XI*, 210–11.

89 *Lancet*, 2 Jan. 1937, 34; 26 June 1937, 1562.

90   PRO MH 55/1326, Minutes of Delegation from BSHC to MOH, 3
     June 1937. Significantly, English members on the BSHC Executive
     were convinced that any inquiry would reveal that 'other factors
     [were] far more important and that compulsory powers [were] left
     largely in abeyance'. However, they urged Colonel L. W. Harrison to
     defer to the wishes of 'compulsionists in the industrial areas of
     Southern Scotland' for an inquiry, in order to prevent 'a serious split'
     in the Social Hygiene Movement. For the subsequent report see,
     Ministry of Health, *Report on Anti-Venereal Measures in Certain
     Scandinavian Countries and Holland* (London: HMSO, 1938).
91   *Lancet*, 2 Jan. 1937, 33.
92   J. Harris, 'Society and the State in Twentieth-Century Britain', in
     F. M. L. Thompson (ed.), *The Cambridge Social History of Britain
     1750–1950, Vol. III: Social Agencies and Institutions* (Cambridge:
     Cambridge University Press, 1990), 69–70; F. B. Smith, *The People's
     Health 1830–1910* (London: Croom Helm, 1979), 418.
93   R. M. MacLeod, 'The Social Role of the Man of Knowledge:
     Expertise and the State', SSRC End-of-Grant Report (HR 4083,
     1978), 3–4, 42–6. Such popular fears were often exploited by the
     general medical profession in their struggle with public health
     doctors over the control of interwar expansion in the personal
     preventive health services. See, e.g., J. Lewis, 'Providers,
     "Consumers", the State and the Delivery of Health-Care Services in
     Twentieth-Century Britain', in A. Wear (ed.), *Medicine in Society:
     Historical Essays* (Cambridge: Cambridge University Press, 1992),
     331–3.
94   *Scotsman*, 3 March 1928; See also, *Scotsman*, 1 March 1928; *The
     Times*, 29 Feb. 1928.
95   *SBH, Ninth Annual Report, op. cit.* (note 46), 118.
96   R. M. MacLeod, 'Law, Medicine and Public Opinion: The
     Resistance to Compulsory Health Legislation, 1870–1907', *Public
     Law* (1967), 107–28, 185–211; *idem*, 'Medico-Legal Issues in
     Victorian Medical Care', *Medical History*, X (1966), 44–9.

9

Combating 'The Great Evil': VD Policy in the Second World War

The Retention of Voluntarism: 1939–1940

During the first year of the Second World War, Scottish health administrators continued to adhere to a strictly voluntary system of VD provisions. While recognizing the arguments in favour of compulsion, the Department of Health for Scotland [DHS] was mindful of the operational and ideological constraints that had frustrated the campaign for VD controls in interwar Scotland. Its medical advisers acknowledged a swing in parliamentary opinion in favour of compulsory notification and treatment but did not consider public opinion was 'yet ripe' for a radical shift in VD policy. Nor did they view the example of overseas controls for VD as a convincing argument for the abandonment of voluntarism in Britain.[1]

In 1939–40, the efforts of the DHS were therefore focused on a reappraisal of existing VD provisions to meet the emergency needs of war, without recourse to controls. Concerned at the likely impact of the 'excitement of war conditions' and the loosening of family ties on promiscuity and the incidence of VD, the Department urged local authorities to review their diagnostic and treatment facilities and, in the interests of public health and manpower, to adjust them to cater for 'new aggregations' of population around munition factories, military camps and aerodromes. Where appropriate, they were encouraged to train general practitioners as replacement venereologists, to consider the provision of mobile treatment units and to extend existing voluntary procedures for contact tracing. Local authorities were also encouraged to extend their programmes of health education, including lectures and film-shows, in collaboration with the Scottish Committee of the British Social Hygiene Council [BSHC].[2]

A number of factors served to reinforce the commitment of the DHS to a voluntarist approach. As in the interwar period, the attitude of the Ministry of Health and of its Special Adviser on VD, Colonel L. W. Harrison, was vital. Throughout the period of wartime planning, the Ministry retained its opposition to VD controls. In the Ministry's view, despite the introduction of new chemotherapy,

205

existing notification procedures were inappropriate for VD with its acute social stigma and its often protracted and poorly defined infectivity. It anticipated considerable public resistance to notification, with patients deterred from seeking medical treatment in the early, most infective stages of their disease. Proposals for compulsory treatment were similarly resisted. In Harrison's view, it would encourage the concealment of infection, and given the wide local variation in clinical procedures, might lead to highly discriminatory practices with the possible alienation of the poorer classes and women's groups from the existing VD services. He considered that the much-heralded success of compulsion in countries such as Sweden in containing the incidence of VD was not a function of compulsion but of 'greater health consciousness' and social deference to medical opinion.[3] Rather than developing new wartime controls, the Ministry therefore concentrated in 1939–40 upon trying to upgrade the existing local authority treatment services by means of a series of administrative guidelines and financial incentives.[4]

The DHS was also sensitive to the continuing lack of agreement within medical circles over the treatment and control of VD. Concern at the legal implications of VD controls remained, particularly in Scotland where health officials were especially vulnerable to charges of defamation under Scots Law. More generally, while many Scottish Medical Officers of Health favoured compulsion during the war emergency, some leading VD clinicians wanted first to exhaust the possibilities for upgrading existing treatment facilities and expanding the use of social workers for contact tracing and follow-up work.[5]

The likely reaction of the women's movement to fresh proposals for VD controls was an added deterrent. Anticipating an attempt to revive the notorious Defence Regulation 40D of 1918 which had sought to criminalize the transmission of VD to the armed forces, the Association of Moral and Social Hygiene [AMSH] and its Scottish affiliates launched a vigorous campaign in the late 1930s against the compulsory notification and treatment of VD. As in the interwar period, a range of medical, ethical and legal objections was advanced, but the strongest concern was that controls would be discriminatory and targeted against working-class women.[6] The Medical Women's Federation also sustained its previous opposition to coercive measures, continuing to advocate improved welfare provisions and social hygiene education along with 'ample arrangements for healthy recreation and amusement' for the forces.[7]

Pressure on the DHS to initiate new controls was also eased in

1939–40 by the fact that the Scottish local authorities which had spearheaded the interwar campaign were temporarily absorbed with the establishment of emergency health and evacuation measures and unresponsive to their erstwhile ally – the Scottish Committee of the BSHC. The latter had, as early as 1938, pressed for wartime defence regulations to include the compulsory treatment of known contacts who refused to seek or sustain treatment or who wilfully exposed others to the risk of infection. However, faced with the temporary reluctance of Scottish health authorities to reopen the campaign for controls, the Scottish Committee was content in 1940 to lobby for improved VD facilities, especially for the establishment of general 'gynaecological' clinics which young women might attend with a minimum of stigma and without 'jeopardising their social and economic position'.[8]

The Genesis of Defence Regulation 33B: 1940–1943

By the summer of 1941, however, the situation had changed dramatically and the issue of VD controls moved once more to the centre of public health debate in Scotland. During the closing months of 1940, there was growing evidence of an increased incidence of VD, especially in early infectious syphilis, in many urban centres. Figures for the first quarter of 1941 indicated a further disturbing rise: in Glasgow, for example, recorded cases of acute syphilis exceeded those for the first quarter of 1940 by 75 per cent.[9]

Clinicians and public health officials attributed the increased incidence of VD to a range of factors, including the breakdown in sexual discipline during the blackout, 'the heightened tension of the population', 'the mobilisation of labour which threw persons of varied outlook, habits and morals into close relationship', and especially the influx of troops, naval personnel and merchant seamen – with particular stress being placed on the role of foreign seamen in inflating VD rates.[10] Some blame was attached to those defaulting from treatment but, as in the First World War, health authorities increasingly identified the critical vector as the 'amateur prostitute' who 'consorted' with servicemen.[11] Once again, the concept of VD became 'militarized'. The casual promiscuity of the 'easy girlfriend', supposedly seeking and dispensing gratuitous and unsafe sex, was singled out for attack, and an official epidemiology was advanced in which such 'good-time girls' were presented as sapping the health and military efficiency of the nation.

In response to the rising incidence of VD, clinicians and Medical Officers of Health called for additional controls. A survey in May

1941 revealed that fourteen out of twenty Scottish health authorities, including Aberdeen, Edinburgh, Glasgow and Lanarkshire, were in favour of additional powers. Some authorities, especially those which lacked adequate follow-up procedures, supported measures to compel defaulters to complete treatment. Others, such as the Edinburgh Public Health Department, which boasted a highly successful almoner system, resisted the intrusion of sanctions into follow-up work as counterproductive. Instead, they argued that, as an emergency measure to cope with *new* sources of infection, there should be 'compulsory powers to investigate all consorts named by two or more patients known to be suffering from venereal disease'.[12] This proposal was strongly supported by the Convention of Scottish Royal Burghs and other local authority associations and was duly urged upon the DHS by the Scottish Committee of the BSHC in the spring of 1941.[13]

Initially, the DHS was unresponsive. It advised local health authorities that, given the political and medico-legal implications of VD controls, compulsory powers were unlikely to be adopted and they must continue to look solely to voluntary procedures.[14] However, by the summer of 1941, under increasing pressure from Scottish local government, from social hygiene organizations and military authorities, the DHS began, in consultation with Medical Officers of Health and venereologists, to formulate proposals designed to 'bring under control the more dangerous disseminators of VD'.[15] Thereafter, in collaboration with the Ministry of Health and the Service departments, the DHS drafted a defence regulation providing for sexual 'contacts' named by two or more infected patients to be notified to Medical Officers of Health, with penalties of a fine and/or imprisonment for such contacts who failed to undergo examination and, where appropriate, a full course of treatment under a suitably qualified practitioner.[16]

Although clauses analogous to Defence Regulation 40D of 1918 were soon dropped as being 'too controversial', the draft regulation was still highly gender-specific. Briefing notes repeatedly stressed the need to target a 'dangerous minority of infected women', identified as casual prostitutes or 'good-time' girls, who were held responsible for the major outbreaks of VD within the forces. In an attempt to forestall the furore that had surrounded the 1918 Regulation 40D, the declared aim of the new regulation was broadened to protect 'all those engaged in essential war work'. Emphasis was also placed less on the punishment of vectors of the disease and more on inducing early and complete treatment. Nevertheless, the social epidemiology shaping the successive drafts of Regulation 33B remained clearly directed towards sexually active *females* and it was assumed that most informants would be male servicemen who had dipped into this 'reservoir' of venereal infection.[17] Indeed, evidence suggests that in certain localities in Scotland, police surveillance of suspected female contacts and, on occasions, physical restraint for examination and treatment using arcane byelaws and the collaboration of medical and military authorities, were already operating.[18]

In the event, Regulation 33B was only introduced in November 1942 after further protracted discussions. In part, the delay resulted from remaining doubts within the DHS as to the wisdom of controls. Issues of confidentiality and enforcement remained problematic, and the Scottish Law Officers questioned both the legal and medical integrity of the draft regulations.[19] In particular, the Lord Advocate doubted the legal immunity from prosecution for malicious accusation of informants with multiple sexual contacts of whom 'only one – perhaps none! – was suffering from VD', and issued the first of many warnings that under Scots Law, as distinct from English Common Law, an alleged contact notified under the Regulation would be entitled to sue informants and Medical Officers for damages 'done to his/her feelings'.[20] Dr I. N. Sutherland, Medical Officer in charge of the DHS Infectious Diseases Section, believed that the regulation would only 'touch the fringe of the problem' and that an improved system of nurse almoners for follow-up work and contact tracing would be more effective, especially as evidence from the Scottish VD services suggested that few contacts would be named more than once.[21] More fundamentally, some senior advisers, such as Sir Alexander Russell, Deputy Chief Medical Officer, feared that the measure 'would introduce too much of the "Gestapo" element into public health work', a view that reflected a common association in official circles of controls with German totalitarianism.[22]

The DHS was also inhibited in 1942 by strenuous opposition to the proposed regulation from a range of women's pressure groups led by the AMSH. To be sure, not all women's organizations were so inclined. In Scotland, local branches of the Women Citizens' Association were prepared, as they had been in the interwar period, to support compulsory notification and treatment.[23] Nonetheless, it was the AMSH's critique of draft government proposals that increasingly defined the agenda for debate within the medical and popular press. With its roots in the British Abolitionist Federation, the AMSH not surprisingly stressed the similarities between the draft regulation and the worst features of the Contagious Diseases Acts and the 1918 Regulation 40D. It argued that, in practice, selective controls would become 'a form of regulated prostitution or promiscuity' with all the associated evils of blackmail, false denunciation and arrest, and concealment of disease. The targeting of alleged 'known women' of the 'prostitute class' and the so-called 'amateur' would, it claimed, serve to reinforce both the 'double moral standard' of sexual conduct and the dangerous fallacy that it was female sexuality rather than 'male demand for sexual indulgence' that had occasioned the rising incidence of VD.[24]

Reservations within the Ministry of Health were also instrumental in delaying the introduction of Regulation 33B. Colonel L. W. Harrison remained unconvinced of the benefits to be gained from compulsion as compared with improved voluntary provisions. He was especially concerned at the lack of legal redress for female contacts against whom false allegations were levelled, and he shared the doubts of the Permanent Secretary, Sir John Maude, as to whether the 'proposed machinery was worth the experiment of putting into being' and would 'ever develop into an operative reality'.[25] The lack of agreement amongst the armed forces as to the most appropriate form of VD control was an additional constraint. The Admiralty and Air Ministry pressed for a regulation on the lines of the 1918 Regulation 40D. Medical advisers within the War Office, however, were more supportive of the draft regulations, although they had serious doubts about the equity of the proposed procedures for identifying and reporting contacts. The War Office finally agreed to back the health departments in their proposals, but only under extreme pressure from the Canadian Corps Commander, who was appalled at the lack of VD controls on 'known sources of infection' in the United Kingdom.[26]

However, as 1942 progressed, the DHS and Ministry of Health came under increasing pressure from public and professional opinion to implement a new regulation. In Scotland, faced with continuing high levels of new VD cases, Medical Officers of Health, such as Dr W. G. Clark of Edinburgh and Dr W. L. Burgess of Dundee, urged the DHS to introduce the necessary statutory orders.[27] Concern was expressed that VD controls had not been introduced along with the Scabies Order (Scotland) in December 1941 which had given public health authorities far-reaching powers to examine and treat the residents of verminous premises. At a series of conferences organized by the Scottish Committee of the BSHC during the spring and summer of 1942, local health authority representatives pressed for the compulsory notification and treatment of 'hardened offenders' who were responsible for Service infections. When this did not produce action from the DHS, the West of Scotland public health committees launched a major press and political campaign, culminating in a conference in Dunoon on VD controls in early October. As in official discussions, the campaign focused on specific groups of 'sexual offender' – pre-eminently the 'harpies who prey[ed] on Service men' and the 'black-out girls whose moral delinquency was threatening the war effort and the national moral fibre'.[28]

Meanwhile, the Ministry of Health was also facing an increasing demand for VD controls from English local health authorities and war emergency committees, and from the medical directorate of the American armed forces.[29] In addition, the Ministry was sensitive to the swing in medical opinion during 1942 in favour of controls. There was a growing consensus amongst venereologists that the existing voluntary system of provisions was inadequate to deal with the VD epidemic and that, in the words of the resolution of the Medical Society for the Study of Venereal Diseases, there was an urgent need 'for further powers, legislative and administrative ... to deal with sources of infection, contacts and defaulters'.[30] Similarly, the BMA and the medical press were increasingly receptive to selective controls.[31] More generally, a poll undertaken in September 1942 by the British Institute of Public Opinion indicated that the majority of the public were sympathetic towards a more interventionist policy for the sexual health of the nation.[32]

Despite continuing reservations over issues of enforcement, the Ministry of Health was persuaded that the rising incidence of VD *was* having a real impact upon war production and service efficiency and that there *was* a compelling need to reduce the exposure of allied troops.[33] In October, it attempted to prepare the ground for controls by a major publicity campaign initiated by a pioneering broadcast on the BBC by the Chief Medical Officer, designed to dispel the traditional taboo on the public discussion of VD and to raise public awareness of its threat to the war effort.[34] Shortly thereafter, on 5 November 1942, Defence Regulation 33B was introduced by statutory rules and orders.

The regulation provided that 'special practitioners' (officially recognized as specialists in venereal diseases) should notify Medical Officers of Health of all 'contacts' voluntarily named by infected patients attending VD clinics as being the source of their infection. In addition, where a contact had been notified as the source of more than one infection, the Medical Officer of Health was empowered to require him/her to submit to medical examination and to remain under medical treatment by a special practitioner until pronounced free from VD 'in a communicable form' by means of a clearance certificate. Failure to comply with a 'treatment notice' constituted a contravention of the Defence of the Realm Act [DORA] and was punishable by a fine and/or imprisonment. To protect informants and Medical Officers from legal proceedings for defamation, information communicated under the regulation was deemed to have been furnished 'in pursuance of a statutory duty', although proffering malicious and 'deliberately false information' would constitute an offence.[35]

A powerful but varied social response was provoked by the regulation. It was vigorously attacked by women's organizations in a wide-ranging press and political campaign culminating in deputations to the DHS and the Ministry of Health on 18 November 1942.[36] The women's groups stressed the deterrent effect of controls on those voluntarily seeking early treatment, the illogicality of regulating 'contacts' but not informants who might well be defaulters, and the likelihood that, as with the licensing of prostitutes in regulationist countries, 'clearance certificates' would encourage a 'false sense of security' and actually promote increased promiscuity. They also objected to the creation of a new class of secret common informer, 'the Medical Officer of Health's nark' – alien to the principles of British law and 'Nazi–Germanic to the very core' – who would be legally protected against proceedings for libel whilst the alleged contact would have no redress either for mistaken accusations or for the indignity of a compulsory medical examination. Above all, it was argued that the regulation would be discriminatory as it omitted contacts of patients seeking private treatment and would inevitably penalize female contacts but not their male 'customers'.[37]

Women's organizations called instead for a range of 'constructive measures' designed to improve the quality and accessibility of treatment, especially for women, and to engender sexual restraint. Significantly, the only control measures advocated were targeted at working-class, adolescent 'problem girls' who, it was widely alleged, were beyond parental and local authority control, and were sexually harassing servicemen. Thus, the Scottish branches of the National Vigilance Association and the National Council for Equal Citizenship advocated a more rigorous use of detention centres and the appointment of more women police patrols as a means of monitoring and disciplining 'vicious girls'.[38]

Most Church leaders in Britain also opposed Regulation 33B.

Particular concern was expressed at the danger that State controls would obscure the sinfulness of promiscuous intercourse and the fundamental need for personal continence and self-control.[39] Significantly, in 1942, the Church of Scotland remained non-committal on the issue, but the United Free Church and the Baptist Union of Scotland both opposed compulsory VD controls. They viewed the growing incidence of VD as essentially a moral problem that demanded an educational campaign to instil 'self-reverence' and a 'high view of the sacredness of sex' among the young.[40]

Meanwhile, the introduction of Regulation 33B reopened long-standing divisions within the BSHC. The English Council was prepared to support compulsory measures only after existing voluntary provisions had been radically improved, including increased resources devoted to the treatment and after-care of young, unmarried women.[41] In contrast, the Scottish Committee was committed to comprehensive wartime controls. Indeed, a prime consideration of the Committee in pressing for a separate Scottish Council for Health Education in 1942 was to ensure that the long-established commitment of the Scottish hygiene movement to compulsion continued to be recognized in government circles.[42] While it lobbied MPs in favour of Regulation 33B, the Committee regarded it as 'a belated and partial response' to the long-standing demands of Scottish health and police authorities, and regretted that more general powers of compulsory notification and treatment had not been introduced.[43]

This ambivalence towards Regulation 33B was representative of Scottish public opinion during the winter of 1942–3. Editorials welcomed official recognition that the threat to public health outweighed libertarian considerations, but viewed the regulation as only a temporary palliative for the problem of VD.[44] The *Glasgow Herald* regarded 'its immediate purpose as [being] a preliminary to some more drastic and effective system of control and prevention'. Similarly, a Mass Observation survey revealed that while approving of the regulation's objectives, 'a considerable body of opinion ... saw it only as the beginning of a campaign, and hoped that the government would take further and wider measures to tackle the problem', including compulsory notification and treatment, the penalization of 'infective intercourse' and conception, and the sterilization of incurables and habitual defaulters.[45]

Predictably, when Parliament debated Regulation 33B in December 1942, opposition came from both compulsionists such as Edith Summerskill and Robert Boothby *and* from long-standing anti-regulationists such as Viscountess Astor. In response, the DHS and Ministry of Health stressed the need for the regulation to be viewed as complementary to its existing policy of upgrading health education, treatment facilities and a range of welfare and surveillance machinery designed to discourage promiscuity.[46] The health departments sought to reassure libertarian and women's groups that a voluntary strategy towards VD was not being abandoned but merely being supplemented by selective emergency controls designed to neutralize the 'anti-social' sexual conduct of all key vectors of VD (male *and* female) within the community who constituted a threat to the war effort. They denied that a new class of 'informer' was being created, pointing out that contact tracing was already an established procedure in many of Britain's clinics. They stressed that action by medical authorities under Regulation 33B would only be taken where information was consistent with the medical evidence, and that where an alleged contact was found to be free of infection, an official review would be instituted to assess whether informants should be prosecuted for furnishing false evidence. Health officials vigorously denied that the regulation sought to proscribe female sexuality and emphasized that the thrust of the measure was to induce recourse to treatment rather than to punish sexual offences.[47] At the same time, government spokesmen were equally concerned to placate pressure groups within the forces and local health authorities which demanded comprehensive powers of compulsory notification and treatment, and they conceded that, if the regulation proved inadequate, additional powers might have to be considered.[48]

The Campaign for Additional Controls: 1943–1944

Despite such assurances, during 1943–4, VD policy came under increasing attack from Scottish local government, which was determined to obtain more stringent controls with which to contain the continuing high incidence of acute VD in all the major ports and cities, as well as the ominous revival of congenital syphilis in centres such as Glasgow.[49] Throughout 1943, the DHS was bombarded with resolutions in favour of various forms of compulsory notification and treatment. The campaign was supported not only by the major public health and joint VD committees but also by virtually all the leading Medical Officers of Health and venereologists, by the Scottish local authority associations and Convention of Royal Burghs, and by the newly formed Scottish Council for Health Education.[50]

Separate initiatives by Edinburgh and Glasgow Corporations continued to put pressure on the DHS during the winter of 1943–4.

Edinburgh Public Health Department considered the Government's attempts to steer a middle course between voluntarism and compulsion as 'misconceived' in that it 'left unreported the hard core of unreported and untreated infection'.[51] In December 1943, after repeated representations to the DHS for additional powers, the Public Health Committee called a major conference of Scottish local authorities on VD controls which unanimously endorsed a resolution that, in view of the failure of Regulation 33B to control the 'relatively small but pernicious class of patients' who were immune to propaganda and persuasion, the Government 'should introduce immediately legislation to provide for the compulsory notification and treatment of VD'.[52] In addition, in an attempt to maintain pressure on the DHS, a conference committee was established in February 1944 to formulate specific proposals. These were subsequently to include the compulsory notification and prosecution of defaulters and their detention in hospital until non-infective, and a general legal requirement that any person with reason to believe that they were venereally infected should submit to medical examination.[53]

Meanwhile, since the summer of 1943, the City of Glasgow had also been making representations to the Government on the issue. In October 1943, a special sub-committee had been appointed to review the incidence of VD and its implications for new control strategies. Evidence suggested that, despite new forms of chemotherapy, there had been a rise in Glasgow of over 200 per cent in recorded cases of female acute gonorrhoea and of 173 per cent in cases of early syphilis since the outbreak of war, and a trebling since 1941 in the incidence of congenital syphilis. However, as was revealed in their subsequent meeting with the Secretary of State for Scotland in March 1944, councillors and their medical advisers were divided over the policy implications to be drawn. Lay members of the Committee were markedly more extreme in their demands. Bailie Stewart 'wished to go the whole way and have those who would not seek and continue treatment detained in prison and compulsorily treated there, even with the risk of the patient dying'. Likewise, Bailie Hunter favoured detention in hospital by order of the Sheriff for six months or a year, if necessary. In contrast, the Medical Officer of Health, A. S. M. Macgregor, and his infectious disease officer, W. A. Horne, stressed the benefits of Regulation 33B in raising public consciousness of VD and of the importance of contact tracing. They considered the physical imposition of treatment to be both medically and socially unacceptable, but did support legal penalties for those who evaded or defaulted from treatment (including parents of children with congenital disease) and a system of notification for VD for purposes of epidemiology and contact tracing. Subsequently, the Glasgow sub-committee increasingly identified with the proposals of the Edinburgh conference committee and with the campaign of Scottish local authorities in the summer of 1944 to obtain unilateral action on VD controls from the Scottish Office.[54]

Throughout 1943, in line with the Ministry of Health, the DHS resisted pressure for additional legislation. Within the departments, key advisers such as Sutherland and Harrison continued to stress the medical and ethical objections to compulsory detention and treatment.[55] In their view, compulsory notification would deter patients from seeking prompt and professionally qualified treatment and, given the moral stigma attached to VD, might fail to secure the co-operation of medical practitioners.[56] They were also sensitive to the continuing campaign of the women's movement against Regulation 33B, fuelled by growing evidence that it was being enforced overwhelmingly upon female contacts. The efforts of AMSH to mobilize public opinion south of the border were paralleled in Scotland by the Scottish Women Citizens' Association and the National Vigilance Association for Scotland, with the backing of the United Free Church and the Baptist Union.[57] The DHS therefore restricted itself in 1943 to urging local health authorities to make greater use of Exchequer grants to improve treatment provisions, and to launching a fresh publicity campaign, with posters, advertisements and films, to heighten public awareness of VD and the importance of early and continuous treatment.[58] The campaign included a series of newspaper homilies based upon supposed extracts 'From a Doctor's Diary',[59] and the issue of one of the most potent and discriminatory images of twentieth-century government health propaganda – the 'Hello boy friend, coming MY way?' poster – in which VD was depicted in the form of a lurid female skull *(see Plate 9.1).*[60]

As it soon became evident that formal proceedings under Regulation 33B based upon two or more notices were to be rare, clinicians and policy-makers increasingly focused on the value of the information gained on *all* contacts under the regulation for enhancing existing voluntary procedures of contact tracing.[61] Indeed, by July 1943, the Ministry of Health was encouraging health authorities to take informal action to secure the voluntary examination and appropriate treatment of contacts named only once, and in December, a circular recommended this procedure as

216

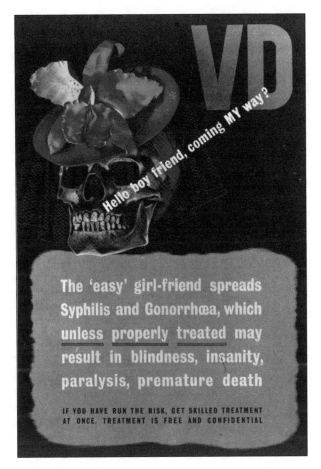

VD

Hello boy friend, coming MY way?

The 'easy' girl-friend spreads Syphilis and Gonorrhœa, which unless properly treated may result in blindness, insanity, paralysis, premature death

IF YOU HAVE RUN THE RISK, GET SKILLED TREATMENT AT ONCE. TREATMENT IS FREE AND CONFIDENTIAL

Plate 9.1
Wartime VD propaganda poster
(courtesy of Imperial War Museum)

providing 'the best immediate prospect of controlling the incidence and spread of venereal disease'.[62] In Scotland, however, although the procedure was vigorously acted upon by VD departments, the DHS legal counsel were not persuaded that such action would be immune from prosecution for libel and defamation of character under Scots Law, and the DHS was therefore unwilling to issue similar guidelines to Scottish health authorities.[63]

However, by January 1944, the pressure from Scottish local authorities was such that the DHS felt compelled to reopen the issue of additional VD controls. The Department's discussions were informed by three sets of proposals: one from the Joint Committee on VD, one from the Scottish Medical Advisory Committee and one from the Ministry of Health. The Joint Committee on VD, an inter-departmental committee appointed in 1943 and including representatives from the Canadian and American forces, had declined to recommend any form of general compulsory notification and treatment for VD on the grounds that it would lead to the concealment of disease and might prejudice the success of existing voluntary procedures. It did, however, recommend that parents of infected children should be compelled not only to secure treatment for their offspring but also to undergo medical examination and treatment themselves in order to prevent any further transmission of disease. It also proposed that prostitutes and 'good-time girls' passing through the hands of the police on solicitation and other moral charges should be required to undergo examination and treatment for VD.[64]

Meanwhile, after canvassing the views of clinicians and health administrators, the Scottish Medical Advisory Committee reported on policy options for containing the incidence of VD. It emphasized the need for a clearly defined national strategy of medico-moral education backed by the Churches and the medical establishment, and for a more integrated and better-resourced VD service with adequate training for clinicians and contact tracers. Although the Committee acknowledged that compulsory notification might inhibit early treatment and contact tracing by introducing 'an atmosphere of accusation or censure', it recommended, in the medium term, legislation to secure the notification and treatment of all cases of VD, with anonymity preserved for patients who co-operated with medical advice but disclosure and penal sanctions for defaulters. In addition, the Committee recommended that parents of children with congenital syphilis or gonococcal ophthalmia neonatorum should be required to submit to examination and treatment.[65]

Senior medical advisers within the Ministry of Health also began to reconsider the possibility of more stringent measures under a new defence regulation to contain the rising incidence of VD in England and Wales. Armed with growing evidence of public support for additional controls, the Chief Medical Officer, Sir Wilson Jameson, advocated a frontal attack upon the 'grave anti-social conduct' of infected persons who evaded or discontinued treatment. Along with the Scottish Medical Advisory Committee, he accepted that contact tracing should 'remain primarily a matter of social work and persuasion' but he believed that Regulation 33B should be retained to control the 'promiscuous contact'. While he agreed that education rather than compulsion should remain the major strategy for securing early treatment, Jameson was prepared to consider making it an offence for an infected person knowingly not to seek qualified medical advice.[66]

However, as 1944 progressed, the DHS began to receive conflicting signals from the Ministry of Health. By March, Sir John Maude, the Permanent Secretary, under the influence of Harrison's dedicated defence of voluntarism, was fast retreating from his initial support for Jameson's position. While he supported compulsory notification for congenital syphilis, he feared that any broader measure would 'drive VD underground' and breach public confidence in the confidentiality of existing VD provisions. More generally, at a time when consensus was imperative for the negotiations surrounding the establishment of a new health service in Britain, Maude was reluctant to introduce health controls that might lead to social and professional friction. When it was suggested that the DHS might consider a unilateral defence regulation introducing additional VD controls for Scotland, the Ministry delayed a decision by referring the issue to a sub-committee of the English Medical Advisory Committee.[67]

Despite residual doubts about the medical effects of compulsion, the DHS was keen to implement the recommendations of its Medical Advisory Committee. Informal canvassing of Scottish public opinion in the spring of 1944 revealed strong support for VD legislation, including support from the Church of Scotland. In the view of its Church and Nation Committee, while the 'clear, reverent teaching of the true function of sex in human life, and the intimate and sacred relationship between body and spirit' was vital, there was also an urgent need to 'secure compulsory notification and complete treatment of VD in the interests of the individual, the future family, and the community'.[68] Senior DHS officials rejected the notion of a regional defence regulation as implying that VD was a peculiarly Scottish problem. They considered that the issue of VD controls was of 'wide and controversial interest' and required full legislative debate with clear and decisive backing from the War Cabinet.[69] At his meeting with the Glasgow Public Health Sub-Committee on VD in March, the Secretary of State, Tom Johnston, stated that while powers to administer compulsory treatment were neither desirable nor realistic, and while compulsory detention of those who failed to seek or to sustain treatment remained problematic, he was prepared to support compulsory notification with sanctions to regulate defaulters and parents of infected children. Thereafter, he determined that 'if he [got] strong support in Scotland for more control, [he would] put a paper to the Lord President's Committee and have the policy thrashed out by the Government'.[70]

Consultation and Conflict: 1944–45

Accordingly, during the summer of 1944, the DHS consulted a range of institutions on the Scottish Medical Advisory Committee's report with a view to achieving consensus over the introduction of VD controls. While some health authorities pressed for more emphasis on the enhancement of moral and religious values and others wanted more stringent sanctions on the sexual behaviour of proven contacts, the majority supported its recommendations.[71] The Scottish Churches were somewhat more divided. The Church of Scotland strongly endorsed proposals for compulsory notification but, after intensive lobbying from women's organizations, many ministers within the Episcopal Church and the United Free Church opposed it on the grounds that it would lead to the concealment of disease, to avoidance of early diagnosis and treatment and to greater recourse to quack remedies. The Roman Catholic Church in Scotland regarded the Medical Advisory Committee report as a 'limited and narrow' medical view of what was essentially a moral problem. While the Catholic Church had no serious objection to VD controls on doctrinal grounds, Archbishop McDonald maintained that the first priority was for the state 'purification' of entertainment and the media.[72]

The Scottish branch of the BMA believed that 'persuasion' rather than compulsion should remain 'the mainstay in any system designed to secure continuous treatment'. They expressed concern that universal notification might deter patients from reporting venereal symptoms and that the operation of controls might be monopolized by specialists and marginalize general practitioners. They rejected any proposal to criminalize failure to seek treatment that went beyond the existing powers of Regulation 33B. Nonetheless the BMA in Scotland *were* strongly in favour of the compulsory notification and prosecution of defaulters.[73]

The DHS shaped its legislative proposals in August 1944 so as to obtain maximum support from community leaders and the medical profession. A statutory requirement to seek treatment was rejected as unenforceable. Given that forcible treatment was neither legally nor medically acceptable and might undermine public confidence in the hospital system, powers of detention were not pursued. According to DHS officials, what was needed were sanctions on the 'sexual

220

'misconduct' of defaulters rather than their infectivity *per se*, and Tom Johnston preferred to rely upon the deterrent of prosecution and the 'moral suasion' of 'good neighbourhood courts' which he hoped would eventually develop in Scotland on similar lines to those operating in the USSR. In deference to BMA opinion, notification was limited to defaulters, with practitioners required only to make aggregative returns for epidemiological purposes. In addition, in order not to alienate the medical profession, the DHS resisted pressure from local health authorities to exclude general practitioners from providing VD treatment carried out under new controls.[74]

However, when in the autumn of 1944 the DHS sought the support of the Ministry of Health in Cabinet for the compulsory notification and prosecution of defaulters along with a requirement on all practitioners to provide returns on the incidence of VD – recommended as 'the minimum provisions that [would] satisfy informed Scottish opinion' – it met with a negative response.[75] The corner-stone of the Ministry's resistance to Scottish proposals was the report of the English Medical Advisory Committee's Sub-Committee on VD. While the Sub-Committee advised that the general notification of VD, with sanctions for non-compliance with treatment, was 'a desirable long-term policy', it argued that public opinion was not yet ready for such a comprehensive measure. They should therefore wait for both 'the more widespread enlightenment of the profession itself' and the provision of a more universal 'consultant and specialist service'. The Committee also opposed selective notification for defaulters on the grounds that, with modern chemotherapy, few defaulters were still infectious, that they no longer constituted 'a large source of venereal infection', and that such notification would be ineffectual in the absence of a fully developed system of social workers for follow-up work. More stringent controls for congenital VD were deemed 'a reasonable and desirable proposal' but the Committee was not satisfied that 'the elaborate legal and administrative arrangements necessary would be justified by the results obtainable'. Instead, it highlighted the need for improved social work facilities and especially the development of more pro-active contact-tracing procedures in line with the American public health services.[76]

The Ministry of Health's reluctance to support the DHS over the issue of VD controls in 1944–5 has also to be placed within the wider context of the health politics of the period. As G. H. Henderson, Secretary of the DHS, observed:

The Ministry of Health are not unsympathetic to the idea of notification and compulsion as a long-term policy. They feel pretty strongly, however, that it would be a mistake to embark on legislation on venereal diseases (which would be bound to be controversial) at a time when our energies are bent to securing agreement on the much bigger issue of the National Health Service. I think they feel that the controversy on venereal diseases might create an atmosphere which would make the Health Service discussions more difficult by suggesting that more Government control for doctors is a likely outcome of the new Service.[77]

Nonetheless, Tom Johnston was determined to press the Scottish case for VD legislation, and the Scottish Secretary and Minister of Health duly argued out the issue before the Lord President's Committee in November 1944 and March 1945.[78] The health departments were agreed on the seriousness of VD as a threat to public health, on the existence of an anti-social group of sexual recidivists who were not amenable to education or persuasion, and on the wartime shift in public opinion in favour of compulsion. However, the Ministry of Health insisted that English local authorities were divided over the issue of VD controls and that English private practitioners appeared far less willing to co-operate with a system of notification than their Scottish counterparts. It argued that Scottish proposals understated the possible damage that compulsion might do to existing voluntary procedures while they exaggerated the problem of 'default'. In view of the widespread debate that had accompanied the introduction of Defence Regulation 33B, the Minister of Health decided against further controversial legislation.

In the event, an expert report on the medical aspects of the issue in April 1945 by Sir Henry Dale, chairman of the War Cabinet's Scientific Advisory Committee, proved decisive. Dale's central conclusions were that new forms of chemotherapy were likely to render default a 'negligible problem' in the case of gonorrhoea and that, although there was a *prima facie* case for the notification of defaulters known to be suffering from infective syphilis, such a measure should be delayed until the effects of penicillin on infectivity had been properly assessed. In view of Dale's evidence and the lack of parliamentary time in which to introduce a separate Scottish bill, and despite continuing pressure from Scottish local authorities and the backing of his all-party Council of State, Johnston felt compelled to concede that further consideration of VD controls should be deferred.[79]

The Demise of DORA 33B

The end of the war and demobilization brought a renewed increase in acute syphilis and gonorrhoea, and Medical Officers of Health in the major Scottish cities continued to press for the implementation of fresh controls.[80] However, by April 1947, the Ministry of Health had decided not to recommend any extension of the emergency powers contained in Defence Regulation 33B after its expiry in December 1947.[81] The Ministry considered that with 'its implications of an "informer" system as the starting point for applying compulsory powers', it would be difficult to justify its retention as a permanent peace-time measure. Health officials in Whitehall claimed that there was little evidence of its renewal 'being called for by public opinion' in England and Wales and that its real value had been in facilitating voluntary procedures of contact tracing which would be better consolidated by means of more vigorous administrative guidelines.[82] The growing tendency of women's groups to discredit such procedures as part of their ongoing campaign against discriminatory VD controls was an added incentive to return to a purely voluntary system of VD administration.

The DHS found Scottish medical opinion divided on the issue of post-war controls. Venereologists in Edinburgh, Dundee, and Lanarkshire favoured the retention and extension of powers under Defence Regulation 33B. For example, R. C. Batchelor, VD Medical Officer for Edinburgh, considered that its operation had underlined the value of notification in enabling 'the tracing and identification of some of the most dangerous and persistent spreaders of infection'. In his view, some form of legal compulsion was needed to underpin contact tracing if the community was to be protected 'against moral imbeciles or persistent and cynical procurers'.[83] Similarly, the VD Medical Officer for Dundee welcomed the resolution of the Union Internationale Contre le Péril Vénérien that 'compulsory powers should be sought nationally and internationally to treat those in a contagious state who refused to submit themselves voluntarily for treatment'.[84] VD clinicians in Glasgow and Aberdeen, however, were less enthusiastic about its retention, stressing that the regulation had been little used by civilian VD centres and that the threat of legal proceedings had had little to do with the wartime development in contact tracing.[85] They believed that the unwillingness of patients to divulge information, the difficulty of clearly establishing the identity and location of contacts, and the elaborate procedures required of health officials, had all conspired to render Regulation 33B largely inoperative.[86] This was a view endorsed by I. N. Sutherland, in charge of infectious disease control at the DHS, and after further consultations and taking into account the reduced incidence of recorded VD in Scotland during the first quarter of 1947, the Department declined to press for legislation to replace Regulation 33B on its expiry. They did, however, warn the Ministry of Health that the Department was 'still liable at any time to be exposed to further pressure in favour of legislation dealing with defaulters ... if not with compulsory notification of new cases' and that it might still be forced to reopen the issue in Cabinet.[87]

As predicted, Scottish local authorities launched yet another campaign for VD controls in the early months of 1948. In February, Edinburgh Town Council endorsed the recommendation of its Public Health Committee in favour of statutory powers of compulsory notification and treatment, and in the following months the DHS received a range of similar resolutions from civic leaders across Scotland.[88] VD Medical Officers such as R. C. L. Batchelor in Edinburgh and D. M. Keay in Dundee urged that Regulation 33B be replaced by some other means for 'controlling the incorrigibles'.[89] As in 1944, local campaigning became subsumed within more general lobbying by Scottish local government organizations, with added support from the hardcore of former BSHC activists within the Scottish Council for Health Education.[90]

Taking its cue from the Ministry of Health's vigorous opposition to the VD controls contained within the 1948 Salford Corporation Bill, and from the growing resentment of public and parliamentary opinion at the continuation of wartime emergency powers, the DHS declined to reopen the debate over compulsory notification and treatment, and focused instead upon trying to strengthen voluntary procedures of contact tracing and follow-up counselling for defaulters as a means of containing the incidence of VD in post-war Scotland.[91]

The Implications

An analysis of Scottish VD policy during the 1940s has a range of implications for the history of public health and, in particular, of the response of British government to sexually transmitted diseases. Despite the consensus for VD controls claimed by Scottish health authorities, and the greater community tolerance during the emergency to State intervention, wartime proposals aroused extensive public debate. They raised a set of fundamental and contentious issues relating to the liberty of the individual, the sexual status of women, the role of the medical profession and the State in the control of sexual behaviour, the medico-legal implications of compulsory notification and treatment, and the constitutional autonomy of Scottish health policy.

Underlying the opposition to compulsory VD controls was a continuing concern to ensure that the health and manpower needs of the wartime emergency should not permanently endanger British civil liberties. As Davenport-Hines has noted: 'Medical people were conscious of the correlation between a nation's form of government and its legislation on social hygiene: the fact that Fascist Italy and Nazi Germany had reintroduced state regulation discredited medical dirigisme in British judgement in the 1940s.'[92] Similarly, other exemplars, such as Scandinavian VD controls, were commonly dismissed as reflecting a culture of social deference and discipline alien to the British ethos.

Clearly, the strength of concern over sexual discrimination was also a powerful constraint upon policy-makers, and the operation of Defence Regulation 33B during the period 1943–7 served to reinforce it. In practice, as in England and Wales, and as with similar wartime controls elsewhere,[93] the measure was operated overwhelmingly against women. Its main purpose was to protect the health and efficiency of the male troops. In the years 1943–7, 83 per cent of multiple notifications in Dundee and 96 per cent of those in Glasgow applied to women.[94] In the few prosecutions that were held, health authorities and magistrates continued to endorse a double moral standard, with infected men being depicted as 'victims' and their female consorts as sexual predators.[95] Female defendants had their alleged 'promiscuity' paraded before the courts and media without any opportunity to establish their innocence beyond submitting to medical examination, while male informants, who might often be highly promiscuous, were neither legally required to attend court proceedings nor to submit to a prescribed regime of treatment.[96] Moreover, although a significant minority of alleged contacts were found not to be infected with gonorrhoea and syphilis, they had no direct recourse in law to raising proceedings for damages against their accusers.[97]

The successful development of voluntary contact-tracing procedures during the war employing information gained on 'single-notice' contacts under DORA 33B also weakened support for the retention of emergency powers. In Edinburgh, an estimated 44 per cent of the 679 'single-notice' contacts received during the years 1942–7 had been informally traced, 'tactfully interviewed' and induced to attend clinics by nurse almoners, of whom 72 per cent were found to be suffering from gonorrhoea and/or syphilis.[98] Over the same period in Dundee, 71 per cent of the 306 cases with single notifications had been contacted and examined, of whom 97 per cent had been infected with VD.[99] In some cities, such as Glasgow, a special branch of health visitors had been created to cope with the expansion in tracing work, including, as in the celebrated Tyneside Scheme south of the border, the tracing of unnamed suspects in cafés, bars, lodging-houses and dance-halls, even when only a vague description of their looks and 'haunts' was available.[100] In the opinion of many Medical Officers of Health and VD Medical Officers, the cumulative effect of such contact tracing, 'in preventing the spread of communicable disease, and in thereby avoiding loss of working time and conserving man-power, must have contributed in no small measure to the national war effort'.[101]

Public health officials, bred in a strong Scottish tradition of civic authoritarianism and intent on maintaining a Scottish identity in health politics, tended to exaggerate the strength of consensus for VD controls. As in the interwar campaign for compulsory notification and treatment, the issue of wartime controls became increasingly viewed as an acid test of the autonomy of Scottish health administration. In local government circles, frustration was aired at the apparent deference of the DHS to the libertarian 'fears and feelings of the cathedral cities south of the border', and the failure of subsequent attempts to introduce more stringent VD measures was regarded as both a slight to Scottish public opinion and a denial of its health needs and agenda.[102] Certainly, Tom Johnston continued to pursue the issue after demitting office and would later single it out in his autobiography as a notable failure of Scottish administration to assert the newfound 'spirit of independence' engendered by his tenure at the Scottish Office.[103] It was also to figure in the evidence of the Scottish Covenant Association to the Royal Commission on Scottish Affairs in 1953 as an illustration of the frustration of 'Scottish aims and aspirations' under a constitutional structure that denied adequate administrative and legislative devolution to Scottish affairs.[104]

Such a view ignored the significant disagreements within Scottish public and professional opinion over the medical, legal and social implications of coercive VD controls. Clinicians continued to hold disparate views on the content and desirability of controls and often harboured serious reservations about the more extreme proposals of their public health committees. Health authorities in major cities such as Edinburgh and Glasgow continued to differ on the value of compulsion in the notification and treatment of VD. Moreover, pressure groups such as the Scottish branches of the BMA and of the

Medical Society for the Study of VD and the Scottish Committee of the BSHC also brought differing professional agendas to the debate. Above all, within the DHS, there remained a wide spectrum of opinion on the issue, and a reluctance on the part of both medical officials and generalist administrators to being pressed into ill-conceived measures by moral panic in the press and local government offices. While they resented having to defer to the views of the Ministry of Health, Whitehall's resistance to compulsory measures was not infrequently used by DHS officials as a cover for their own reservations. For in trying to regulate for sexually transmitted diseases, wartime policy-makers faced a cluster of intractable and potentially divisive issues: how to target allegedly high-risk groups without sexual discrimination; how to impose controls without infringing medical rights and civil liberties; how to provide specialist facilities to underpin compulsory procedures at a time of scarce medical resources while maintaining the co-operation of the general medical profession; and above all, how to implement controls without alienating the public from existing voluntary procedures for diagnosis, treatment, and contact epidemiology. These were not, of course, issues specific to wartime policy-making. Debates on these issues had shaped the outcome of the previous campaign for VD controls in interwar Scotland and similar debates would re-emerge surrounding the call for public health legislation to protect society against the threat of AIDS.

Notes

1 National Archives of Scotland [NAS], HH 65/116/87–9, Minutes by I. N. Sutherland and A. Davidson, Sept. 1940.

2 NAS, HH 48/65/2, *Circulars 113/1940, 6 June 1940; 223/1940, 4 Sept. 1940; 275/1940, 26 Oct. 1940; 284/1940, 6 Nov. 1940.*

3 L. W. Harrison, 'Anti-Venereal Measures in Denmark and Sweden', *British Journal of Venereal Diseases [BJVD]*, 15 (1939), 1–17; Public Record Office [PRO], MH 55/1386, Minute L. W. Harrison, 23 Sept. 1939; MH 55/1326, Papers relating to VD: Compulsory Notification and Treatment, 1934–43.

4 See especially, PRO, MH 55/1333; MH 55/1334, Wartime Treatment Services, Papers and Correspondence.

5 See especially, Medical Society for the Study of Venereal Diseases Scottish Branch [MSSVDSB], Minutes, 29 March 1933, 22 Feb. 1939; D. H. Kitchin, 'Medico-Legal Aspects of Venereal Disease', *Practitioner*, 143 (1939), 177–84.

6 See, e.g., Editorial, 'Venereal Disease: Proposals for a New

D.O.R.A.', *The Shield,* VII, no. 2 (Oct. 1939), 50–3.

7 Contemporary Medical Archives Centre [CMAC], SA/MWF/A12, Minutes of Medical Women's Federation [MWF] Standing Committee on VD, 23 Feb. 1940; *British Medical Journal [BMJ],* 20 July 1940, 96.

8 NAS, HH 65/126/2, Memoranda and Correspondence on Proposed Legislation 1939–42.

9 NAS, HH 65/126/7, N. Wattie, 'The Incidence of Venereal Disease in Scotland', 15 May 1941. New cases of early infectious syphilis and acute gonorrhoea at Scottish civilian treatment centres for the year 1941 exceeded those recorded for 1940 by 116% and 45% respectively (NAS, HH 65/119/24; HH 65/126/78).

10 NAS, HH 65/126/7, N. Wattie, *op. cit.* (note 9); *Dundee Medical Officer of Health [MOH] Annual Report (1941–5),* 114; *Edinburgh Public Health Department [EPHD] Annual Report (1940),* 18; *Glasgow MOH Annual Report (1941),* 37; *Aberdeen MOH Annual Report (1940–45),* 37.

11 See, e.g., NAS, HH 65/126/7; *EPHD Annual Report (1940),* 18.

12 NAS, HH 65/126/7, Survey of Local Authority Views on the Incidence and Control of VD; *EPHD Annual Report (1940),* 19.

13 Edinburgh City Archives [ECA], Minutes of Convention of Scottish Royal Burghs, 1 April 1941; NAS, HH 65/126/7, Minutes of Delegation to Department of Health for Scotland [DHS] from Scottish Committee of the British Social Hygiene Council [BSHC], 26 May 1941.

14 NAS, HH 65/116/87–9, Minutes by A. Davidson [Deputy Chief Medical Officer] and I. N. Sutherland [Medical Officer] 1940–1.

15 NAS, HH 65/126/12, DHS to Office of Secretary of State for Scotland, 2 June 1941.

16 NAS, HH 65/126/17–18, 23, Correspondence relating to VD Regulations, 1941–2.

17 NAS, HH 65/126/18, 23, 33, Correspondence relating to VD Regulations 1941–2. Similar views shaped VD policy in the USA and Australia. See A. M. Brandt, *No Magic Bullet: A Social History of Venereal Disease in the United States since 1880* (Oxford: Oxford University Press, 1985), ch. 5; M. Sturma, 'Public Health and Sexual Morality: Venereal Disease in World War II Australia', *Signs,* XIII (1988), 725–40.

18 NAS, HH 65/126/33; Fawcett Library, 3/AMS/46, Minutes of Association for Moral and Social Hygiene [AMSH] Executive Committee, 12 March 1942.

19 NAS, HH 65/126/37, Minute on views of Law Officers, 5 Feb.

1942.

20 NAS, HH 65/126/43, Minute on 'Proposed VD Regulation', 5 March 1942; HH 58/66, Minute on Legal Advice.

21 NAS, HH 65/126/53, Minute by I. N. Sutherland, 30 July 1942. In Glasgow, in 1941, not one alleged source of infection out of 400 had been named by two or more patients.

22 NAS, HH 65/126/18, Notes on meeting in Chief Medical Officer's room, 3 July 1941. R. Davenport-Hines, *Sex, Death and Punishment: Attitudes to Sex and Sexuality in Britain since the Renaissance* (London: William Collins, 1990), 270.

23 See, e.g., NAS, HH 65/116/94, Resolution of Dunoon Women Citizens' Association.

24 Editorial, 'Compulsory Methods and the Treatment of Venereal Diseases', *The Shield*, IX, no. 2 (June 1942), 55–8; Open letter to Medical Officers of Health, 'Venereal Diseases: The question of some compulsory action being taken', *BJVD*, 18 (1942), 95; NAS, HH 65/116/99, AMSH to Secretary of State for Scotland, 3 Nov. 1942.

25 NAS, HH 65/126/23, Report on Interdepartmental Meeting on Draft Regulation, 16 July 1941.

26 NAS, HH 65/126/33, Memo. by W. Dalrymple Champneys on 'Proposed Venereal Disease Regulations', 23 Jan. 1942.

27 Despite a levelling off in the number of new cases of gonorrhoea in Scotland in 1942, they still exceeded recorded cases for 1939 by 40%. New cases of syphilis attending treatment centres in 1942 represented a 31% increase compared with 1941 and 101% increase compared with 1939 (NAS, HH 65/117/64, Statement of New Cases Attending Treatment Centres 1938–43).

28 NAS, HH 65/126/42, Minutes of DHS Consultative Committee of MOHs, 5 March 1942; Dundee City Archives [DCA], H38, Minutes of SCBSHC, 23 April, 4 June 1942; *Glasgow Herald*, 17 Oct. 1942. In addition to health controls, night curfews and identity cards were advocated as a means of restricting the movement of 'sexually promiscuous girls', especially in the vicinity of railway stations.

29 PRO, MH 55/1326, Papers relating to Compulsory Notification and Treatment.

30 PRO, MH 55/1326, MSSVD to Ministry of Health, 16 May 1942.

31 See, e.g., BMA Scottish Office, Edinburgh, Minutes of Scottish Committee of BMA, 16 Sept. 1942.

32 *News Chronicle*, 16 Sept. 1942.

33 NAS, HH 65/126/49, 59, Draft Regulation for Home Policy

Committee, April 1942.

34 *Summary Report of the Ministry of Health for 1942–3, PP 1942–3 (Cmd. 6468) IV*, 10.

35 NAS, HH 65/119/11, *Statutory Rules and Orders, 1942, No. 2277.*

36 NAS, HH 65/117/31, Memo. on Representations to DHS by Associations against Compulsory Notification and Treatment of VD, 1942–3. Protesting organizations included Alliance of Honour, AMSH, Married Women's Association, Mothers Union, National Council of Equal Citizenship, National Council of Women and Women's Freedom League.

37 NAS, HH 65/119/38, Representations of Women's Organisations to DHS, Nov.–Dec. 1942; 'Regulation 33B', *Time and Tide*, 21 Nov. 1942; PRO, MH 55/1347, Venereal Disease General Regulation 33B, Resolutions.

38 NAS, HH 65/117/31, Representations to DHS, 6 Nov. 1942, 2 Dec. 1942.

39 See, e.g., the speeches of the Archbishop of Canterbury and the Bishop of Norwich, *Hansard [HL]* 125, 8 Dec. 1942, cols 445–51, 459–63.

40 NAS, HH 65/117/31; United Free Church of Scotland, *Report of Committee on Temperance and Public Morals (1942)*, 87–93.

41 NAS, HH 65/119/38, BSHC pamphlet, '33B and the VD situation', Nov. 1942; CMAC, SA/BSH/F10/1, Minutes of BSHC Social Implications of VD Sub-Committee, 12 Nov. 1942.

42 DCA, H38, Scottish Committee BSHC Files, Memo. by W. E. Whyte, March 1942.

43 PRO, HH 55/1347, Scottish Committee BSHC to Ministry of Health, 18 Nov. 1942; *The Times*, 7 Dec. 1942.

44 See, e.g., *Glasgow Evening News*, 10 Nov. 1942; *Glasgow Herald*, 11 Nov. 1942; *Forward*, 12 Dec. 1942.

45 *Glasgow Herald*, 16 Dec. 1942; University of Sussex, Mass Observation Archives, File Report 1599, 'The Public and VD', 23 Feb. 1943. For views of individual Scottish respondents, see especially, DR 2568, 2741, 2932, Boxes DR 59, DR 60, Nov. 1942; DR 2799, 3263, Box DR 61, Dec. 1942.

46 *Hansard [HL]* 125, cols 435–73, 8 Dec. 1942; *[HC]* 385, cols 1808–86, 15 Dec. 1942.

47 NAS, HH 65/119/23–4, Briefing Notes for Debate on Defence Regulation 33B, 7 Dec., 11 Dec. 1942.

48 NAS, HH 65/119/23, Briefing Notes.

49 NAS, HH 65/119/27, Statistical Abstract of New Cases of Syphilis and Gonorrhoea in Scotland, 1939–42. Cases of congenital syphilis

in Glasgow rose by 37% between 1942 and 1943. There was also a significant rise in the percentage of positive ante-natal blood tests (*Glasgow MOH Annual Report (1943)*, 41).

50 NAS, HH 65/117/31, Statement of Representations by Local Authorities and Associations, Aug. 1943. A similar campaign, although less co-ordinated, was undertaken by English local authorities. See, PRO, MH 55/1326, VD: Papers on Compulsory Notification and Treatment.

51 *EPHD Annual Report (1942)*, 7, 35; *Edinburgh Evening News*, 7 Jan. 1944, 10 Feb. 1944. The recorded incidence for early syphilis in Edinburgh for 1942 exceeded 1941 by 45% and pre-war levels by 500%.

52 For the conference papers, see ECA, EPHD Papers, Box 36, file 15/14.

53 ECA, Minutes of Town Council, 6 July 1944. Draft proposals on 'Venereal Diseases: Compulsory Notification and Treatment'.

54 Glasgow City Archives [GCA], Minutes of Glasgow Corporation, 6 Aug. 1943; Minutes of Sub-Committee on Clinical Services, 22 Oct. 1943, 3 Dec. 1943, 14 April 1944, 9 June 1944; NAS, HH 65/117/65, W. A. Horne, 'Incidence of Venereal Disease in Glasgow', 3 Dec. 1943; HH 65/117/70, Note of Secretary of State's meeting with Glasgow Public Health Committee, 31 March 1944.

55 They did, however, favour the introduction of powers to compel the parents of congenital syphilitics to undergo medical treatment until certified free of infection. See PRO, MH 55/1341, Correspondence Relating to the Spread and Control of VD.

56 NAS, HH 65/117/25, Minute by I. N. Sutherland, 21 July 1943; PRO, MH 55/1326, Minute by L. W. Harrison, 21 April 1943.

57 NAS, GD 333/11, Edinburgh Women Citizens' Association Papers, Minutes of Executive Committee, 4 Feb. 1943; Fawcett Library, 3/AMS/310 Pt 2, AMSH Papers, Memo. of Standing Conference of Women's Organisations of Edinburgh on VD, 27 July 1943; *Proceedings of the General Assembly of the United Free Church of Scotland (1943)*, 37.

58 NAS, HH 65/119/42, *DHS Circulars 2/1943, 18 Jan. 1943; 56/1943, 7 June 1943*.

59 See *Scotsman*, 31 July, 17 Sept., 6 Nov., 20 Nov., 11 Dec. 1943.

60 Female images were also central to the demonology of VD portrayed in many other countries during World War II. See especially, R. R. Pierson, 'The Double Bind of the Double Standard: VD Control and the CWAC in World War II', *Canadian Historical Review*, 62 (1981), 50; Brandt, *op. cit.* (note 17), illustrations 14, 18–20.

231

61 In Scotland in 1943, only 43 contacts were named twice as
    compared with 827 single notices. Legal proceedings were taken in
    only one instance (*Summary Report by DHS, PP 1943–44 (Cmd.
    6545) III,* 19–20).

62 PRO, MH 55/1353, Minute by L. W. Harrison, 1 May 1943; MH
    55/1354, Ministry of Health Questionnaire, 7 July 1943; *Ministry of
    Health Circular 2896, 28 Dec. 1943.*

63 NAS, HH 58/66, Minute by G. A. Birse, 31 Jan. 1944; HH
    65/120/87–8. For a full discussion of the impact of Regulation 33B
    on contact tracing in Scotland, see R. Davidson, '"Searching for
    Mary, Glasgow": Contact Tracing for Sexually Transmitted Diseases
    in Twentieth Century Scotland', *Social History of Medicine,* 9 (1996),
    195–214.

64 PRO, MH 102/1149, Report of Joint Committee on Venereal
    Diseases, 10 Dec. 1943.

65 *Medical Advisory Committee (Scotland), Report on Venereal Diseases,
    PP 1943–44 (Cmd. 6518) IV.*

66 NAS, HH 65/123/3, Memorandum on 'Venereal Diseases' by Sir
    Wilson Jameson, 12 Jan. 1944; HH 65/124, Minutes on
    Negotiations between Ministry of Health and DHS, Jan.–March
    1944; PRO, RG 23/56, P. J. Wilson and V. Barker, *The Campaign
    against Venereal Diseases, Social Survey Report for Ministry of Health,*
    Jan. 1944.

67 NAS, HH 65/124/5, Minutes by G. H. Henderson [Secretary,
    DHS], 6 March, 24 March 1944; PRO, MH 55/1327, L. W.
    Harrison to H. K. Ainsworth, 21 March 1944.

68 *Report of the Church and Nation Committee to the General Assembly of
    the Church of Scotland (1944),* 280–1.

69 NAS, HH 65/124, DHS Minutes Feb.–March 1944.

70 NAS, HH 65/117/70, Note on Proceedings of Meeting, 31 March
    1944; HH 65/124, Minute by G. H. Henderson, 4 April 1944.

71 NAS, HH 48/65/6, *Circular 54/1944, 3 May 1944;* HH
    65/117/71–7, Local Authority Responses.

72 NAS, HH 65/122/11, Minutes of Conferences of Secretary of State
    with Scottish Protestant Churches and with Representatives of the
    Roman Catholic Church in Scotland, 30 June, 17 July 1944; *Report
    of Committee on Temperance and Public Morals, United Free Church
    (1944),* 69.

73 NAS, HH 65/122/11, Note of Meeting of Secretary of State and
    BMA (Scottish Branch), 17 July 1944.

74 NAS, HH 65/122/13, Note by G. H. Henderson, 3 Aug. 1944; HH
    65/122/17, Note of Meeting of Secretary of State and Scottish Local

Authority Associations, 3 Aug. 1944.

75 NAS, HH 65/122/18, DHS to Ministry of Health, 31 Aug. 1944; HH 65/122/19, Ministry of Health to DHS, 6 Sept. 1944.

76 PRO, MH 71/104, Reports and Papers of English Medical Advisory Committee Sub-Committee on Venereal Disease.

77 NAS, HH 65/122/23, Minute G. H. Henderson to T. Johnston, 28 Sept. 1944.

78 PRO, War Cabinet Papers, CAB 71/18, Papers of Lord President's Committee, L.P. (44) 184, 8 Nov. 1944; (44) 52nd meeting, Minute 4, 14 Nov. 1944; CAB 71/20, L.P. (45) 62, 12 March 1945.

79 PRO, War Cabinet Papers, CAB 71/20, L.P. (45) 98, 26 April 1945; (45) 106, 15 May 1945.

80 *Glasgow MOH Annual Report (1946)*, 78; *EPHD Annual Report (1946)*, 96–7.

81 NAS, HH 65/121/79a, 81, Ministry of Health to DHS, 10 April, 16 April 1947. In contrast, in many other countries such as Holland, wartime ordinances involving the compulsory regulation of likely vectors of VD were retained into the 1950s. See A. Mooij, *Out of Otherness: Characters and Narrators in the Dutch Venereal Disease Debates 1850–1990* (Amsterdam/Atlanta: Rodopi, 1998), ch. 3.

82 In fact, a survey of Medical Officers of Health in England and Wales undertaken by the BSHC in March 1948 revealed that two-thirds of their sample 'wanted some form of compulsory powers in dealing with VD – as a last resort'. See PRO, MH 55/1385, Report of Ad Hoc Sub-Committee on Regulation 33B, 31 March 1948.

83 *EPHD Annual Report (1947)*, 90.

84 *Dundee MOH Annual Report (1947)*, 21.

85 Throughout the operation of DORA 33B, only 169 contacts in Scotland were notified more than once. In only 17 cases were formal notices served requiring medical examination or treatment, and only 4 contacts were reported to the Procurator-Fiscal for evading the Regulation (*DHS, Annual Report for 1947, PP 1947–8 (Cmd. 7453) XII*, 74).

86 *Aberdeen MOH Annual Report (1940–45)*, 38; NAS, HH 65/121/84, Summary of Views of VD Medical Officers, April 1947.

87 NAS, HH 65/121/84, Minute by I. N. Sutherland, 29 April 1947; HH 65/121/85, DHS to Ministry of Health, 21 May 1947.

88 See, e.g., ECA, Convention of Royal Burghs, Minutes of Law Committee, 7 April 1948.

89 *EPHD Annual Report (1947)*, 90; *Dundee MOH Annual Report (1947)*, 129.

90 BMA Scottish Committee Papers, Communication from Scottish

Council for Health Education, 5 Jan. 1948.

91 NAS, HH 58/66/7; HH 65/121/94; HH 58/66, Papers and Correspondence on VD policy, 1944–62.

92 Davenport-Hines, *op. cit.* (note 22), 270.

93 See, e.g., Pierson, *op. cit.* (note 60), 31–58; Sturma, *op. cit.* (note 17), 725–40.

94 *Dundee MOH Annual Report (1947)*, 128; *Glasgow MOH Annual Report (1944)*, 52; *(1945)*, 78; *(1946)*, 81; *(1947)*, 110. For comparative data relating to England and Wales, see *Hansard [HC]* 396, cols 1529–30, 4 Feb. 1944; *Ministry of Health Summary Report to 31 March 1947, PP 1947–8 (Cmd. 7441) XII*, 47.

95 See, e.g., *Glasgow MOH (1947)*, 109; *Paisley Daily Express*, 9 May 1944; *Scotsman*, 9 May 1944.

96 NAS, HH 65/120, National Vigilance Association of Scotland to DHS, 1 April 1943. Magistrates compounded the problem by wrongly assuming that they were bound to commit offenders under Defence Regulation 33B to prison in order to receive treatment, and that the sentence should reflect the period required to affect a cure. In practice, however, women imprisoned under the Regulation often received inadequate medical treatment for their infections. In addition, although in law they could not be compelled to undergo medical examination and treatment, in the experience of health officials, solitary confinement 'on grounds of infection to others' usually brought 'the obstinate ones to heel'. See PRO, MH 55/1366, Venereal Disease: Treatment in Prisons; MH 55/1341, Correspondence Relating to the Spread and Control of VD. See also, F. Henriques, *Prostitution and Society: A Survey, Vol. 3: Modern Sexuality* (London: MacGibbon and Kee, 1968), 295.

97 During the period 1942–7, some 25% of contacts attending VD clinics in Edinburgh under Regulation 33B were found to be uninfected with gonorrhoea or syphilis (*EPHD, Annual Report (1947)*, 90). The Secretary of State *was* authorized, where appropriate, to refer any case brought under DORA 33B that was found to be free of venereal infection to the Procurator-Fiscal for possible proceedings by the Crown against the informants. For the recollections of one venereologist of false accusations under the Regulation, see *Lancet*, 11 Feb. 1967, 328.

98 *EPHD Annual Report (1943)*, 24; *(1944)*, 27–8; *(1945)*, 37; *(1946)*, 100; *(1947)*, 90.

99 *Dundee MOH Annual Report (1947)*, 128. In view of the problem of 'false positives' and the variability in the quality of diagnosis and testing within the Scottish VD services, such figures are highly

speculative.

100 GCA, Minutes of Corporation of Glasgow, Sub-Committee on
Clinical Services, 4 June 1943; Fawcett Library, AMSH Papers,
3/AMS/310, Pt 2, National Vigilance Association for Scotland to
AMSH, 12 Dec. 1944. For developments in England, see especially,
H. M. Johns, 'The Social Aspect of the Venereal Diseases – 3:
Contact Tracing', *BJVD*, XXI (1945), 17–21.

101 *EPHD Annual Report (1945)*, 37; *(1946)*, 100; *Aberdeen MOH
Annual Report (1940–45)*, 38; *Dundee MOH Annual Report (1947)*,
21; NAS, HH 65/117/65, Memo. on 'Incidence of Venereal
Diseases in Glasgow', W. A. Horne, 3 Dec. 1943.

102 See, e.g., NAS, HH 65/126/77a, Press Cuttings. For the broader
constitutional implications of such tensions, see I. Levitt, *The
Scottish Office: Depression and Reconstruction: 1919–1959*
(Edinburgh: Scottish History Society, 1992), ch. 1.

103 NAS, HH 65/122/60, T. Johnston to J. J. Johnstone, 13 March
1948; T. Johnston, *Memories* (London: Collins, 1952), 152, 164,
167.

104 NAS, HH 65/122/60, Observations of DHS on Supplementary
Memorandum from Scottish Covenant Association, 22 Oct. 1953.
See also, Levitt, *op. cit.* (note 102), 19–21.

10

'The Price of the Permissive Society': The Incidence and Epidemiology of VD, 1948–80

The Incidence of VD and STDs

Any attempt to measure the incidence of VD/STDs in post-war Scotland is fraught with difficulties. In the absence of any system of notification, it was impossible to establish precisely what proportion of those infected within the community presented themselves for treatment at the clinics. In the 1950s, there was evidence that, with the aid of new forms of chemotherapy, a significant amount of VD work was being undertaken by general practitioners. Indeed, concern was expressed by venereologists that this was depressing official statistics and 'delaying necessary epidemiological action'.[1]

Moreover, shifts in the incidence of VD/STDs as reflected in the case-loads of the clinics were often more apparent than real. In the late 1940s and early 1950s, demobilization and the subsequent recruitment of young men for National Service almost certainly distorted civilian VD figures.[2] The long-term upward trend in the level of female infection was in part a function of improvements in diagnosis and contact tracing and of changes in the social and medical status of women and their willingness to seek treatment for genital infections. Similarly, the emergence of a new generation of STDs was in part a reflection of shifts in medical awareness and technology and in the taxonomy of health statistics. Thus, non-specific urethritis [NSU] and trichomonas infection were only recorded separately after 1956. The subsequent rise in reported NSU was partly due to improvements in the diagnosis of gonorrhoea, by means of culture in addition to microscopy.[3] Likewise, the increased reported incidence of unspecified STDs after 1965 partly reflected a new awareness of the sexual origins of a range of diseases hitherto classified as 'non-venereal conditions', such as genital herpes.[4]

Nonetheless, even allowing for such caveats, the data produced by the clinics can provide valuable indicators of the incidence and social prevalence of VD/STDs in post-war Scotland.[5] They reveal a dramatic and sustained decline in the number of cases of syphilis from the peaks associated with wartime and post-war demobilization. Some 80 per cent of this decline occurred in the period 1948–56, and the Scottish trend clearly paralleled that experienced in England and Wales *(see Figure 10.1)*.[6]

Scottish gonorrhoea figures also reveal a sharp decline in the immediate post-war years – some 42 per cent over the period 1948–52. Thereafter, the most significant feature was their relative stability until the mid-1960s. This was in marked contrast to the sharply rising trend in the incidence of gonorrhoea elsewhere in the United Kingdom and overseas from the mid-1950s onwards. Indeed, this aspect of the Scottish health experience was one that the Scottish Home and Health Department [SHHD] was at pains to stress,[7] and it had, as we shall see, a decisive impact on the shaping of VD/STD policy and resourcing. Between 1968 and 1974, Scotland did experience a significant upswing in the number of gonorrhoea cases (some 58 per cent) but they then levelled off for the remainder of the decade and, although some convergence took place, new cases per 100,000 population remained well below the level for England.[8]

However, as in England, there was a dramatic rise in the incidence of the 'newer' venereal infections in Scotland after 1965, with a 156 per cent rise in the number of cases of male NSU over the following decade, along with rises of 63 per cent in female trichomoniasis and 288 per cent in other sexually transmitted diseases, including chancroid, genital

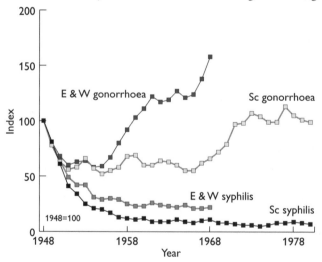

Figure 10.1
Index of New Cases of Syphilis and Gonorrhoea
for Scotland, England and Wales
(*Source:* see note 5)

'The Price of the Permissive Society'

candidosis, genital scabies, pubic lice, genital warts, genital herpes and molluscum contagiosum.[9] As a result, the 'classical venereal infections' of syphilis and gonorrhoea came to occupy only about one-quarter of the case load of the special clinics by 1980 compared with three-quarters prior to the Second World War *(see Table 10.1)*.

Table 10.1:
Proportion of Infected VD/STD Cases Diagnosed as Syphilis and Gonorrhoea in Scottish Clinics: Selected Dates

Year	Per Cent
1937	76
1950	61
1960	47
1970	31
1980	27

A breakdown by sex of VD/STD cases attending the Scottish clinics between 1948 and 1980 reveals a slow but steady rise in the male share of syphilis cases from an annual average of 57 per cent for the 1950s, which was very much in line with the pre-war period, to 63 per cent in the 1960s and 68 per cent in the 1970s. There was a particularly marked rise in the proportion represented by male cases in the later 1970s to an average of 73 per cent, which clinicians attributed largely to an emerging pattern of 'homosexually acquired infections'.[10]

In contrast, statistics for gonorrhoea *(see Table 10.2)* show that, although in absolute numbers, male cases continued to far exceed female cases, there was a significant convergence in their respective shares after the mid-1960s, with female cases representing over one-third of the total workload for gonorrhoea in the clinics by the 1970s.[11] Ominously, this shift was coincident with a sharp resurgence in the incidence of gonococcal ophthalmia neonatorum.[12]

These trends attracted widespread attention in the medical press and the media and were to figure prominently in contemporary debate on the state of public health and morality. Moreover, the age-specificity of much of the rising incidence of VD/STDs tapped into a deep well of concern over the moral decadence and sexual promiscuity of youth culture and in particular of girls and young women. Contemporary health statistics *(see Tables 10.2–10.4)* revealed that a growing proportion of VD/STDs was contracted by the 15–24 age-group and that female teenagers represented the fastest growth area for infections such as gonorrhoea.[13]

239

Figure 10.2
Scottish Clinics: Percentage Breakdown
of Gonorrhoea Cases by Sex: 1948–80
(*Source: Scottish Health Statistics*)

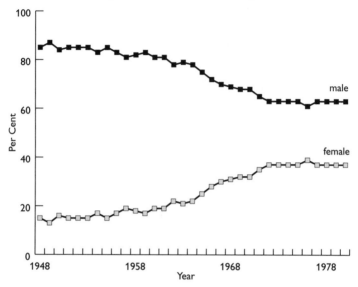

Table 10.2:
Sexually Transmitted Diseases:
New Male Cases in Scotland by Age,
Rate per 100,000 Population

Age	1960	1965	1970	1975	1980
15–19	463*	548*	571	688	606
20–24	463*	548*	1466	2110	2052
25–34	562	684	957	1113	1258
35–44	273	271	385	351	401
45+	78	74	89	55	55

* Figures only available for 15–24 age-group.
Source: Scottish Health Statistics (1980), 29.

240

Table 10.3:
Sexually Transmitted Diseases:
New Female Cases in Scotland by Age,
Rate per 100,000 Population

Age	1960	1965	1970	1975	1980
15–19	244*	361*	639	801	770
20–24	244*	361*	745	1211	1268
25–34	186	213	343	436	523
35–44	59	72	96	92	130
45+	12	10	10	10	14

* Figures only available for 15–24 age-group.
Source: Scottish Health Statistics (1980), 29.

Table 10.4:
New Cases of Genital Gonorrhoea at Scottish Clinics
by Age and Sex (%)

Year	Male			Female		
	15–24	25–34	35+	15–24	25–34	35+
1948	30	46	25	40	33	22
1958	29	43	28	53	30	15
1968	47	36	17	61	29	9
1978	51	37	12	68	26	6

Source: Scottish Health Statistics

To contemporary observers and epidemiologists, one of the most striking contrasts between the incidence of VD/STDs in Scotland and in England and Wales was the 'racial' distribution of infection. Whereas in England and Wales a significant number of VD/STD patients, and especially male patients, were born outwith the United Kingdom, in Scotland the overwhelming majority were native-born. Thus, in the 1960s, whereas around 90 per cent of Scottish male patients and 98 per cent of Scottish female patients with gonorrhoea were born within the United Kingdom, the comparable figures for England and Wales were 54 per cent and 83 per cent.[14] According to the British Cooperative Clinical Group, in 1968, some 17.3 per cent of male and 6.9 per cent of female gonorrhoea patients in England

and Wales were 'West Indies (Negro)' while in Scotland the same category accounted for only 1.5 per cent of male and 0.2 per cent of female patients.[15]

It is difficult to establish the class and occupational distribution of VD/STD cases in post-war Scotland. In many instances, case registers have been destroyed and where, as in Edinburgh, they have been preserved, access to more recent records is restricted for reasons of confidentiality. It has been possible to sample the VD registers of the Edinburgh Royal Infirmary and Leith Dispensary for the period up to 1951. In addition, there is a scatter of published reports on the social distribution of cases in Edinburgh, Glasgow and Aberdeen for the 1960s and early 1970s. However, given the vague and often inaccurate information supplied by patients, and the regional and chronological variances in the recording and classification of data, especially in the social classification of housewives and the unemployed, only very tentative conclusions can be drawn from these studies.

For male cases at VD/STD clinics *(Table 10.5)* there were clear indications in the Edinburgh data of a growing use of the clinics by professionals in social class II,[16] and computer mapping confirms the social dispersion of patients after the Second World War. Time series are not available for the other Scottish cities, but qualitative evidence would suggest that this was a feature of all the major clinics.[17] Moreover, if student cases are included within this class, this trend becomes even more pronounced.[18] The proportion of male cases in social class III remained remarkably constant over time and region, as did its under-representation compared with the Census returns. Whether or not this reflected, as Schofield surmised, 'the dwindling remnants of "middle class morality"', is hard to tell.[19] The fall in the proportion of male patients in social class IV is perhaps the most notable feature of the Edinburgh data. As in Glasgow and Aberdeen, part of the explanation may have been the marked decline in the proportion of patients who were seamen, due in part to a contraction in the labour force and to the increasing administration of antibiotic treatment on board ship.[20] However, it is also likely that a significant proportion of the cases recorded as 'economically inactive' in the 1970s were in social classes IV and V.[21] Certainly, contemporary estimates of rates of gonorrhoea in each electoral ward indicated that the highest incidence of disease was still located in the least affluent parts of the city, and strongly correlated with areas of social deprivation.[22]

Information on the social class distribution of female patients

(Tables 10.6–10.7) is even more intractable given the number of patients whose occupation was recorded as 'housewife'. In Edinburgh, there does appear to have been a significant rise in the proportion of cases from social classes I–III, from *c.*20 per cent in the early 1950s to nearer 50 per cent in the early 1970s, with a correspondingly sharp decline in the proportion of women describing themselves as 'housewives'. According to Edinburgh venereologists, 'it [was] probable that this represent[ed] a genuine change, rather than simply a greater willingness on the part of nurses, teachers and secretaries to admit their occupation'.[23] The significant representation of female students in Aberdeen's VD/STD case-load by the early 1970s may also be indicative of a more general trend in the university cities. In Glasgow, there was a marked excess of women in class V in the late 1960s and 1970s, especially of the unmarried, 'an increasing proportion of whom appeared to have no means of gainful employment',[24] but there is no strictly comparable data available for other periods or Scottish cities.

Despite the continuing importance of 'prostitution' to the socio-medical discourse surrounding VD/STDs, it was not recorded routinely as an occupation in the VD registers. For a brief period, Edinburgh Public Health Department did report the share of female patients who were known to be "prostitutes" (averaging 9.5 per cent for the period 1955–65), on the basis of the patient's own statements or 'on facts verified by the department's social worker'. However, the

Table 10.5:
Male Cases (Economically Active) at Scottish VD/STD Clinics:
Social Class Distribution (%)[27]

Class	Edinburgh 1951	Edinburgh 1970–76a	Glasgow 1972b	Aberdeen 1972
I	2(6)*	5(8)**	3(3)**	3(5)**
II	3(13)	21(17)	13(10)	12(14)
III	40(56)	40(50)	42(54)	41(48)
IV	37(12)	20(16)	20(19)	27(21)
V	18(13)	14(9)	22(14)	17(12)

a. cases defined as heterosexuals only
b. gonorrhoea cases only
* Census distribution 1951
** Census distribution 1971

Table 10.6:
Female Cases at Scottish VD/STD Clinics:
Social Class Distribution (%)[28]

Social Class	Edinburgh 1951	Edinburgh 1976	Glasgow 1972a*	Glasgow 1972b*	Aberdeen 1972
I	-	3	4	0.5	1
II	2	14	8	8	8
III	18	36	41	40	22
IV	15	5	17	12	12
V	6	1	30	40	13
Housewives, Students & Unemployed	59	41	n.a.	n.a.	44

* gonorrhoea only
a. married
b. unmarried

Table 10.7:
Female Cases at Scottish VD/STD Clinics:
Occupational Distribution (%)[29]

Occupation	Edinburgh 1951	Edinburgh 1962	Aberdeen 1972
Clerical Worker	7	17	16
Domestic Worker	8	13	4
Factory Worker	12	23	22
Waitress	5	4	5
Shop Assistant	5	7	4
Hairdresser	–	2	1
Bus Conductress	–	1	–
Student	1	1	14
Housewife	51	17	16
Nurse	2	–	3
Teacher	1	–	–
Cook	1	–	1
Unemployed	7	15	14

practice was subsequently discontinued.[25] It had arisen less from a concern for the health risks to sex workers than from a desire to publicize the fact that, contrary to prevailing sexual folklore, 'the professional [prostitute][was] *not* safe', and constituted a major and often careless vector of disease. Certainly, the evidence sat at curious odds with the blithe assertion of the senior venereologist that his sample indicated 'no obvious occupational hazard'.[26]

The Epidemiological Debate

The central explanatory concepts informing medical and public debate over the rise of VD/STDs in post-war Scotland were 'sexual promiscuity' and 'permissiveness'. The role of prostitution, with its epidemiological mind-set of a small cluster of feckless and vicious vectors, remained a *leitmotiv* of public health reports,[30] but it was steadily superceded by the spectre of widespread casual sex and an endless chain of infection. Evidence on the source of venereal infection in Edinburgh and Glasgow revealed a significant fall in the proportion of male infection attributed to prostitution with a commensurate increase in the proportion contracted through non-commercial casual sex *(see Table 10.8)*.[31] Interviewed in 1970, the Consultant Venereologist for Glasgow, C. B. S. Schofield, remarked that: 'A few years ago one man in five said he caught his infection from a prostitute; now the figure is one in fifteen.'[32] Information from female patients indicated a similar rise in disease arising out of so-called 'promiscuous amateur contact'.

Many strands of the pre-war medico-moral discourse surrounding VD survived well into later twentieth-century Scottish society. There is a notable similarity between the language and assumptions of the social hygiene and purity literature of the

Table 10.8:
Percentage Breakdown of Sources
of Infection of Edinburgh VD Patients 1955–65

Year	Prostitution male	Prostitution female	Casual Sex male	Casual Sex female	Marital Partner male	Marital Partner female
1955	32	5	55	42	13	53
1960	27	12	58	56	15	32
1965	19	8	66	60	15	32

Source: EPHD Annual Reports.

245

interwar period and those articulated in Public Health Department reports of the 1950s and 1960s. In particular, there was a continuing identity in the media and professional journals between VD/STDs and moral degeneration.

As in the 1920s, it was widely believed in the 1950s that war had seriously eroded familial and community controls and that its disinhibiting effects on patterns of sexual behaviour had profoundly 'demoralised' the nation.[33] Scottish venereologists were always sceptical of the more sensational claims for moral decadence, including those of the British Medical Association, but they shared the sentiments of Ambrose King, Adviser in VD to the Ministry of Health, that 'venereal disease was but one symptom of the general breakdown of moral order'.[34] Especial concern attached to the decline in the influence of religious values and commitment to the sanctity of marriage. Indeed, Robert Lees, Physician-in-Charge of Edinburgh's VD services in the period 1954–67, saw a clear connection between venereal infection and 'unions' that were only 'temporary and unblessed by Church!'.[35]

The long-established association between alcohol and promiscuity also resurfaced in post-war attempts by public health and Church authorities to explain the incidence of VD.[36] Thus, in the view of the Temperance and Morals Committee of the Church of Scotland, VD was one of many social problems arising from the influence of drink upon 'the censor of the conscience'.[37] A UK survey in 1956 found that 77 per cent of male and 25 per cent of female gonorrhoea patients had been drinking prior to intercourse from which they claimed to have contracted their infections.[38] Similarly, evidence from Glasgow in the late 1960s indicated that some 90 per cent of all VD cases had frequented a public house as a prelude to infective intercourse, while 35 per cent of infected male cases had picked up their contacts in public houses.[39] Seasonal fluctuations in the incidence of disease were also viewed in part as a function of drinking patterns, with the late December/early January peak commonly attributed to 'drunken parties at the festive season'.[40]

Meanwhile, fresh concerns were emerging about the impact of new chemotherapies on sexual behaviour. While venereologists had no wish to return to the draconian regimes of the early twentieth century, they were acutely aware of the moral dilemma posed by the widespread application of antibiotics. As Dr R. C. L. Batchelor (Physician-in-Charge of Edinburgh's VD services 1934–54) observed as early as 1949:

Gonorrhoea has lost its terrors, and the public may no longer bother

246

about something which it reckons is less difficult to cure than a common cold. Thus modern treatment, by creating a belief that sexual indiscretion is comparatively safe, may actually promote an increase in promiscuity and so conduce to the spread of venereal disease.[41]

In his view, 'the myth of the miracle drug' with the prospect of a cure at State expense 'without discomfort or inconvenience', and with a much reduced opportunity for the clinician to regulate behaviour as part of therapy, had trivialized venereal infection in the minds of patients and undermined the impact of social hygiene propaganda.[42] This association between VD, promiscuity, and 'over-confidence in antibiotics' was to be frequently asserted in both the Scottish press and official circles throughout the 1950s and early 1960s.[43]

As in other countries, from the late 1950s, venereologists and public health officials in Scotland increasingly adopted a more sociological approach to the epidemiology of VD.[44] Its incidence was explained less in terms of individual moral deficiencies and more in terms of the impact of a range of cultural, institutional and economic factors upon general patterns of sexual morality and behaviour. In the view of many social commentators, it was 'the price of the Permissive Society'.[45] In particular, certain 'high risk' groups were identified who were socially isolated due to marital or family disharmony, who were alienated from traditional values, and prey to a range of disinhibitants including alcohol, drugs such as cannabis and LSD, new forms of contraception, and a media 'obsessed with sexual permissiveness and gratification'.[46]

Although attitude surveys on sexual issues continued to reveal a younger generation in Scotland that was 'conformist rather than permissive or hedonistic',[47] the burden of blame was commonly attached to teenage promiscuity.[48] VD figures were widely presented as part of a wider 'social pathology' of youth culture including violence, drug-taking, illegitimacy and sexual deviancy.[49] In the view of a BMA Committee, VD among young people was 'a symptom of an underlying malaise affecting the social and sexual life of our society'.[50] As Weeks aptly remarks: 'What was clearly taking place was a displacement of the anxieties aroused by the nature of the social changes, especially expressed in the growing autonomous styles of the various youth cultures, on to the terrain of sexuality, where hidden fears and social anxieties could most easily be stirred.'[51]

Scottish public health and church reports in the late 1950s and 1960s frequently identified the rise in teenage VD/STD cases with adolescent alienation from a morally bankrupt, acquisitive society. Concern was expressed at an emerging 'cult of sexual sensuality' amongst juveniles in the absence of 'parental and community restraint' and adequate health education, and with the decline of spiritual values in personal and civic relationships. Venereologists welcomed the erosion of the secrecy and hypocrisy with which 'the older "Victorian" morality' had surrounded sexual issues, but lamented the health costs associated with the ensuing 'sensual license' of Scottish youth, inflamed, it was claimed, by exposure to an increasingly permissive leisure and media culture.[52] Concern was also expressed at the link between juvenile infections and the disinhibiting effects on sexual behaviour of alcohol at so-called 'necking sessions' and all-night parties.[53]

In addition, the casual attitude of teenagers towards venereal infection and towards medical therapy and surveillance was identified as a major factor in the increase in the number of carriers and penicillin-resistant strains in the community. While it was reluctantly conceded that there was little evidence 'that the teddy boy cult ... or Rock'n Roll' had any significant influence on the incidence of VD/STDs, its addicts were typified as 'uncooperative in treatment' and lacking in 'the self-discipline necessary for cure'. Similarly, there were serious doubts as to the value of contact tracing among teenagers given that 'a fair proportion of infected cases [were] already delinquents who resist[ed] any kind of control'.[54] Such non-compliance with medical authority was often viewed as part of a broader breakdown in civil and moral order amongst Scottish youth.[55]

However, as in the interwar period and the Second World War, post-war moral panic surrounding the sexual hygiene of the young centred on the sexual promiscuity of teenage girls. The potent image of asymptomatic, promiscuous girls as 'reservoirs of infection' haunting cafés, pubs, cinemas and dance-halls was widely projected in the media and public health literature.[56] The language of public health epidemiology still presented a largely passive role for male sexuality. According to senior venereologists in Edinburgh and Glasgow, it was female adolescent promiscuity that constituted 'the real danger' and a 'considerable nuisance and danger to seamen, servicemen, and mildly intoxicated youths'.[57] This asymmetry in perceptions of sexual behaviour and disease was powerfully reflected in contemporary analyses of the sources of infection, which enshrined the concept of women as the pro-active polluters well into the 1960s. Thus, Edinburgh's Public Health Department reports tabulated these sources as follows:[58]

Male Infection	Female Infection
prostitutes	prostitution
'amateur types'	promiscuous 'amateur' contact
marital partner	marital partner

Any reference to male 'clients' or 'consorts' was significantly absent. Equally notable is the retention of a taxonomy that retains the highly stigmatic term 'amateur' [prostitution] for non-marital female sexual encounters. Within the socio-medical ideology of venereologists such as Robert Lees, sexually active girls continued to be viewed as deviant and regressive.

Moreover, the emergence of a more social scientific interpretation of sexual behaviour and disease in the 1960s and 1970s served in many ways to reinforce this pathological view of female adolescent sexuality. Sexual promiscuity and VD/STDs among teenage girls became increasingly identified with a syndrome of distinctively female juvenile delinquency and revolt.[59] Whereas boys indulged in drink, vandalism and gang violence, girls were deemed to manifest their 'anti-social urges' primarily through promiscuity, with 'the ever-willing teenage girl' being 'the female equivalent of the skinhead in his bovver boots'.[60] Social psychologists also resurrected the linkages between VD, sexual permissiveness and mental instability that had so powerfully shaped interwar responses to 'problem girls'. According to personality studies of VD patients, promiscuous females attending the clinics displayed a 'high degree of neuroticism and psychoticism'.[61]

Inevitably, the debate surrounding female sexuality and the incidence of VD/STDs gave prominence to the increasing use by girls and young women of the 'pill'·and its implications for promiscuity and reduced protection from disease. Several research investigations in the early 1970s, while revealing a dramatic rise in the number of patients using contraceptive techniques, found little correlation between the use of the oral contraceptive pill, the number of sexual partners, and a positive diagnosis for VD/STDs. In part, this was attributed to the fact that the use of such contraception implied 'a degree of responsibility and care not widely observed by those at risk'.[62] However, the broad consensus amongst social commentators and medical practitioners was that the pill had radically altered patterns of female sexual behaviour, thus promoting sexual promiscuity and disease. In its annual report for 1969, the Scottish Home and Health Department acknowledged it to be a contributory factor in the rising incidence of venereal infection.[63] According to Robert Morton, President of the Medical Society for the Study of Venereal Diseases, for the single, the pill could 'be classified with the most dangerous of the polluting pesticides' and 'its use' was 'more calamitous than anything precipitated by thalidomide'.[64] In his view, which was shared by the BMA and other medical authorities, it made the 'permissive society' a practical reality and was the primary factor in bringing the male–female ratios of recorded infection, especially of gonorrhoea, more towards unity.[65] Likewise, C. B. S. Schofield, consultant venereologist at Glasgow Royal Infirmary, viewed the rise in VD/STDs as largely a function of the disinhibiting effects of the pill on female sexuality, in that 'women as well as men [could] sow their wild oats without fear of pregnancy'.[66]

In Scotland, the linkage between the pill and the rise in STDs was central to the broader campaign of the Churches against the extension of family planning provisions for single women and girls. According to the Free Church's Committee on Public Questions, Religion and Morals, increasing sexual disease was due to 'Her Majesty's Government ... throwing open the flood-gates to fornication, adultery and promiscuity, making them risk-free on the NHS'.[67] In similar vein, it argued that in promoting 'a permissive life style', the ready availability of the contraceptive pill had 'violated the sanctity and beauty of sex' and, in the crisis of escalating VD rates, 'reaped the whirlwind for having sown to the wind'.[68] Such views echoed the concerns and assumptions not only of the other Scottish churches but also of the 'Moral Right' within Scottish public health debates of the early 1970s.[69] The Chairman of Edinburgh's Public Health Committee used similar arguments in her campaign to frustrate the extension of family planning provisions, as did the Scottish Tory Conference in endorsing a motion denouncing what it perceived to be a general breakdown of public order and public morality.[70]

Epidemiological debate drew on a similar mix of social concern and moral outrage in its treatment of the role of homosexual behaviour in the spread of VD/STDs. Hitherto, it had been virtually ignored in medical texts and only emerged in the medical press and public health reports after the mid-1950s. The 'homosexual' failed to surface within the post-war demonology surrounding VD in Scotland in the same way as it did in the early 1960s in England and European countries such as Holland, and the prominence accorded by the Ministry of Health to 'homosexual practices' in explaining the rising incidence of VD was never matched in the reports of the SHHD.[71]

Early references to homosexual cases in Scottish reports on VD were largely cryptic and/or judgemental asides. Leading venereologists such as Batchelor and Lees did not subscribe to 'the modern view of homosexuality', and viewed it as a 'deviant' and dangerous 'perversion', driven by an 'aberrant instinct'.[72] In many respects, as the Scottish evidence before the Wolfenden Committee on Homosexual Offences and Prostitution had revealed in the mid-1950s, such views were in accord with broad areas of Scottish public and professional opinion.[73] They were certainly in line with grass-roots opinion in the Scottish Churches who viewed parliamentary proposals for homosexual law reform as a blatant attempt 'to stamp the foul brand of Sodom upon the nation's brow'.[74]

The subsequent report in 1973 of the Gilloran Committee on Sexually Transmitted Diseases in Scotland did little to dispel prevailing prejudices when it identified 'passive homosexuals' as 'reservoirs of infection',[75] thus stigmatizing their sexuality as a source of pollution and disease in a fashion traditionally reserved for female prostitutes and 'good-time girls'. Research published by the British Cooperative Clinical Group revealed that some 13.5 per cent of primary and secondary syphilis and 4.1 per cent of gonorrhoea recorded at Scottish clinics was transmitted 'homosexually'.[76] Although these levels were far below those recorded south of the border,[77] they were sufficient to fuel contemporary perceptions of homosexuals as an extremely promiscuous group whose casual sexual behaviour frustrated the best efforts of clinicians and contact tracers to contain the spread of disease.

A marked contrast between the epidemiological debate on VD/STDs in England and Scotland was the notable absence within Scottish health publications of allusions to immigration. This reflected the absence in Scotland of 'coloured, west indian immigrants' who were viewed as major vectors of disease, especially gonorrhoea. Yet, although it lacked the racial imagery of sexual politics in London and the industrial cities of the Midlands and North of England,[78] the discussion of VD/STDs in Scotland was not entirely free of racial prejudice. Public health reports sustained the long tradition of stigmatizing 'foreign infections'. Thus, in the 1950s, Edinburgh's VD Department attributed the survival of syphilis in the city largely to the importation of infection from countries 'where Mars, Bacchus and Venus [were] still a formidable trio'.[79] Moreover, there were powerful xenophobic, if not racial, overtones in the condemnation by Scottish venereologists of the impact on the sexual mores of the younger generation of 'the worst type of American and negro films, booklets, music and dancing'.[80] They surfaced also in several diplomatic incidents when local clinicians and politicians publicly linked the spread of casual 'prostitution' and VD to the presence of American servicemen at the Polaris Base at Holy Loch and at airbases in Midlothian.[81] The blame attached by some commentators to the 'hospitality schemes' of multi-nationals in North-East Scotland and to the sexual behaviour of Irish navvies employed on platform construction sites such as Ardyne during the oil boom of the 1970s had similar connotations.[82]

The epidemiological debate surrounding VD/STDs in Scotland between the Second World War and the onset of HIV/AIDS continued to be shaped by a powerful set of moral fears, assumptions and stereotypes. Gradually there was, as in other countries,[83] a shift in emphasis from diseased 'types' to patterns of individual sexual behaviour and their associated risk, but it was only a very partial shift. Traditional patterns of 'scapegoating' persisted within contemporary 'sociological' analyses of public health and the 'permissive society'. Moreover, in Scotland, Church attitudes on sexual issues remained highly influential and continued to maintain 'the remarkable influence of puritanical religion'.[84] As late as 1980, the General Assembly of the Free Church of Scotland endorsed the view that:

> It will not do for cynical men to scoff at cleanliness as 'Victorian'. The categories of fornication, adultery, bestiality and sodomy are fully as meaningful as ever. To a holy God they are fully as offensive and punishable. *The increased incidence of certain sexually-transmitted diseases bears witness to the reality of God's just judgement.*[85]

Notes

1   British Medical Association [BMA Archive], Venereologists Group Committee, 29 Nov. 1957. Draft paper on 'Occult Venereal Disease'. However, an investigation by the Scottish Medical Advisory Council in the 1960s revealed that only 9% of general practitioners treated patients with VD and that *c.*90% of all cases of gonorrhoea and of male urethritis were treated at the clinics (National Archives of Scotland [NAS], HH 104/35/75, Report of Working Party on the Incidence, Epidemiology and Control of Gonorrhoea in Scotland, 1965).

2   See, *Edinburgh Public Health Department [EPHD] Annual Report (1951)*, 95; Interview with former consultant venereologist, 4 Aug. 1994.

3   C. B. S. Schofield and N. McNeil, 'Venereal Disease in Scotland',

Health Bulletin, 28, no. 4 (1970), 19. Before the early 1970s, lack of clinical awareness and laboratory problems meant that only *c.*10% of trichomonas vaginalis infections in males (a major cause of urethritis) were recorded (N. McNeil and C. B. S. Schofield, 'Sexually Transmitted Diseases in Scotland 1968–71', *Health Bulletin*, 31, no. 2 (1973), 61–2).

4 Schofield and McNeil, *op. cit.* (note 3), 21.

5 Unless otherwise specified, the following account is based on *Scottish Health Statistics, 1948–80*; *Annual Reports of the Ministry of Health/Department of Health and Social Security on The State of Public Health*; Schofield and McNeil, *op. cit.* (note 3), 19–25; J. Hunter, S. Bain and D. H. H. Robertson, 'Sexually Transmitted Diseases in Edinburgh: A Changing Pattern 1961–76', *Health Bulletin*, 36, no. 5 (1978), 251–9; T. S. Wilson, 'The Incidence of Gonococcal Ophthalmia, Syphilis and Gonorrhoea since the inception of the Glasgow Schemes of Prevention and Treatment', *Medical Officer*, CXXI (17 Jan. 1969), 27–30.

6 The percentage of pre-natal blood tests for syphilis found to be positive also fell significantly from 1.46% in 1947 to 0.017% in 1962 (Wilson, *ibid.*, 29; *Glasgow Medical Officer of Health [MOH] Annual Reports*).

7 *Scottish Home and Health Department [SHHD] Annual Report on Health and Welfare Services in Scotland (1962), PP 1962–3 (Cmnd. 1996) XIX*, 14; *(1963), PP 1963–4 (Cmnd. 2359) XV*, 17; *(1964) PP 1964–5 (Cmnd. 2700) XVII*, 20; *(1966) PP 1966–7 (Cmnd. 3337) 61*, 12; *(1968), PP 1968–9 (Cmnd. 4012) 63*, 9.

8 In 1980, the incidences of new male and female STD cases in Scotland per 100,000 population were 124 and 67. The comparable figures for England were 164 and 85.

9 Non-specific genital infections rapidly overtook gonorrhoea as a cause of urethritis in males, and by 1975, the ratio of cases was 3:2 (C. B. S. Schofield and N. McNeil, 'Sexually Transmitted Diseases', *Health Bulletin*, 35, no. 1 (Jan. 1977), 14).

10 Hunter, Bain and Robertson, *op. cit.* (note 5), 252.

11 The sex distribution of cases varied between the Scottish cities. Thus, in 1971, while the female share of gonorrhoea cases in Glasgow was 29%, in Edinburgh it was 39%. However, both cities witnessed the long-term shift in recorded incidence towards women (*Glasgow MOH Annual Reports*; Hunter, Bain and Robertson, *op. cit.* (note 5), 256). In part, this convergence reflected the introduction of better diagnostic techniques.

12 McNeil and Schofield, *op. cit.* (note 3), 61, 66.

13 While teenage girls made up only 11.8% of Glasgow's population in
    1972, they accounted for 30.8% of gonorrhoea patients. See C. B. S.
    Schofield, *Sexually Transmitted Diseases* (Edinburgh: Churchill
    Livingstone, 2nd edition 1975), 39.

14 British Cooperative Clinical Group, 'Gonorrhoea Studies', *British
    Journal of Venereal Diseases [BJVD]*, 36 (1960), 239; 38 (1962), 2, 4;
    41 (1965), 238, 240; 46 (1970), 63, 66.

15 British Cooperative Clinical Group, 'Gonorrhoea Study, 1968',
    BJVD, 46 (1970), 63; Schofield and McNeil, *op. cit.* (note 3), 20.

16 This was especially so for 'homosexual' patients, whose social class
    was significantly higher than that of 'heterosexual' patients. See
    A. McMillan and D. H. H. Robertson, 'Sexually-Transmitted
    Disease in Homosexual Males in Edinburgh', *Health Bulletin*, 35
    (Sept. 1977), 267.

17 See, e.g., C. B. S. Schofield, *Sexually Transmitted Diseases*
    (Edinburgh: Churchill Livingstone, 3rd edition 1979), 38.

18 The share of male students in the Edinburgh case-load rose from 3%
    in 1951 to 12% in 1970–6. In 1972, 15% of male cases at Aberdeen
    clinics were students.

19 Schofield, *op. cit.* (note 17), 38.

20 Schofield and McNeil, *op. cit.* (note 3), 19. In Glasgow, in 1945,
    seamen had accounted for 34% of all male contagious syphilis cases
    and 25% of gonorrhoea cases. By 1970, these shares had reduced to
    20% and 8% respectively (*Glasgow MOH Annual Report (1971)*,
    219).

21 Eight per cent of all male VD/STD cases in Aberdeen (1972) and
    Edinburgh (1970–6) were recorded as being unemployed.

22 D. H. H. Robertson, 'Venereal Diseases', *Synapse: Journal of the
    Edinburgh Medical School*, 21, no. 3 (1972), 29.

23 Hunter, Bain and Robertson, *op. cit.* (note 5), 258.

24 Schofield, *op. cit.* (note 13), 40.

25 *Edinburgh Health and Social Services Department [EHSSD] Annual
    Report (1963)*, 139; *(1964)*, 99.

26 *EHSSD Annual Report (1963)*, 139.

27 Sources: For Edinburgh, VD Registers, Royal Infirmary of
    Edinburgh and Leith Dispensary (1951; 5% sample); McMillan and
    Robertson, *op. cit.* (note 16), 267. For Glasgow, Schofield, *op. cit.*
    (note 13), 39–40. For Aberdeen, Northern Health Services Archives
    [NHSA], GRHB A1/3 [22/1 Pt 3], Aberdeen City VD Statistics
    (1972). Census data from General Register Office, *Census 1951.
    Scotland Vol. IV: Occupations and Industries* (Edinburgh: HMSO,
    1956), Table 6; Office of Population Censuses and Surveys and

General Register Office, *Census 1971, Great Britain: Economic Activity, Part V (10% Sample)* (London: HMSO, 1975), Table 37, 118–20.

28 Sources: VD Registers, Royal Infirmary of Edinburgh and Leith Dispensary (1951; 5% sample); Hunter, Bain and Robertson, *op. cit.* (note 5), 258; Schofield, *op. cit.* (note 13), 39–40.

29 Sources: VD Registers, Royal Infirmary of Edinburgh and Leith Dispensary (1951; 5% sample); *EPHD Annual Report (1962)*, 157–8; NHSA, GRHB A1/3 [22/1 Pt 3], Aberdeen City VD Statistics (1972).

30 See, e.g., *EPHD Annual Report (1960)*, 145; *(1963)*, 139.

31 In Glasgow, Schofield estimated that while prostitutes infected 14% of male gonorrhoea patients in 1967, by 1976 the figure had fallen to 5.2% (Schofield, *op. cit.* (note 17), 39).

32 *Sunday Mirror*, 15 June 1970. See also Schofield, *op. cit.* (note 13), 41.

33 C. Haste, *Rules of Desire: Sex in Britain: World War I to the Present* (London: Chatto and Windus, 1992), 143.

34 *EHSSD Annual Report (1967)*, 73.

35 *EPHD Annual Report (1958)*, 196.

36 See, e.g., *EPHD Annual Report (1955)*, 158.

37 *Report of Committee on Temperance and Morals to General Assembly of the Church of Scotland (1960)* 419–20.

38 British Cooperative Clinical Group, 'Gonorrhoea Study', *BJVD*, 32 (1956), 22.

39 B. P. W. Wells and C. B. S. Schofield, '"Target" Sites for Anti-VD Propaganda', *Health Bulletin*, XXVIII, no. 1 (1970), 76.

40 See, e.g., *EPHD Annual Report (1957)*, 152.

41 *EPHD Annual Report (1949)*, 93.

42 R. C. L. Batchelor, 'Recent Developments in Venereology', *Edinburgh Medical Journal [EMJ]*, 61 (1954), 367–8.

43 See, e.g., National Archives of Scotland [NAS], HH 58/66, *Department of Health for Scotland, Memorandum 74/1961, 'Venereal Disease'*.

44 From 1954, the annual report of Edinburgh's VD Department contained a section on 'sociological investigations'.

45 See, e.g., the lead article by Dorothy Grace Elder in the *Glasgow Herald*, 3 Oct. 1972.

46 See especially, *Report of Joint Sub-Committee on Sexually Transmitted Diseases [Gilloran Report]* (Edinburgh: HMSO, 1973), 14; Schofield, *op. cit.* (note 13), 35–42.

47 See, e.g., *Scotsman*, 28 April 1976. According to this survey, only

16% of a sample of Scots aged 16–20 approved of casual sexual relationships.

48 Significantly, it was in 1966 that the Scottish Home and Health Department first published separate VD statistics for the 15–19 age-group.

49 See, e.g., J. Weeks, *Sex, Politics and Society: The Regulation of Sexuality since 1800* (London and New York: Longman, 2nd edition, 1989), 253; *Glasgow Herald,* 28 Sept. 1971.

50 *BMA Report on Venereal Disease and Young People* (1964), 6.

51 Weeks, *op. cit.* (note 49), 254.

52 See especially, *EPHD Annual Report (1959)*, 142–3; *EHSSD Annual Report (1967)*, 72–3; C. B. S. Schofield, *op. cit.* (note 17), 35–7; . NAS, HH 104/35, Memorandum of Scottish Medical Advisory Committee's [MAC] Sub-Committee on the Epidemiology of Gonorrhoea, Autumn 1965; *Report of Committee on Temperance and Morals to General Assembly of Church of Scotland (1962)*, 442; *Report of Temperance and Social Questions Committee of Congregational Union of Scotland (1962–3)*, 116. For the debate in England, see especially, *BMA Report, op. cit.* (note 50); A. King [Adviser on VD to the Ministry of Health], 'The Adolescent: Promiscuity and Venereal Disease', *Journal of the Royal Institute of Public Health and Hygiene,* 26 (1963), 299–308.

53 *BMA Report, op. cit.* (note 50), 51. The effects of alcohol in reducing awareness of risk in casual sexual encounters was stressed in health education literature targeted at the younger generation. See, Health Education Board for Scotland Library, Scottish Health Education Unit Circular no. 1/70, 5 Jan. 1970.

54 *EPHD Annual Report (1956)*, 157; *(1962)*, 156; NAS, HH 104/35/75, Report of Scottish MAC Sub-Committee on Gonorrhoea in Scotland (1965), 3. See also below, ch. 12.

55 See, e.g., *Glasgow Herald,* 15 May 1971.

56 See, e.g., *EHSSD Annual Report (1969)*, 71; *Gilloran Report, op. cit.* (note 46), 2.

57 *EPHD Annual Report (1956)*, 156; C. B. S. Schofield in *Sunday Mirror,* 15 June 1970.

58 Source: *EPHD Annual Reports (1958–60)*.

59 See, e.g., *EPHD Annual Report (1955)*, 158; *EHSSD Annual Report (1968)*, 66–7; *(1969)*, 71.

60 Schofield, *op. cit.* (note 13), 43–4; Robertson, *op. cit.* (note 22), 35.

61 Schofield, *op. cit.* (note 13), 44–6.

62 *EHSSD Annual Report (1968)*, 69; NHSA, North-Eastern Regional Hospital Board, Film A20, File 22/1, IIIA.

63 Annual Report on Health and Welfare Services in Scotland (1969), PP 1970–71 (Cmnd. 4392) 38, 9.

64 Daily Mirror, 13 Jan. 1972; R. S. Morton, Sexual Freedom and Venereal Disease (London: Owen, 1971), 90–1.

65 R. S. Morton, 'A Short History of the Medical Society for the Study of Venereal Diseases', Sexually Transmitted Infections, 74 (1998), 156.

66 Cited in Reports to the General Assembly of the Free Church of Scotland (1974), 145.

67 Ibid. (1974), 146.

68 Ibid. (1975), 155.

69 See, e.g., Year Book of the Congregational Union of Scotland (1970–1), 85–6; Reports to the General Assembly of the Church of Scotland (1968), 491–2; (1969), 503–8; Glasgow Herald, 14 April 1971, 13 May 1971.

70 Glasgow Herald, 3 Feb. 1971, Editorial on 'Policy on Morality', 19 Feb. 1971, 15 May 1971, 28 Sept. 1971.

71 A. Mooij, Out of Otherness: Characters and Narrators in the Dutch Venereal Disease Debates (Amsterdam/Atlanta: Rodopi, 1998), 181–2, 185–8; Ministry of Health, Chief Medical Officer of Health, Report of the State of the Public Health for 1961, PP 1962–3 (Cmnd. 1856) XIX, 59, 64.

72 Written communication from Dr L. Lees, 20 May 1995; R. C. L. Batchelor, 'Changing Concepts and Changing Patterns in Venereology', Lecture Notes, 21 Oct. 1963, 13–16; EPHD Annual Report (1953), 100; (1961), 144; EHSSD Annual Report (1968), 66. The first reference to the role of bisexuals in the spread of VD was in 1971 with the revealing warning that 'their reservoir effect is not restricted as a hazard to a deviant group' (EHSSD Annual Report (1971), 64).

73 See NAS, HH 57/1287, Papers relating to Wolfenden Committee 1955–7.

74 The Times, 11 Jan. 1967, reporting on the Annual Report of the Glasgow Presbytery of the Free Church of Scotland. See also Glasgow Herald, 10 May 1968.

75 Gilloran Report, op. cit. (note 46), 2.

76 British Cooperative Clinical Group, 'Homosexuality and Venereal Disease in the United Kingdom', BJVD, 49 (1973), 329–34.

77 The comparable figures for England were 45.9% and 10.5% respectively.

78 See L. Bland and F. Mort, 'Look Out for the "Good Time" Girl: Dangerous Sexualities as a Threat to National Health', in Formations of Nation and People (London: Routledge and Kegan Paul, 1984),

145.
79 *EPHD Annual Report (1952)*, 99.
80 *EPHD Annual Report (1959)*, 142–3. Robert Lees, Physician-in-
    Charge of Edinburgh's VD Services, had previously placed on record
    his view that 'coloured' male immigrants, who 'unfortunately ...
    seem[ed] to possess a great attraction for certain types of white girl',
    presented a very acute VD problem, as 'they certainly [had] not the
    moral or social training which would enable them to live as decent
    members of a civilized society' (R. Lees, 'V.D. – Some Random
    Reflections of a Venereologist', *BJVD*, 26 (1950), 162–3).
81 *Ibid.*, 143; *Scottish Daily Express*, 20 Oct. 1960, 'Sex-Shock Doctor
    Meets Grim US Men'; NAS, HH 58/66, Memo. by I. N.
    Sutherland, 31 Oct. 1960; *Scottish Daily Express,* 27 June 1963,
    'Clinic for Girls in Polaris Town'; NAS, HH 104/35, Papers relating
    to Parliamentary Question, 17 July 1963; G. C. Giarchi, *Between
    McAlpine and Polaris* (London: Routledge, 1984), 188–92; *Hansard
    [HC]* 691 (1963–4), col. 1180, 17 March 1964.
82 *Glasgow Herald,* 6 June 1975. Report of Proceedings of United Free
    Church Assembly; NHSA, Grampian Health Board Papers, DF
    5/28; Giarchi, *op. cit.* (note 81), 209.
83 See, e.g., M. Dux, 'Reclassifying the Diseased: Venereal Disease,
    Medicine and Homosexuality, 1970–1982', *Melbourne Historical
    Journal,* 25 (1997), 35–45.
84 C. G. Brown, *The People in the Pews: Religion and Society in Scotland
    since 1870* (Dundee: Economic and Social History Society of
    Scotland, 1993), 44–5.
85 *Reports to General Assembly of Free Church of Scotland (1980)*, 146.
    My emphasis.

11

'A Specialty in Crisis':
The Status and Resourcing of Venereology, 1948–80

The first circular issued to Regional Hospital Boards on the development of specialist services under the National Health Service (Scotland) Act of 1947 stipulated that 'the diagnosis and treatment of venereal diseases constitute[d] a separate clinical specialty and should not be left to become a minor interest of specialists in other fields'.[1] However, from the start, the Boards failed to recognize the specialist status of venereology in their staffing of VD clinics, and throughout the 1950s and 1960s, Scottish venereologists were faced with the erosion of their professional identity by the 'dilution' policies of their health authorities.[2]

As the reported incidence of VD declined after 1948, and the moral panic over wartime sexual behaviour dissipated, venereology was again relegated to 'Cinderella' status among the specialist health services. Within the medical profession, venereologists continued to be treated as 'outcasts' and their work as an excuse for 'ribaldry', the presence of a venereologist commonly providing 'the signal for recounting an obscene yarn or apocryphal tale' of the 'clap' or the 'pox'.[3] Venereologists continued to lack influence on the advisory committees shaping Scottish and regional health policies and resource allocations. Whereas in England and Wales, a Special Adviser in VD represented the interests of the specialty within the Ministry of Health, no such post existed at the Department of Health for Scotland [DHS], where issues relating to VD were administered as part of a wider remit by the Infectious Diseases Unit. Significantly, not one of the 150-strong Scottish Panel of Specialists for Medical Appointments nominated by the Scottish Universities, the Royal Colleges and the Scottish Secretary of State, was a consultant venereologist.[4]

Within the Regional Hospital Boards, the specialty was accorded low status and priority.[5] In part, this stemmed from its historic association with the ethos of interwar public health dispensaries. In part, it may have reflected a continuing perception of VD patients by the medical elite as 'undeserving'.[6] As one leading venereologist lamented in 1968: 'We come right down at the bottom of the list for money because the people who allocate it are still the ones who believe that those who get VD deserve to suffer a bit'.[7] It also reflected the increasing priority accorded to diseases such as diptheria, smallpox and poliomyelitis in post-war public health debate. However, it mainly stemmed from the view of medical administrators that VD no longer presented a serious health problem, given the lack of any dramatic upswing in Scottish VD rates, and the common belief that new forms of chemotherapy, often within the competence of general practitioners, rendered a large specialist clinical establishment redundant.[8]

Indeed, this was a view shared by many officials within the DHS. R. J. Peters, Deputy Chief Medical Officer, agreed with the view of the Ministry of Health in 1958 that 'there was no longer the same justification for VD specialists and that the number of consultants required would decline'.[9] In 1960, W. D. Hood, Principal Medical Officer, questioned the wisdom of David Lees' campaign for 'the continuance of venereology as a specialty *per se*', and raised serious doubts as to whether health authorities would 'ever deliberately try to raise another crop of specialists in the treatment of VD'.[10] Similarly, in 1964, I. M. Macgregor, Senior Medical Officer in the Scottish Home and Health Department [SHHD], opposed the recommendation of the *BMA Report on VD and Young People* that the staffing and resourcing of venereology should be substantially upgraded. 'I would not', he minuted, 'encourage any young doctor to take up this work as the report suggests – it is not a field which could give very much satisfaction to any physician except as a part-time interest.'[11]

As a result, Scottish venereology became chronically under-resourced in the 1950s and early 1960s. As in England and Wales, in contrast to other 'more socially and professionally acceptable specialties', there was little if any increase in the number of consultants despite a steady rise in the workload of the clinics *(see Tables 11.1 and 11.2)*.[12]

Increasingly, senior posts were left unfilled and VD sessions farmed out on a part-time basis to non-specialists and general practitioners. Thus, in Aberdeen, the North-Eastern Regional Hospital Board continued to use a consultant dermatologist to head the VD department until 1962 despite representations that 'career venereologists were essential to plan and implement preventive, diagnostic and therapeutic regimens for an ever-increasing range of sexually-transmitted infections'.[13] Moreover, the Board refused to appoint specialist registrars to training posts 'in view of the

Table 11.1:
Percentage Increase in Consultants in Scotland, 1949–59

All Specialties	28
Medicine	18
Infectious Diseases	57
TB	71
Dermatology	23
Neurology	50
Urology	29
Venereology	0

Source: BMA Archives, 2(2)15(4)14, Papers of Nicholson-Lailey Committee.

Table 11.2:
Scottish Venereology Staffing 1950–65

	Consultants		SHMOs		Senior Reg. & Reg.	
---	WT*	PT**	WT	PT	WT	PT
1950	2	4	4	2	1	–
1965	3	3	3	1	2	–

Source: Scottish Health Statistics. * Whole-time; ** Part-time

uncertainty as to the future of venereology as a specialty',[14] employing instead, on a part-time basis, a Senior Hospital Medical Officer [SHMO] in chest medicine (albeit with extensive wartime experience of VD work in the RAMC) and a SHMO in dermatology, supported increasingly by *ad hoc* assistance from general practitioners in the clinics.[15] The shortage of specialists also led to a lack of peripheral clinics for patients in other centres such as Elgin, Fraserburgh and Peterhead.[16]

Similar 'dilution' took place in the West of Scotland. The post of full-time Consultant Venereologist in Glasgow remained vacant between 1954 and 1963. Instead, the post was fragmented into minor appointments of 2–3 sessions, undertaken by a *mélange* of non-specialists including a consultant cardiologist and a public health officer, who possessed limited experience and often 'a meagre training' in venereology. Moreover, work in the treatment centres was commonly sought by clinicians in other fields of medicine that were overmanned. This lack of specialist appointments to senior posts effectively eroded the career structure and incentives for aspiring venereologists, further threatening the viability of an already ageing specialty.[17] As in Edinburgh, even when posts did become available, it became increasingly difficult to attract young, well-qualified applicants.[18] In practice, in some clinics, as the workload escalated after the mid-1960s, increasing responsibility for diagnosis and injections was placed upon the male orderlies, who were often left effectively in charge during vacation periods.[19]

The problem of staffing was further compounded by the lack of adequate training provisions for venereology and the continued use of antiquated and poorly located accommodation. As VD slipped from the agenda of Scottish health politics in the 1950s, it was increasingly marginalized within both undergraduate and post-graduate medical curricula. Outwith Edinburgh, the exposure of students to lectures and clinical training in venereology was meagre and inadequate, a situation made worse by the continued lack of integration of many clinics with the central teaching hospitals.[20] In Aberdeen and Glasgow, for example, medical students received only three lectures and four hours of clinical training. Given the lack of an appointments system at the clinics, the latter was often of dubious value. Moreover, in the absence of a consultant venereologist on the staff of the teaching hospitals, much of the teaching was undertaken, often perfunctorily, by non-specialists from dermatology, public health, and general practice.[21] Meanwhile, in many clinics, staff recruited from public health departments or from general practice to undertake sessions had access to very limited specialist training.[22]

Working conditions remained an added constraint upon recruitment to venereology in the 1950s and 1960s. Many of the Scottish VD clinics dated back to the early 'cloak and dagger days of VD' in the 1920s, 'when people slunk in basement bolt-holes to get the unspeakable disease dealt with'.[23] Their location and facilities generated an aura of moral stigma and judgementalism. VD departments continued to be 'basement-based' – located in 'unhygienic cellars, or inconvenient corners of hospitals'.[24] Equally demoralizing for medical staff and patients was the siting of many of the surviving *ad hoc* clinics, such as the Market Street clinic in Dunfermline, located in a semi-detached cottage in a cul-de-sac opposite the bus station, exposed to the unremitting gaze and censure of local inhabitants.[25] Although the BMA *Report on VD and Young People* in 1964 stressed the urgent need for the modernization of VD clinics in order to improve professional morale and to create a less stigmatic ambience for patients, little progress was achieved. Given the prevailing budgetary constraints facing health authorities and their already hard-pressed building programmes, the SHHD was unwilling to put pressure on Regional Hospital Boards to reallocate their resources.[26]

However, by the early 1970s, there was a growing crisis of public confidence, widely articulated in the national press, in the ability of the VD services to cope with the rising incidence of VD and in particular the 'newer generation' of sexually transmitted diseases. The system was reported to be at 'breaking point' due to the lack of trained venereologists.[27] According to the *Daily Mirror*, medical experts were agreed that 'Britain [was] facing the biggest crisis over the spread of VD since the war years. Too many patients are chasing too few specialists. And those few are getting fewer.'[28] As *The Sunday Times* concluded: 'If you're going to have sexual liberation, you must budget for its side effects, whether you approve or not.'[29] A 'crisis in venereology' was also declared in the medical press.[30]

At the local level, the steady erosion of staff resource in venereology since the Second World War had led in many areas to the closure of clinics, such as the clinics at the Victoria Hospital, Kirkcaldy and at Bruntsfield Hospital in Edinburgh,[31] or to an unhealthy reliance, as at the Royal Infirmary of Edinburgh, on general practitioner sessions.[32] Meanwhile, clinical workloads were rising dramatically, with gonorrhoea becoming 'the most common infectious disease among persons past the age of puberty'.[33] Not only was there a marked rise in the number of cases.[34] An increasing amount of time had to be spent on patients with non-specific and other refractory infections such as trichonomas vaginalis, vaginitis and candidiasis. The problems of staff resourcing were further increased by seasonal fluctuations in the incidence of STDs and random surges in demand occasioned by TV programmes highlighting the issue.[35]

In-patient and laboratory facilities were also under-resourced. Thus, at the Royal Infirmary of Edinburgh, there was a lack of beds dedicated to the treatment of 'difficult cases of venereal disease'. An *ad hoc* committee reported that 'the patients [were] often young people, social misfits and psychologically disturbed and ... [were] sharing wards with geriatric patients and overflow patients from medical wards'.[36] At the same time, the laboratory service appeared 'to be inadequate in terms of the range of tests done and uneconomical in that clinical staff [were] engaged in microscopy of exodate smears and other "side room" tests when they could [have

263

been] devoting the time to clinical work'.[37] Constraints on the range and frequency of serological testing were also a feature of other Scottish VD centres.[38]

By 1970, the pressure of events was making the comparatively *laissez-faire* stance of the SHHD towards VD policy increasingly difficult to sustain. The media campaign surrounding VD, coupled with new publicity initiatives by the Ministry of Health and the upward convergence of Scottish VD trends with those elsewhere in the UK, precipitated a renewed demand, especially from some leading venereologists and from the Department's Consultative Committee of Medical Officers of Health, for a fresh appraisal of VD services and procedures in Scotland. As a result, a Joint Sub-Committee on Sexually Transmitted Diseases (the Gilloran Committee) was appointed in 1971 to advise on a wide range of issues relating to the epidemiology, treatment and control of VD in Scotland.

In its subsequent report,[39] the Gilloran Committee recommended 'the expansion of all services concerned with the management of sexually transmitted diseases'. Although some additional consultant posts had been established in response to a review of the medical staffing structure in Scottish hospitals in 1963,[40] the Committee considered that the specialist establishment was inadequate to provide a comprehensive venereology service in Scotland. In the light of the dramatic upswing in the incidence of sexually transmitted diseases in Scotland since 1965, it identified an urgent need 'for a new consultant establishment to be defined'. It recommended that even where additional consultant posts could not immediately be filled, they should be created in order to provide an incentive for doctors in the training grades and generally to enhance the appeal of the specialty. The Committee recognized the need to employ staff in training and general practitioners to carry out some of the clinic work, but was fundamentally opposed to the more aggressive dilution policies of some Regional Hospital Boards. In its view, 'as in other clinical specialties, the care of patients with sexually transmitted diseases should be the responsibility of a consultant' and all special clinics should be supervised by a consultant.

The Gilloran Committee also made wide-ranging proposals with regard to staff training. It recommended that instruction in sexual problems and STDs should be provided for all medical undergraduates and that, in order to up-grade postgraduate training facilities, rotation posts in the specialty should be made available to junior hospital medical staff. In addition to postgraduate courses in STDs for all general practitioners, there was also an urgent need for more substantial vocational training for those undertaking sessional work in the specialty. The Committee called for a substantial upgrading in the STD training of nurses and for the introduction of special in-service training for contact tracers. There was also a need to ensure that the equipment and premises of the special clinics were comparable to those of other clinical specialties, and that the services of microbiological technicians were available for diagnostic work, wherever possible. In addition, the Committee recommended that *ad hoc* clinics should be phased out and in future integrated within the out-patient departments of the district general hospitals.

The Gilloran Report, coming as it did in the middle of a period of severe financial restraint and a major reorganization of the National Health Services, received a dismissive response from the new Area Health Boards. They were prepared neither to commit new resources to the VD services nor, as the SHHD tentatively and somewhat disingenuously suggested, to reallocate their existing health budgets in order to try and eliminate some of the future medical costs of STDs. While they acknowledged that a shortage of specialists existed, they remained unconvinced of the case for comprehensive consultant cover.[41]

Scottish venereologists viewed this response as part of a broader neglect by the Health Boards of the importance of the problem and of the role of the specialty within the health services. Accordingly, in the late 1970s, in an effort to obtain urgent action on the Gilloran Report, the Scottish Branch of the Medical Society for the Study of Venereal Diseases [MSSVD] made vigorous representations to the Specialty Sub-Committee for Medicine of the National Medical Consultative Committee. In addition, in what was admitted by the SHHD to be a 'critical and rather disturbing report', D. H. H. Robertson, Consultant Venereologist at the Royal Infirmary of Edinburgh, sought to expose what he regarded as a systemic under-resourcing of the Scottish STD services.[42] Gross inadequacies were revealed in the recruitment and training of medical, nursing, technical and social work staff, including contact tracers. The Specialty Sub-Committee was critical of the lack of progress in implementing the Gilloran Report and urged the SHHD to press the Scottish Area Health Boards to give greater priority to the STD services in their resource allocations. However, given the continued public expenditure cuts, the Department remained reluctant to press the issue, although it did request the Health Boards in 1978 to review their provisions.[43]

Yet, clear evidence remained of an urgent need to upgrade STD facilities in many areas of Scotland. The process of integrating *ad hoc* clinics into regional general hospitals was laboured and incomplete and some consultants still had to work 'in old, decaying, isolated premises', which, as with Black Street Clinic in Glasgow, continued to attract considerable stigma.[44] As the report of Glasgow's Department of STDs stressed in 1978, the retention of such clinics was 'an anachronism' as they took 'no account of the changed pattern of infection or in the public attitudes to such diseases'.[45]

In addition, there continued to be serious gaps in the consultant establishment of the service. Thus, although in principle six consultant posts had been agreed for the Glasgow Area, in 1982 there were still only four consultants serving a population of three million people.[46] The situation was also critical in Grampian and Tayside.[47] In 1982, the consultant venereologist for Tayside reported that: 'He had been trying for four years to get further staff but to no avail. He had to run male and female clinics, do his own slide work and teach students single-handedly, and he also had to attend the clinic at Perth. He had, in addition, the administrative work of the clinic to do.'[48] He had no laboratory or clerical assistance and no contact tracer. Similarly, in Aberdeen in the late 1970s, there was still an urgent need for a second consultant appointment. In addition, despite the recommendation of the Gilloran Report that all STD clinics should have a qualified microbiological technician, technical support at the Aberdeen clinic was 'minimal', and it remained 'entirely dependent on a self-trained technician' for the preparation and interpretation of slides.[49] Even in Edinburgh, the quality of diagnosis, treatment and follow-up was seriously constrained by the lack of clinical and support staff.[50]

Moreover, training in STDs was still fragmentary in many areas of Scotland. In the late 1970s, medical students in Dundee had no regular clinical training in STDs. The situation in Glasgow had actually regressed. In contrast to Edinburgh, liaison between the STD Department and the University Medical Faculty in Glasgow was poor. Formerly, students had received a clinical lecture at the STD ward at Belvidere Hospital, but when the ward closed, attempts to negotiate a new clinical component in STD proved abortive.[51] Even in Edinburgh, lecture time devoted to STDs was minimal and the statutory attendance at one session of a male and female clinic still meant that 'most medical students graduate[d] without ever having taken a sexual history ... or examined a patient who may have acquired an STD'. As a result, most were largely ignorant of venereology as a specialty.[52]

In-house training for nurses in STDs was equally lacking.[53] The location of many treatment centres in *ad hoc* clinics had served to isolate the mainstream nursing profession from the specialty and to inhibit any perception of it as a career option.[54] Nursing and midwifery administrators regarded the recommendations of the Gilloran Report for post-basic training courses in STDs as 'extravagant'.[55] Moreover, one traditional source of supply, the nurse-technicians, who had received their training in the armed forces, had virtually disappeared as the forces ceased to undertake STD work on their own account.[56]

Thus, although STDs figured prominently in the moral panic surrounding sexual permissiveness in the late 1960s and 1970s, venereology as a specialty continued to struggle for professional status and identity. In some ways, it was a vicious circle. Poor resourcing led to poor morale and career prospects and a chronic shortage of new recruits, which in turn reinforced the dilution mentality of the Health Boards. As *The Listener* observed in 1971: 'The field is not inherently very attractive and the fate of the chest physician robbed of pulmonary tuberculosis discourages the young doctor from committing his professional career to so narrow a field'. Physicians still tended to view venereology as 'a dirty, unpleasant subject beneath their notice' and unworthy of their skills as 'members of the Senior Service of Medicine'.[57] At best, it was regarded as a specialty to which clinicians gravitated by default after promotion had eluded them in other medical fields such as obstetrics or gynaecology.[58] The media also attached a moral dimension to the recruitment crisis in venereology, arguing that many doctors displayed 'the ingrained puritanism' of their quintessentially middle-class upbringings and disapproved of the promiscuous lifestyles of those contracting VD. Moreover, venereology, it was argued, was not a specialty that their wives wished their husbands to espouse.[59]

But the continuing problems of venereology also lay in its institutional weakness. It lacked clout and credibility as a distinct specialty among the Scottish medical establishment and senior health administrators.[60] Despite the best efforts of the Scottish Branch of the MSSVD, it failed to secure for Scottish venereology representation on medical committees at all levels, including the National Medical Consultative Committee, or even permission to establish a specialty sub-committee for advisory purposes.[61] Whatever the broader social implications of a rising incidence of STD, within the SHHD there were growing reservations as to how far it was desirable to resource a distinct STD consultant establishment given what it perceived to be the relatively trivial nature of the day-to-day running of a clinic. As one medical official remarked in 1979, an emerging view on the

Consultative Committee was 'that venereology as a specialty was probably not viable as a separate entity and *it may be that this view is correct*'.[62]

Notes

1 National Archives of Scotland [NAS], HH 48/65/007, Department of Health for Scotland [DHS] Circulars, 1947.

2 British Medical Association [BMA] Archive, Minutes of Venereologists Group Committee, 26 Oct. 1948, 28 Jan. 1949, 26 Feb. 1953, 29 Nov. 1957, 26 June 1959.

3 A. S. Wigfield, 'The Emergence of the Consultant Venereologist', *British Journal of Venereal Diseases [BJVD]*, 48 (1972), 550; R. Lees, 'Some Random Reflections of a Venereologist', *BJVD*, 26 (1950), 157.

4 NAS, HH 104/35/84, Minute W. Bain, 21 Dec. 1965.

5 This was duly reflected in the very low incidence of venereologists holding distinction awards. See *Scottish Health Statistics*.

6 D. H. H. Robertson, 'Venereal Diseases', *Synapse: Journal of the Edinburgh Medical School*, 21, no. 3 (1972), 38; Interview with consultant venereologist, 9 April 1997.

7 *The Observer*, 18 Feb. 1968.

8 See, e.g., NAS, HH 65/128/9, Venereal Diseases: Staffing of VD Clinics, Minutes of Senior Administrative Medical Officers [SAMO] Committee, 20 March 1958. In 1958, the main out-patient area for VD at the Royal Infirmary of Edinburgh [RIE] had been 'given up when it was believed that the level of VD appeared to be diminishing and when venereologists were fearful for their future!' (Robertson, *op. cit.* (note 6), 27). For an analysis and spirited critique of regional hospital board staffing policy in England and Wales, see *The Lancet*, Vol. I (1958), 651–7, 962, 1073, 1127, 1177, 1229.

9 NAS, HH 65/128/9, Minutes of SAMO Committee, 20 March 1958.

10 NAS, HH 58/66, Minute W. D. Hood, 6 Oct. 1960.

11 NAS, HH 104/35/39, Minute I. M. Macgregor, 14 July 1964.

12 For contemporary press coverage of the shortage of specialists nationwide, see *Daily Mirror*, 27 Oct. 1961, 'More VD – but few experts to fight it'. In 1955, while the ratio of consultants to Senior Hospital Medical Officers [SHMOs] in all the specialist services in the UK was 73.5%, in venereology it was only 54.1% (*Lancet*, Vol. 1 (1958), 656).

13 I. Levack and H. Dudley, *Aberdeen Royal Infirmary: The People's Hospital of the North-East* (London: Bailliere Tindall, 1992), 123.

14 The lack of 'attractive training posts' and its repercussions for 'the

image of the specialty' was also an issue in Edinburgh (Lothian
Health Services Archives [LHSA], LHB1/61/39/3, Report of Ad
Hoc Committee on Venereology, 17 June 1971).

15 Northern Health Services Archives [NHSA], North-Eastern Regional
Hospital Board [N-ERHB] Minutes, 25 July 1950, 7 Nov. 1956, 8
July 1958; Admin. Files, 22/1, Film A 20, BMA to SAMO, 9 Feb.
1961; NAS, HH 65/128/9, Minutes of SAMO Committee, 20
March 1958; BMA Archive, BMA Venereologists Group
Committee, 29 Nov. 1957, Memo. by David Lees on 'Staffing of
VD Clinics: Scotland'.

16 NHSA, N-ERHB Admin. File 22/1, Film 29, SAMO to DHS, 1
Feb. 1952.

17 *Glasgow Medical Officer of Health [MOH] Annual Report (1952)*, 12;
(1954), 120; BMA Archive, Minutes of Venereologists Group
Committee, 29 Nov. 1957, 26 Nov. 1960, 30 Nov. 1962; *Lancet*, 29
March 1958, 656.

18 *BJVD*, 42 (1966), 224, Editorial; LHSA, LHB1/80/174,
Correspondence on Staffing Requirements: Venereal Diseases, RIE,
1968–74.

19 Interview with consultant venereologist, 9 April 1997.

20 *Lancet*, Vol. I (1958), 656.

21 BMA Archive, Minutes of Venereologists Group Committee, 26
June 1959, 26 Nov. 1960; NHSA, N-ERHB Minutes, 8 July 1958.

22 Interview with consultant venereologist, 9 April 1997; Interview
with former general practitioner involved in VD work, 7 April 1997.

23 Robertson, *op. cit.* (note 6), 28–9.

24 *The Observer*, 10 May 1970; R. Lees, *op. cit.* (note 3), 157.

25 Interview with former consultant venereologist, 21 June 1995.

26 NAS, HH 104/35/39, Minute A. F. Reid, 2 June 1964.

27 See, e.g., *Glasgow Herald*, 3 Oct. 1972. One consultant venereologist
was quoted as describing medical provisions as 'utterly inadequate',
reflecting the low priority accorded to STDs within health politics
compared with other diseases.

28 *Daily Mirror*, 31 March 1970.

29 *Sunday Times*, 9 Aug. 1970.

30 See especially, R. D. Catherall and R. S. Morton, 'Crisis in
Venereology', *British Medical Journal [BMJ]*, Vol. III, 1970,
699–702.

31 Staff shortages were also in part responsible for the closure of the
Seamen's Dispensary at Leith in 1968 (LHSA, Pamphlet Box FS-
GR, L. Scarth, 'Notes on VD Out-Patient Clinics' (1971), 2).

32 *Edinburgh Health and Social Services Department [EHSSD] Annual*

Report (1971), 64; LHSA, LHB 1/80/174, Memo. by D. H. H. Robertson, 11 March 1971. In 1971, at RIE, the Medical Assistant, the Registrar and the Senior House Officer posts remained vacant 'for lack of suitable applicants' and the funds for their salaries were used to pay for 22 sessions by general practitioners and others (Robertson, *op. cit.* (note 6), 29).

33 *Glasgow Herald,* 22 Oct 1971. In some instances, it was claimed that the 'pressure of service work' had 'brought research to a halt' (LHSA, LHB 1/61/39/3, Report of Ad Hoc Committee on Venereology, 17 June 1971).

34 The VD Department at RIE experienced a 30% rise in its case-load over the period 1965–70 (*ibid.*).

35 *EHSSD Annual Report (1970),* 56; LHSA, LHB 1/81/228, Report of RIE VD Department (1973), 6.

36 LHSA, LHB 1/61/39/3, Report of Ad Hoc Committee on Venereology, 17 June 1971. There was increasing demand for in-patient facilities to provide intensive treatment for cases with resistant strains of gonorrhoea (Robertson, *op. cit.* (note 6), 30).

37 LHSA, LHB 1/61/39/3, Report of Ad Hoc Committee on Venereology, 17 June 1971.

38 NHSA, N-ERHB Admin. File 22/1, Film A20, correspondence between Aberdeen City Hospital Laboratory and Consultant Venereologist, Woolmanhill, 23 June 1960.

39 *Report of Joint Sub-Committee on Sexually Transmitted Diseases* (Edinburgh: HMSO, 1973).

40 *Report on Medical Staffing Structure in Scottish Hospitals* (Edinburgh: HMSO, 1964).

41 NAS, HH 104/36/136, Correspondence and Papers relating to the Gilloran Report. Thus, the Services, Planning and Resources Committee of Grampian Health Board considered that the recommendations of the Gilloran Report were 'to a very large extent' met by existing services and that no increase in staffing was justified (NHSA, Grampian Health Board Admin. File 22/1, Part IIIA: Correspondence on Gilloran Report, 13 May 1974).

42 Medical Society for the Study of Venereal Diseases Scottish Branch [MSSVDSB] Minutes, 5 May 1979, 6 Oct. 1979; NAS, HH 104/36, Memorandum by D. H. H. Robertson, June 1977, 'Sexually Transmitted Disease Facilities in Scotland'.

43 NAS, HH 104/36/136, Minutes of meeting of National Medical Consultative Committee, Specialty Sub-Committee for Medicine, 15 Sept. 1977; Minutes of Department of Health and Social Security Policy Group, 19 Jan. 1978.

44 NAS, HH 104/36/199, Sexually Transmitted Diseases: Information from Health Boards, 25 April 1979; *Glasgow Herald*, 23 Nov. 1978.

45 *Ibid.*

46 MSSVDSB, Papers, Draft letter to Secretary of State for Scotland, 8 May 1982.

47 *Ibid.*, Minutes, 2 Oct. 1981; D. H. H. Robertson, 'Sexually Transmitted Diseases: Notes on Facilities in Scotland', 9 April 1984.

48 MSSVDSB Minutes, 8 May 1982.

49 NHSA, Grampian Health Board Admin. File 22/1, Pt IV: VD Arrangements 1977–81, H. G. Robinson to W. B. Howie, 30 Nov. 1978; Memorandum by Chief Administrative Medical Officer [CAMO] on Clinic for Sexually Transmitted Diseases, 31 May 1979.

50 LHSA, LHB 1/81/228, D. H. H. Robertson, Report on 'RIE, Department of Genito-Urinary Medicine: Sexually Transmitted Diseases, Part 1: The Present Problem' (1983).

51 NAS, HH 104/36, Memorandum by Robertson, *op. cit.* (note 42), 6, appendix 4.

52 LHSA, LHB 1/81/228, Robertson, Report, *op. cit.* (note 50); MSSVDSB Minutes, 6 Oct. 1979. See also Schofield, *Sexually Transmitted Diseases* (Edinburgh: Churchill Livingstone, 2nd edition 1975), 26.

53 See especially, MSSVDSB Minutes, 17 May 1980.

54 Greater Glasgow Health Board Archive, HH 55/T88 Chief Area Nursing Officer's [CANO] Files, Policy and Planning Committee Paper V4/7, 'Sexually Transmitted Diseases', 6 May 1974. The Board for Clinical Nursing Studies did not recognize work in a VD clinic as 'a suitable area for training purposes' (NHSA, Grampian Health Board Admin. File 22/1, Part IIIA: VD Arrangements 1974–6, Note by CANO, 24 March 1974).

55 See, e.g., *ibid.*, Minutes of Nursing and Midwifery Committee, 6 June 1974.

56 NAS, HH 104/36/199, Sexually Transmitted Diseases: Information from Health Boards, 25 April 1979.

57 *The Listener*, 28 Oct. 1971.

58 Interview with former general practitioner involved in VD work, 7 April 1997.

59 *Sunday Times*, 9 Aug. 1970; *BJVD*, 'Correspondence: The Future of Venereology', 52 (1976), 208. In 1972, on average, only 1.7 applications were received for every consultant's post in the UK (*Guardian*, 3 July 1972).

60 Thus, in 1979, Grampian Area Medical Committee was determined that venereology should be integrated with other clinical services

(NHSA, Grampian Health Board Admin. File 22/1, Pt IV: VD
Arrangements 1977–81, G. Innes to G. Stone, 11 Dec. 1979).
61 NAS, HH 104/36; MSSVDSB Papers, Draft letter to Secretary of
State for Scotland, 8 May 1982.
62 NAS, HH 104/36/199, Memorandum by G. Gilray, 25 April 1979.
His emphasis. The identity of venereology as a specialty was also
eroded by the decision of Whitehall in the 1970s to try and create a
less stigmatic and more socially acceptable image for VD and STD
work as 'Genito-Urinary Medicine'. See, A. J. King, 'The Future of
Venereology', *BJVD*, 52 (1976), 208.

12

'Breaking the Chain of Infection': Treatment and Control Strategies 1948–80

Legal Compulsion

The issue of legal controls for regulating sexual contacts and defaulters continued to surface in the reports of Scottish VD medical officers in the late 1940s and early 1950s, with active support from the Scottish Council for Health Education [SCHE].[1] In the 1960s, prompted by the rising incidence of gonorrhoea and non-specific STDs, the debate was re-opened in the *Lancet* and in the House of Commons.[2] As late as 1968, Sir Myer Galpern, MP for Glasgow Shettleston, sought to introduce a bill 'to provide for the compulsory examination and treatment of persons suspected of suffering from venereal diseases by the restoration of provisions similar to those formerly contained in Defence Regulation 33B'.[3]

Particular attention was drawn to the variety of VD controls operating in other European and Commonwealth countries. Thus, in post-war Sweden, the transmission of VD or sexual behaviour likely to expose others to a venereal infection was an offence and treatment was compulsory for all patients. In Italy, all contagious cases of VD were notifiable. In France, persons suspected of communicating VD were compelled by health authorities to undergo medical examination. In New Zealand, those infected were by law required to undergo treatment, while in Canada, it was the duty of medical practitioners to notify VD cases and to secure their isolation and appropriate treatment if contagious.[4]

However, the Ministry of Health, the Department of Health for Scotland [DHS], and its successor from 1962, the Scottish Home and Health Department [SHHD] remained opposed to new legislation. In their view, the traditional arguments against legal controls still held good. They considered that the operation of Defence Regulation 33B had not demonstrated the value of compulsion and that the reintroduction of similar powers would merely undermine the confidence of patients and contacts in existing voluntary tracing procedures. It was feared that patients, especially homosexual patients already in fear of the law, would be deterred from obtaining prompt and professional treatment. Concern was also

273

expressed that it would revive an informer system with the danger of blackmail and with 'totalitarian' implications that were inimical to civil liberties, especially those of young women.[5] Moreover, by the late 1960s, a new generation of Scottish venereologists were in post who broadly rejected legal compulsion as a control strategy for VD. They viewed it as 'panic legislation' that would prove inoperable in a society where casual sex was increasingly prevalent and a 'target group of "culpable" vectors' no longer so clearly identifiable. They also feared that such proposals would divert attention from the fundamental need for more adequate medical resources.[6]

Yet, significant strands of socio-medical control did persist in post-war Scottish VD administration. During the 1950s, Scottish venereologists such as Robert Lees campaigned for comprehensive screening for VD on lines analogous to contemporary mass radiography for TB. They echoed the views of the Chief Medical Officer of the Ministry of Health that the application of penicillin to a wide variety of non-syphilitic conditions had masked significant pools of hidden infection and that routine serological testing should be undertaken of hospital in-patients and out-patients, of candidates for insurance, and of personnel demobilized from the Services.[7] As in England, such proposals encountered opposition on the grounds that they would infringe civil liberties and the medical confidentiality so central to public confidence in any VD service.[8]

At the same time, there were particular groups of female vectors within Scottish society whom venereologists and health officials sought to regulate in the interests of public health; namely infected pregnant women, convicted prostitutes, and so-called 'moral delinquents'. In order to combat the stubborn persistence of congenital syphilis in the community, the major Scottish health authorities had all introduced routine ante-natal VD testing by the 1960s, with long-term surveillance of women found to be infected.[9] In addition, there is evidence that, in Edinburgh at least, with the encouragement of epidemiologists, wider screening and prevalence testing was done from the late 1950s employing information from the Blood Transfusion Service, a procedure rejected in England.

There was also a continuing anxiety to ensure that prostitutes were adequately treated. R. C. L. Batchelor, Physician-in-Charge of Edinburgh's VD Services, had considerable sympathy with the prophylactoria of interwar Russia in which prostitutes were institutionalized for treatment and moral rehabilitation.[10] Along with other clinicians whose ideology was shaped by pre-war eugenics and the Social Hygiene Movement, he continued to identify promiscuity and prostitution with mental deficiency and to advocate the notification and confinement of 'moral defectives' for the purposes of reducing the reservoir of infection within the community.[11] His successor, Robert Lees, also advocated a more vigorous policy towards prostitution in the interests of social hygiene, observing to the Medical Society for the Study of Venereal Diseases that:

> The problem of prostitution is not insoluble and toleration is the reason for its flourishing. It has been attacked on moral and religious grounds, and even on economic grounds without much effect. If it is tackled as a public health problem and every painted street-corner wench is recognised as a carrier of disease rather than as an unfortunate victim of society, then the 'racket' can be broken.[12]

In his view, police authorities, clinic social workers and prison medical officers should liaise in order to ensure the detention and intensive treatment of prostitutes.

In contrast, to the disappointment of many leading venereologists, the proceedings and debates surrounding the *Wolfenden Report on Homosexual Offences and Prostitution* focused almost exclusively on issues of 'public order and decency' rather than public health, and reference to VD was notably absent.[13] The Committee favoured the Scottish law on street offences and solicitation and recommended that the Scottish practice of referring girls cautioned for prostitution to a 'moral welfare worker' be extended to England.[14] It also recommended that young prostitutes be automatically remanded for social and medical reports.[15]

In fact, it was already common practice in Scotland for 'habitual prostitutes' appearing before the courts to be remanded in custody for medical examination under Section 26 of the 1948 Criminal Justice Act. Indeed, public health officials and clinicians were concerned that, by driving prostitutes from the streets and reducing their contact with the law, fresh legislation might actively impair such efforts to monitor the sexual health of this 'reservoir of venereal disease'.[16] However, the Scottish Law Officers subsequently ruled that such powers had been intended as an aid to sentencing and not infectious disease prevention and could not be used purely as a public health measure.[17] In some Scottish cities, all women convicted of prostitution continued to be referred to the VD clinics, irrespective of whether they had any symptoms.[18] However, as the focus of epidemiological debate surrounding VD/STDs shifted in the 1960s and 1970s from prostitution to the effects of greater sexual permissiveness within society, calls for the closer regulation of prostitution on public health grounds became less strident.

Meanwhile, the regulation of the sexual behaviour of 'problem girls' that had so exercised health officials and clinicians in inter-war Scotland remained an integral part of VD/STD administration after the Second World War. Prior to the 1970s, girls committed to remand homes and approved schools under the Children and Young Persons (Scotland) Act of 1937 were routinely examined for VD/STDs on their first admission and on any readmission after absconding or after returning from a holiday or home visit.[19] Whereas young persons of either sex might be brought to the juvenile courts for suspected promiscuity, in practice it was girls deemed to be promiscuous or 'falling into bad associations or exposed to moral danger' who were targeted and referred to the clinics.[20] In the late 1960s, some 56 per cent of female patients under eighteen years of age attending the Edinburgh clinic were referred by approved schools and remand homes, and about 9 per cent of the work of the clinic was devoted to ensuring 'that adolescent girls committed to custodial institutions [were] free from sexually transmitted infections' and to ensuring 'continued medical care in promiscuous girls'.[21] Evidence would suggest that, while physical compulsion was never contemplated, formal permission was rarely sought from the girls for vaginal examinations as they were perceived as 'rebellious and unco-operative' and 'impervious to argument' as to the medical risks of their sexual behaviour.[22]

However, by the late 1960s, there was growing unease amongst Scottish venereologists; firstly, that it was 'possible for a group of girls to be continuously segregated because of sexual behaviour which [was] not in itself punishable in other persons', and secondly, that the medical expertise of venereologists was being deployed as part of coercive procedures of social work departments designed to control juvenile promiscuity.[23] The recommendation of the Latey Committee on the Age of Majority that the age of consent for medical treatment should be lowered to sixteen, coupled with the introduction of children's panels under the Social Work (Scotland) Act (1968), altered the situation. Girls might still be subject to supervision orders and residential care for moral offences and sexual promiscuity but the VD services were no longer an integral part of such procedures. Thus, by 1977, only 5 per cent of referrals to the Edinburgh clinic for females under eighteen were from the assessment centres.[24]

For the most part, post-war Scottish VD administration did not rely on compulsion but on the traditional strategies of voluntary medical treatment, health education, and a developing system of contact tracing.

Diagnosis and Treatment

The late 1940s and 1950s witnessed dramatic changes in the treatment of VD in Scotland with penicillin as the central therapy. It was initially introduced for the treatment of civilian cases in the autumn of 1944 and its use rose dramatically thereafter. Thus, during the course of 1945, the allocation of penicillin to the VD Department of the Royal Infirmary of Edinburgh rose from thirteen to 150 million units a month.[25] As with the introduction of Salvarsan earlier in the century, penicillin was initially received with some caution by clinicians. For several years, its use for early contagious syphilis continued to be supplemented by courses of arsenic and bismuth, in part to prolong the treponemicidal activity of the therapy, and in part as a means of impressing upon patients the seriousness of the disease.[26] There were also marked variations between treatment centres in the duration and intensity of dosages administered.[27] Nonetheless, by the mid-1950s, significant advances had been made in the development of 'prolonged action' preparations such as PAM [procaine penicillin suspended in arachis oil with aluminium monostearate] which enabled speedy, cost-effective, out-patient treatment for early syphilis with a comparatively low incidence of toxic side-effects. The impact of penicillin on the incidence of acute syphilis was such that the clinics might 'operate for months without seeing a single chancre'.[28] According to R. C. L. Batchelor, 'the foundations of the old syphilo-therapy [were] rocking under the impact of PAM' and 'the vision' of 'a one-shot cure for syphilis' had 'taken definite shape'. As he enthused in 1954:

> all this goes to show that 'Ehrlich's silver bullet, his therapia magna sterilans' which would wipe out syphilis at one blow, if not actually in our hands is at any rate very nearly within reach.[29]

The treatment of other forms of syphilis was also radically improved by the introduction of penicillin chemotherapy. It proved 'infallible' in protecting the foetus of pregnant syphilitic mothers from the disease.[30] In cases of tertiary syphilis, such as general paresis or tabes, penicillin also became the keystone of treatment, but in conjunction with more conventional preparations of bismuth and iodide and a continued use of fever therapy, albeit with a less drastic frequency of 'rigors'. Malarial therapy for neurosyphilis was still being employed by the Western and Northern Regional Hospital Boards as late as

1959.[31] Elsewhere, it had been gradually abandoned in favour of intensive penicillin therapy, although pyrexial treatment using the inductotherm was still employed in resistant cases of GPI.[32]

The late 1940s and 1950s witnessed a similar transformation in the treatment of gonorrhoea. In the early 1940s, although less toxic derivatives of the sulphonamides had become available, the proportion of failures and relapses had steadily increased, with disturbing evidence of the emergence of resistant strains of gonococci.[33] As a result, after 1944, sulphonamides were quickly abandoned in favour of penicillin, which was then '95–98 per cent effective, cheap, quick in action (twelve to twenty-four hours) with few immediate or delayed reactions'.[34] By 1950, one single injection of PAM was confirmed as the standard treatment for cases of uncomplicated gonorrhoea in men, women receiving a higher dosage as typically they sought treatment at a later stage of the disease when it was more intractable.[35] More complicated cases, with conditions such as epididymitis or salpingitis, hitherto addressed with the imprecise and often dangerous technology of fever cabinet therapy, were increasingly treated with multiple injections of aqueous penicillin.[36] However, periodic instrumental dilation had to be retained for the many victims of the 'old discredited and discarded syringings' who still suffered acutely from its 'dreaded sequel' – stricture of the urethra.[37]

Trials also took place of penicillin compounds for oral use for gonorrhoea. In general, this was resisted by venereologists on the grounds that patients would not administer the drugs properly and that injections enabled the clinician to monitor patients more effectively. Evidence suggested that, where oral therapy was employed, patients were more prone to cease their medication prematurely, to 'share their supply of the drug with their sexual partner', or to keep some of the drug 'for the next time'.[38] It was common knowledge that antibiotic tablets became an alternative form of currency in some dock areas.[39]

Despite the dramatic advances in venereology in post-war Scotland, there remained significant technical, institutional and cultural constraints on the ability of new forms of chemotherapy to contain the incidence of VD/STDs. As in the interwar period, the quality of treatment varied markedly between regions and between urban and rural areas. In the more remote areas of the borders and the Highlands and Islands, the bulk of treatment continued to be undertaken by family practitioners with a predictable focus on male cases. Contact tracing was rarely undertaken and a significant amount of asymptomatic female infection, especially gonorrhoea, remained undetected. Take-up of the more modern clinic facilities by patients living outwith the major cities was also inhibited by the process of local authority means-testing of travel expenses which operated in Scotland, which was thought to undermine the confidentiality of treatment.[40]

Another important constraint was the continuing lack of standardization and quality control in diagnostic techniques. Treatment centres employed a 'bewildering variety' of reagin tests for syphilis, using either 'home-made' antigens or those obtained from a number of commercial sources. Given the difference of opinion within the specialty over the relative merits of the newer flocculation and complement fixation tests and the limited resources of some of the smaller laboratories, official guidelines tended to cater for 'simplicity in procedures' rather than optimum standards, a weakness reinforced, it was claimed, by the lack of a separate reference laboratory in Scotland.[41] Efforts to counter the rising incidence of gonorrhoea were also constrained by weaknesses in diagnostic procedures. In the early 1960s, even the best laboratory examinations missed about 20 per cent of female infections.[42] The bacteriological diagnosis of gonorrhoea was often impaired by the 'indifferent collection' of specimens by general practitioners, by delays in their delivery to central laboratories, or by the reliance of clinicians on the routine application of complement fixation tests rather than on the isolation of the organism by cultural methods.[43] Moreover, a shortage of laboratory facilities regularly forced VD clinicians to undertake their own diagnostic tests 'in-house', for which they were often ill-equipped and ill-qualified.

A third area of constraint was the limited impact of penicillin and other antibiotics such as streptomycin upon the non-specific and trichonomal infections such as non-specific urethritis [NSU] in men and trichonomas vaginalis in women, which came increasingly to occupy the attention of the treatment centres. Despite extensive trials of new drugs, very little real advance was made in the 1950s, a problem compounded by the tendency of general practitioners to frustrate effective diagnosis by the premature and promiscuous use of penicillin 'just to be on the safe side'.[44] In the early 1960s, pioneering research by venereologists at the Royal Infirmary of Edinburgh facilitated the introduction of metronidazole (Flagyl), an effective specific drug for trichonomas vaginalis, and identified more clearly its linkages with NSU in male patients.[45] In addition, the major laboratories had significantly improved their diagnosis of the infection by implementing cultural as well as microscopic procedures for all specimens submitted to them by the clinics and general practitioners.[46]

However, unless such technical advances were accompanied by the continued investigation of sexual partners, there was a systemic problem of 'repeated mutual reinfestation'. Equally serious was the widespread coexistence of trichonomal infection and gonorrhoea in female patients. Treatment often eliminated the former while masking latent gonococcal infection which remained undetected until either a consort became infected or complications ensued.[47] Moreover, although many cases of NSU did respond to treatment with broad-spectrum antibiotics, and diagnostic procedures for acute cases of urethritis were improved,[48] a specific remedy for NSU continued to elude clinicians. Meanwhile, fever therapy, using either the inductotherm cabinet or the injection of a special TAB vaccine, remained a common treatment for complicated cases, such as those displaying symptoms of Reiters disease, into the 1960s.[49] Thereafter, the use of new drugs for NSU such as tetracyclines did obtain better results but levels of relapse remained high, constituting some 40 per cent of male NSU cases in Edinburgh in 1972.[50]

A further significant factor in inhibiting the success of treatment as a control strategy was the development of resistant strains of gonococci coupled with continuingly high levels of default *(see Figure 11.1)*. As early as 1952, R. C. L. Batchelor drew attention to the possible links between the arrest of the declining incidence of gonorrhoea and the emergence of resistant strains. He lamented that:

> In present-day medical practice penicillin is commonly given for all sorts of ailments .... The danger of its promiscuous use producing penicillin-resistant types of bacteria has long been foreseen and feared, and now this deplorable denouement may actually have arrived.[51]

The problem was compounded by the 'familiarity and scant respect' paid to gonorrhoea – the 'one-shot mentality' that encouraged patients to refuse further tests and treatment once the initial symptoms had diminished, leaving many such defaulters as asymptomatic carriers of partially resistant strains.[52]

In fact, the evidence on the sensitivity of gonorrhoea to penicillin and other antibiotics in Scotland was far from clear-cut. In Glasgow, the proportion of resistant strains appeared to be fairly stable, although the degree of resistance of such strains became more acute.[53] The Department of Health for Scotland [DHS] assured the public that available antibiotics were more than sufficient to cope with the problem and were privately of the opinion that Edinburgh venereologists were exaggerating the issue in order to secure resources and more public recognition for their specialty.[54] Nonetheless, there was growing concern at the implications for disease control, and throughout the 1960s, the major VD departments in Scotland strove to develop a single-injection, high-dosage, long-acting preparation for gonorrhoea that would both combat resistant strains and eliminate the effects of default on VD administration.[55]

Such efforts were undoubtedly restricted by lack of research funding, in part a function of general financial constraints, but also a reflection of the low status of venereology and of contemporary professional concerns over the likely impact of easier cures or preventive vaccines on sexual promiscuity. As a number of medical researchers and journalists pointed out, 'moralistic attitudes still prevail[ed] to some extent in the medical establishment', which did not universally welcome new methods of treatment and was not 'whole-hearted in its desire to eliminate the disease [VD]'.[56]

In the event, the medical innovations of the 1940s and 1950s

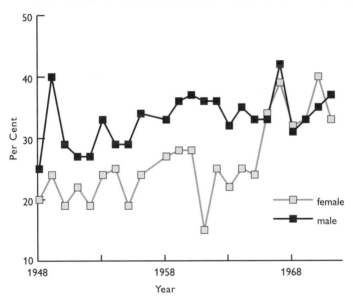

Figure 12.1
Percentage of Gonorrhoea Cases at Scottish
VD/STD Clinics Defaulting 1948–72
(*Source: Annual Reports DHS/SHHD; Scottish Health Statistics*)

remained at the heart of treatment regimes for the 'classical' venereal diseases into the 1970s.[57] Venereologists and medical commentators had long ago abandoned their more euphoric predictions of eradicating the 'great scourge', aired in the immediate post-war years.[58] Methods of increasing the resistance of individuals to venereal infection by immunization still eluded medical science, nor had there emerged an acceptable method of using prophylactic drugs. In 1968, one of Scotland's leading venereologists conceded that, given the changing pattern of sexual behaviour and relationships in Britain, it was 'unlikely that any improvement in treatment [would] reduce substantially the occurrence of venereal disease'. In his opinion, the only hope lay in improved health education and more systematic tracing and surveillance of the chain of infection.[59]

Health Education

In the immediate aftermath of the Second World War, the rising incidence of VD occasioned by demobilization led to a renewed propaganda campaign. Under the aegis of the Scottish Council for Health Education [SCHE], which had inherited much of the agenda and personnel of the former Scottish Committee of the British Social Hygiene Council, health authorities launched a series of press and poster campaigns in the late 1940s, supplemented with public filmshows and exhibitions devoted to social hygiene and VD. Despite concern at the 'unruliness and levity' of the younger elements in the audiences, health officials were impressed by the degree of public interest in the issue. Thus, in 1949, a screening in Edinburgh of the VD film, *The People at No. 19*, followed by a public discussion between the Medical Officer of Health and local venereologists, attracted a mixed audience of over 2,000.[60] In addition, despite a suspension of press advertisements due to public expenditure cuts, a cluster of new posters was issued by the DHS and the SCHE from 1950 to 1953 stressing the disastrous effects of untreated VD on fertility, parenthood and family life and the importance of early treatment.

The VD posters and literature distributed in the late 1940s and 1950s continued to enshrine many of the assumptions and stereotypes that had shaped interwar propaganda.[61] There was a less overt moralistic tone to VD posters, but a continuing stress on VD as a racial pollutant. VD continued to be depicted as 'a great evil and a grave menace to the whole nation and to the future of our race' and 'clean living' to be advocated as 'the only safeguard' *(see Plates 12.1 and 12.2)*. Likewise, VD continued to be identified in propaganda

SIXTEEN-SHEET POSTERS
exhibited by the Government

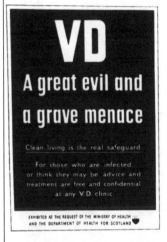
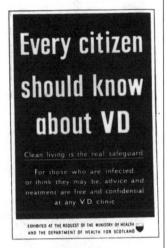

Above are reproductions of the Sixteen-Sheet Posters (size 10 feet
by 6 feet 8 inches), printed in red and white on a black ground,
which are already being exhibited in all parts of England, Wales
and Scotland by the Ministry of Information on behalf of the
Ministry of Health and the Department of Health for Scotland.

SOUND FILMS (in 35mm. and 16mm. sizes).

" Subject for Discussion " (35mm. only).	(Venereal Diseases)	(17 mins.)
" Subject Discussed " (just issued).	(Venereal Diseases)	(12 mins.)
" Sex in Life."	(Sex Education—Reproductive Systems from amœba to human)	(25 mins.)
" Human Reproduction."	(Sex Education)	(12 mins.)

Local Authorities who can make their own arrangements for showing these films
should apply for loan copies (postage only charged) to the Scottish Central Film
Library, 2, Newton Place, Glasgow, C.3.

Plate 12.1
Department of Health for Scotland VD posters displayed in the late 1940s
and early 1950s (courtesy of National Archives of Scotland)

materials with dysfunctional extra-marital sex in which moral and
physical degeneracy were intimately related. As before, infidelity and
infection were conflated, with syphilis and gonorrhoea the
'homebreakers, bringing suspicion and danger to family life' *(see Plate
12.3)*. Lectures delivered in schools by the Scottish Council of The
Alliance (formerly the Alliance of Honour), which remained grant-
aided by the Scottish Education Department [SED] for the purposes
of social hygiene education as late as the early 1960s, sustained a

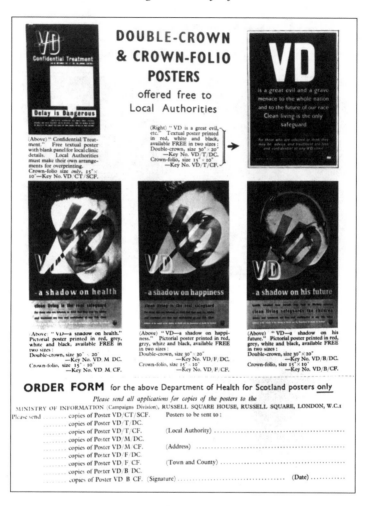

Plate 12.2
Official VD posters displayed in the late 1940s and early 1950s
(courtesy of National Archives of Scotland)

similar conflation between medical risk and moral culpability.[62]

Moreover, their representation of the epidemiology and social repercussions of venereal infection remained strongly gendered. The prevailing assumption that VD was a disease that 'develops in women and is then passed onto men' was explicitly attacked in some of the literature. Nonetheless, female sexuality remained at the core of the demonology that surrounded VD and the discourse of VD propaganda still represented young women as the primary

284

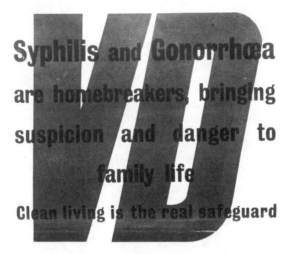

These venereal diseases can be cured if treated early. For those who are infected, or think they may be, advice and treatment are free and confidential at any V.D. Clinic

The addresses of nearest clinics may be obtained from the Office of the Medical Officer of Health or from local posters

V.D. CAN BE CURED 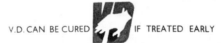 IF TREATED EARLY

BUT CLEAN LIVING IS THE REAL SAFEGUARD

Issued by the DEPARTMENT OF HEALTH FOR SCOTLAND

Plate 12.3
Official VD poster issued in the 1950s
(courtesy of National Archives of Scotland)

protectors/destroyers of the moral health and efficiency of the nation. Thus, central to the plot of *The People at No. 19*, which was frequently screened in Scotland in the late 1940s, was the infidelity of the young wife during the war leading to syphilitic infection. Typically, the overriding concern was less for her health *per se* and more for the health of the unborn child and the peace of mind of her husband. Even the natural sexual attraction of a chaste girl had the 'power' to pollute for, according to the SCHE's pamphlet, *Women in*

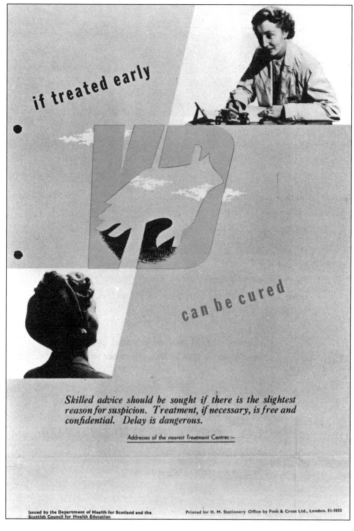

Plate 12.4
Official VD poster issued in the 1950s
(courtesy of Edinburgh City Archives)

War and Peace: 'She should remember that a man whose desires have been excited without being satisfied may be driven to that type of woman who merely gratifies the man's physical sex hunger which has been so unfairly aroused' and who 'too often give him venereal disease'.[63] Similarly, again echoing interwar representations, while

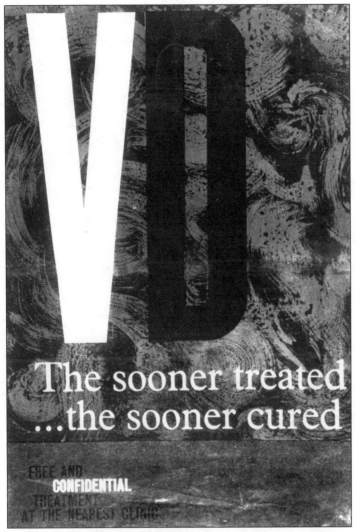

Plate 12.5
Official VD poster issued from 1962
(courtesy of National Archives of Scotland)

male VD was depicted as a 'shadow on health', female VD was 'a shadow on happiness', a lasting degradation of social reputation and domestic fulfilment with wide-ranging moral overtones *(see Plate 12.2)*.[64] Posters also continued to re-affirm the power and authority of medical expertise, although hierarchy was increasingly depicted in

287

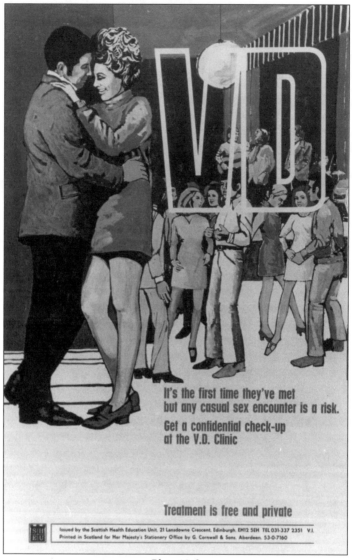

Plate 12.6
Scottish Health Education Unit poster issued in 1970
(courtesy of Health Education Board for Scotland)

terms of class rather than gender *(see Plate 12.4).*

Although markedly less acute than in England, the rising incidence of gonorrhoea in Scotland in the late 1950s prompted

288

fresh initiatives in the field of social hygiene education. A DHS Circular in 1960 urged local health authorities to review their publicity arrangements and to 'intensify their efforts'.[65] New posters were produced for the department *(see Plate 12.5)*. The SCHE also upgraded its materials on VD and sexual relationships, and films relating to VD rose from under 5 per cent to 15 per cent of its public screenings by 1968. Posters and leaflets continued to stress the importance of early treatment where 'a sexual risk' had been taken. Although their tone was less censorious and intimidating than that of earlier VD propaganda, they continued to imply a model of infection that located blame within the female body. Thus, a leaflet issued in 1962 warned that the 'sexual adventurer' was:

> sooner or later ... bound to come into contact with the infectious, and so runs a continuing risk. Many a man has said: 'But she was a clean girl!'. Such a belief is worthless, since a girl may be perfectly clean in the ordinary sense of the word and yet have in her body millions of the invisible germs of gonorrhoea or syphilis, or perhaps both.[66]

Meanwhile, local initiatives were also being undertaken. In Edinburgh, Robert Lees persuaded the Public Health Committee to introduce a new propaganda campaign to counter the widespread ignorance of 'doctors, nurses and laymen' surrounding VD, and the prevailing belief that gonorrhoea was 'a trivial infection easily cured'.[67] A local survey found that some 62 per cent of male patients were referred to the clinics by their GPs with the remainder attending mainly on the basis of information gleaned through peer-group gossip. Posters, leaflets, and health education in school were rarely the source of their knowledge.[68] Accordingly, Lees advocated a new set of VD notices targeted at public houses, dance-halls and washrooms and – to 'avoid offence' – associated with a series of poster campaigns directed at a range of 'avoidable diseases associated with personal habits' including obesity and food hygiene.[69] In addition, in response to the recommendations of the Cohen Committee on Health Education in 1964 that more priority be given to education in human relationships, including sex education, other Scottish cities introduced a range of courses on 'personal relationships'.[70]

Yet, only limited progress in raising public awareness of VD and in affecting patterns of sexual behaviour appears to have been achieved. As early as the mid-1950s, the issue of VD had become increasingly overshadowed in local health education programmes by mass radiography for TB, dental health, food-handling and home safety. Thereafter, health education remained a low priority within the National Health Service and, in particular, VD continued to attract meagre funding and resources compared with campaigns addressing issues such as smoking, air pollution and polio immunization. Significantly, STDs did not figure in the list of priorities identified by the Cohen Committee.[71] In addition, there was considerable resistance from publicans and ballroom owners to displaying literature and posters relating to VD, on the grounds that it was offensive to their clientele and would attract obscene graffiti. As a result, both spatially and symbolically, VD continued to be 'thought of and dealt with' mainly 'on a lavatorial level'.[72]

The whole area of sex education was regarded by the SHHD, the SED, and local public health committees as highly contentious, especially in areas with sectarian differences.[73] There was a lack of professional and public consensus on the role of local education authorities in matters relating to sexuality, and on the appropriate content, timing and methods of sex instruction.[74] Many parents and teachers feared that it would actively promote promiscuity.[75] As the Dundee Medical Officer of Health warned in 1966, 'there [were] probably few more vexed questions in ... the world of education'.[76] In reviewing publicity and curriculum developments, officials at the DHS and SED were predictably cautious.[77] Caution was also advised by the Scottish Medical Advisory Committee's Sub-Committee on Gonorrhoea. In their view, the experience in Denmark, where gonorrhoea among young people had steadily increased despite well-developed health education facilities, suggested 'that infection [was] not likely to be controlled in this way'.[78]

However, with rising public concern with sexual promiscuity and sexually transmitted diseases, and with the establishment of a new Scottish Health Education Unit [SHEU] in 1968, a more pro-active stance was adopted by Scottish health administrators.[79] Using research by venereologists in Glasgow into the socio-sexual behaviour patterns of patients attending VD clinics, a new set of posters and information materials was prepared focusing on the dangers of casual sex and targeted at the venues of youth culture.[80] The main poster depicted youngsters in a dance-hall setting with the wording 'It's the first time they've met, but any casual sex encounter is a risk' *(see Plate 12.6)*.[81] It reflected the shift in epidemiology from a pre-occupation with a few critical vector groups, such as prostitutes, radiating disease, to the endless chain of infection created by the casual sex of a promiscuous generation. The central message of the new materials was that 'people who [were] too easy [were] too dangerous' because of their previous sexual contacts. There was also more gender symmetry in their wording, albeit the hidden threat of vaginal infection still retained some of its former sinister overtones. Thus, two posters designed for lavatories in public houses read respectively:

> Sex–and her. Is she easy? – Then she's dangerous. Women often don't know when they have VD – but they can give it to you during intimacy. You don't know who she was with last.

> Sex–and him. Does he want it right away? – His sort can give you VD – and you wouldn't know you've got it – the germs work inside. You don't know who he was with last.[82]

There were also fresh local initiatives in the late 1960s and early 1970s. In Edinburgh and Aberdeen, sex education in schools and further education colleges was further extended with the aid of TV documentaries.[83] Such efforts were strongly endorsed by the SED's working party on health education in schools in 1974. It recognised that VD/STDs had only recently been 'considered a suitable topic' for the school curriculum, but concluded that, with the rising incidence of juvenile infection, it was essential that children be informed as to their origin, transmission, symptoms and wide-ranging medical and social effects.[84]

In Edinburgh and Glasgow, new information procedures, including a telephone advice service, were introduced. In addition, a shift in public awareness of the health hazards of VD/STDs elicited a more receptive response to the display of publicity materials. Public lavatories remained the main venue for posters, but increasingly, they were also displayed in dance-halls, libraries, colleges, hostels, public houses, voluntary welfare agencies, and on municipal information boards and vehicles (although predictably only those of the cleansing department).[85]

Nonetheless, although health education was viewed by many health administrators as 'the best hope of halting the increase in STDs', its impact remained limited. Health education budgets were under intense pressure in a period of public expenditure cuts and the SHHD was reluctant to put pressure on the Scottish Health Boards in this area. For much of the 1970s, VD/STDs were not accorded high priority by the Scottish Health Education Unit in comparison with issues such as smoking, alcoholism, immunization and family planning.[86]

The extent and quality of sex education in schools remained highly variable. In some areas, such as the East of Scotland, educationalists believed that sex education should be undertaken by

291

the teaching profession and the role of medical staff and health visitors was limited to *ad hoc* visits. Yet, teachers were often inadequately trained and reluctant to address issues relating to sexuality. An Edinburgh survey in 1977 revealed situations varying from 'biology taught but reproduction not mentioned' to occasional discussions led by a guidance teacher.[87] In Glasgow and the West of Scotland, the issue remained highly contentious. In some schools, talks and counselling by medical officers and health visitors were regularly integrated into the curriculum, while in others, as late as the mid-1980s, teachers were banned from involvement in sex education.[88] Elsewhere, as in Grampian and Dundee, provision was 'very sporadic and poor'. There was a lack of coordination between health and education authorities and ignorance of 'how or even if any sexuality content of any health education programme [was] being carried out'. Although the majority of parents appeared to favour sex education in schools, many heads of staff and teachers were unresponsive.[89] As a result, quantitative research on the knowledge of patients attending clinics in 1978 revealed that school education on STDs in Scotland was 'practically non-existent'.[90]

The SED viewed sex education as a peculiarly 'sensitive and delicate' issue, shaped by a range of contesting 'personal, sectional and public attitudes'. Although they issued curriculum guidelines on health education in 1974, they still believed that the initiative in sex education should be left with individual schools. They were fearful that any attempt to 'prescribe a sex education programme' would alienate many parents and much of the community, and that the media would misinterpret such efforts as 'an encouragement to permissiveness'.[91] They resented the intrusion of the SHHD and the Scottish Health Education Unit in curriculum issues and were resistant to the introduction of specialist teachers for health education.[92] Pressure from the SHHD to develop a more aggressive educational approach to the problems of STDs and teenage pregnancy, and to undertake research into professional and parental attitudes to the issue, also received a cool response.[93] Better liaison between the departments was attempted by means of a working group on sex education, established in 1976, but new initiatives were prevented by 'other priorities and the manpower situation'.[94] Issues relating to sexual behaviour were always viewed by officials as 'politically sensitive', and the group 'took fright' following a heated debate in the House of Lords in which recent sex education materials were roundly condemned as socially and morally subversive.[95]

The attitude of the Scottish Churches towards sex education in schools was an additional constraint. While acknowledging the need for educational initiatives to reduce levels of juvenile VD, they were acutely concerned that sexual issues should only be taught as part of broader instruction in Christian values of moral chastity and social responsibility. There was a continuing fear of corrupting youth and of 'assaulting the comparative innocence of the young' and increasing anger at what was perceived as the 'permissive' content of sex education materials issued by secular organizations such as the SHEU and Family Planning Association.[96] In the words of the Free Church of Scotland's Committee on Public Questions, Religion and Morals in 1980:

> We deplore those types of sex education teaching which omit to stress that God has permitted marriage as the only legitimate context within which physical coitus may take place .... The responsible in our society should be telling the young, not to 'make it happy', but to make it holy.[97]

Meanwhile, posters and leaflets had a limited success in educating the general public, and the main points of referral to the clinics continued to be general practitioners and friends, and in the case of women, contact tracing.[98] Much of the publicity material was unsuitable for social groups who were often semi-illiterate and resistant to health messages that were frequently 'coded' both to avoid public offence and to secure ministerial approval.[99] As the SHEU's annual report for 1978–9 concluded, they were too often:

> couched in middle-class terms and language, often relying on a play on words for the punchline. It may be that social classes III, IV and V reject the material because it does not relate to their own lives and experiences, the language is too formal, and the negative message creates a defensive reaction.[100]

Some venereologists also argued that health education materials were insufficiently targeted upon high-risk groups and failed to take into account the personality traits of VD/STD patients. Thus, according to Schofield, allowances had to be made in 'all instructions and propaganda' for the fact that female patients and male defaulters did not 'necessarily think as [did] the normal or non-promiscuous population' and they could not be 'expected to react favourably to advice that would be accepted by more normal groups'.[101]

Much of such consumer resistance may also have been due to the moral conservatism that continued to inform VD posters and information leaflets in post-war Scotland. Amidst the rising panic over promiscuous sex and disease, their representations were 'part of the continuing legacy of medical discourse which linked moral health to national concerns' and which regulated 'by establishing powerful norms around sex and health and by reaffirming the social and cultural divisions between the respectable and the unrespectable, the normal and the deviant, defined in medico-moral terms'.[102] Many venereologists, such as Robert Lees, viewed health education as very much a moral crusade in which the Churches had a central role to play. In Lees' view, sex education had to be not only factual but also 'idealistic', so as 'to present the association of "sex" with morality, spirituality, and inspiration to discover that "love" is not a dirty game or a transient and largely meaningless satisfaction of a physical appetite'.[103]

As in the interwar period, moral issues and taxonomies significantly shaped post-war VD literature, with its concern for the social costs of casual sex, and endorsed a highly normative view of sexuality and sexual behaviour. Thus, the information leaflets of the 1970s focused as much on social behaviour as on medical symptoms, with the key vectors identified as those who 'had intercourse without the *normal* courtship'.[104] Concepts of 'virtue' and 'vice' and 'deviance' still figured prominently in the warnings that venereologists sought to convey in public health reports.[105] As Weeks has noted: 'Even the most liberal texts tended to endorse a "stages" view of sexual development, which was either to be happily resolved in heterosexual monogamy or unhappily resolved in sadness and isolation',[106] and this ideology was very much at the heart of the operational philosophy of the SED and SHHD in their handling of health education.[107]

Moreover, within the context of post-war sexual health education, girls were still accorded the prime responsibility for civic virtue and social hygiene. As Dundee's Medical Officer of Health reflected in 1966: 'Sexuality has far more profound influence in girls than in boys, and conversely, girls exert a far greater effect upon sexual morals than do boys. They are indeed virtually the custodians of our sexual morals.'[108] His advocacy of 'systematic instruction in mothercraft' was entirely consistent with an official discourse that continued, despite the more 'permissive' society of the 1960s, to view 'safe' female sexual activity as primarily a procreative duty rather than a recreational pleasure.[109]

Meanwhile, ignorance and stigma continued to surround the discussion of homosexual behaviour and its implications for VD/STDs, and the subject remained notably absent from official health education materials. SHEU circulars were clearly worded for an exclusively heterosexual audience. From the mid-1970s, Scottish venereologists made increasing efforts to publicize the risks of casual gay sex in liaison with the Scottish Minorities Group, but it is significant that, when writing or lecturing on the subject, they often felt compelled to use a pseudonym for fear of attracting adverse publicity or offending the medical establishment.[110]

Perhaps the most revealing testimony to the moral agenda underpinning post-war VD information campaigns in Scotland was the absence of any reference to prophylactic techniques, and in particular, to the use of condoms. A few venereologists had advocated the wider availability and use of condoms and self-disinfection packets in the early years of the Second World War.[111] Similarly, while making no specific recommendations, the Scottish Medical Advisory Committee had in 1943 stressed the potential of greater public awareness of prophylaxis as a means of controlling the incidence of VD.[112]

However, such views had not reflected the consensus of Scottish professional and public opinion. The Scottish Churches had regarded prophylactic measures as an offence against 'the social and moral code' and an incentive to sexual licence and 'moral lawlessness', and this was a view broadly endorsed within Scottish women's associations and moral welfare agencies.[113] Moreover, throughout the war, the Scottish Committee of the British Social Hygiene Council and its successor, the SCHE, had continued a long-standing resistance to the social hygiene propaganda of the Society for the Prevention of VD [SPVD], with its advocacy of condoms and self-disinfection packets. The former believed that such 'preventive measures' would be ineffective for the civilian population, and that they would only serve to legitimize 'irregular' sex and promote immorality. Officials within the DHS had broadly shared this view and concluded that, while compulsory notification and the penalization of defaulters might enjoy considerable support within Scotland, prophylactic measures beyond the conventional appeal to moral restraint would prove highly contentious and widely unacceptable.[114]

This continued to be the case after the Second World War. Brief references to 'early preventive treatment' were retained in leaflets distributed to seamen and lorry drivers, but Scottish health authorities resisted fresh overtures from the SPVD for a publicity campaign to promote the civilian use of self-disinfection and condoms.[115] The Scottish Churches also sustained their opposition to the freer public availability of condoms, arguing that while this might reduce the incidence of VD, it would create 'unnecessary temptation' and merely reinforce the 'growing dissociation ... of sex relationships from the sanctities and responsibilities of married life'.[116] Many leading post-war venereologists sympathized with this view, maintaining a broadly conservative and at times judgemental attitude towards what they regarded as a 'new permissiveness'. They considered that, in practice, the State promotion of condoms as a prophylactic measure for VD might engender a 'false sense of security' and further erode the moral self-restraint that could alone ensure sexual health and fulfilment. Oral history evidence suggests that from the 1960s some clinicians and contact tracers routinely advocated protected sex in their confidential advice to patients. However, mindful of the censorious attitude of the media, of church and civic leaders, and of the medical establishment, such advice remained strictly off-the-record.[117]

The DHS did consider the issue of contraceptive advice in its VD publicity in the early 1960s, but decided that such an initiative would provoke widespread opposition and might render health education even more of a sectarian issue in the West of Scotland. Some officials doubted the protective value of sheaths and concurred with the Ministry of Health's view that 'physical barriers to infection or inunction with chemicals before or after intercourse, through misuse or for other reasons, [had] not proved to be reliable safe-guards'.[118] Others, such as I. N. Sutherland, Head of the Infectious Diseases Section, were adamant that the use of mechanical contraceptives would 'in general reduce the risk of acquiring VD'. However, he felt compelled to warn the Chief Medical Officer that: 'Objections to publicising such information have in the past been based on the supposition that Health Departments must not "encourage promiscuity" and I shall be surprised if these objections do not still hold.'[119]

They did indeed, and were to become increasingly strident as the whole issue of contraceptive advice and facilities for single girls and women moved to the forefront of Scottish civic debate in the early 1970s.[120] As a result, health education continued to rely on moral prophylaxis in its approach to VD. The concept of 'safe sex' as articulated in VD posters and literature remained firmly associated with concepts of courtship and marriage and sexual fidelity rather than with the use of 'precautions'. As many clinicians and health administrators increasingly recognized, given this ideology of prevention and the evident shift in the pattern of sexual behaviour within British society, there were severe limits to the degree to which health education might contain the rising incidence of VD/STDs. Any real success in VD/STD control would have also to depend on tracing the chain of infection and identifying infected contacts for treatment.

Contact Tracing

After the Second World War, the DHS felt unable to emulate the Ministry of Health and to issue new guidelines on contact tracing to the local health and hospital authorities designated under the National Health Service (Scotland) Act of 1947. While the Department confidentially advised VD Medical Officers that 'contact tracing should be conducted as vigorously as ever', open encouragement remained inhibited by the continuing advice of the Law Officers that existing Statute would not protect health authorities from action for damages under Scots Law for slander or for 'injury done to feelings', should information be divulged for the purposes of contact tracing.[121]

Concern over the legal status of contact tracing under Scots Law continued to inhibit the VD policy of the DHS throughout the late 1940s and 1950s, with officials unable to formulate a set of guidelines that incorporated legal safeguards while not actively discouraging local health authorities. In 1950, the Under-Secretary, T. D. Haddow, urged that the Department should place the needs of public health before legal caveats and openly encourage contact tracing, but no further action was taken on the issue until the end of the decade.[122]

Lack of central government initiative was reflected in a decline in contact tracing by local health authorities in the 1950s. The division of responsibilities for VD under the National Health Service (Scotland) Act 1947, with diagnosis and treatment the responsibility of the Regional Hospital Boards and issues of epidemiology and prevention remaining within the remit of the Local Authority Health Departments, served to disrupt existing contact-tracing services and to perpetuate deficiencies in staff resourcing and the standardization of procedures. This tendency was reinforced by lack of consensus over the appropriate role of social workers in VD work, and a growing belief on the part of some medical officers that the rapid impact of antibiotics on patient infectivity had reduced the urgency of 'follow-up' procedures.[123] In Edinburgh, with the repeal of Regulation 33B, the number of contacts traced fell dramatically and, during the 1950s, tracing was primarily restricted to female contacts identified by the armed forces or by 'the principal municipal protective organizations'.[124] Meanwhile, the Senior Venereologist for the City of Glasgow reported a similar failure to broaden the scope of contact tracing. On average, only 10 per cent of the contacts of men diagnosed with acute VD during the years 1948–60 were followed up, of whom only one half of those defined as 'consorts' subsequently attended for treatment. Tracing was conducted in a very *ad hoc* and uncoordinated fashion with little support from health administrators who continued to adopt a 'Calvinistic' judgementalism towards those infected with VD.[125]

The DHS was put under renewed pressure to review its policy on contact tracing by the issue in 1959 by the Ministry of Health of fresh guidelines on the prevention of VD. Concerned at the rise in the incidence of gonorrhoea in England and Wales and the spread of resistant strains of the disease, the Ministry urged local health authorities to 'intensify their efforts to trace contacts' by the use of specially selected health visitors or social workers, with particular emphasis on locating promiscuous female contacts who, it was argued, formed the major vectors of the disease.[126] Once again, the DHS's medical advisers were resistant to issuing similar guidelines for Scotland. In their view, substantive legal objections still remained. Moreover, they argued that, while in some regions there had been a recent rise in the incidence of female gonorrhoea, it was far less dramatic in Scotland, and there was actually a small decrease on trend in the incidence of male gonorrhoea.

Action was also inhibited by the lack of administrative coherence in existing contact-tracing services and by the low status accorded to venereology by many of the Hospital Boards. In some areas, as in Edinburgh and Glasgow, health visitors were seconded to the VD clinic from the Public Health Department to undertake contact tracing and there was a close liaison between the clinical and preventive services, but in others, the liaison was tenuous and contact tracing became very marginalized. For their part, the Regional Hospital Boards did not feel that additional measures or resourcing were justified and considered the issue to be the responsibility of local health authorities. The latter were keen to upgrade contact tracing but were concerned at the ability of their tracers to obtain adequate information from hospital authorities and at the legal status of almoners and health visitors who might act upon it.[127]

However, by late 1959, senior medical advisers within the DHS were conceding the need for a Scottish circular. In the face of new publicity releases by the Ministry of Health in collaboration with the women's media, and several television exposés of the worsening problem of gonorrhoea, the DHS felt compelled to act. Senior Scottish venereologists such as Robert Lees urged the Department to adopt a more pro-active line on contact tracing before the recent increase in recorded female gonorrhoea in parts of Scotland 'fed through' to the male incidence of the disease. DHS officials were also concerned that unless they took the initiative, the Scottish Council for Health Education and Scottish Local Authority Associations might revive their more extreme campaign for the compulsory notification and treatment of VD. Accordingly, after further protracted discussions with Medical Officers of Health, with the Hospital Boards and with its legal advisers, the Department eventually issued a circular to health authorities in September 1960.[128]

Compared with its English counterpart, the Scottish Circular was extremely tentative. Priority was given to vague exhortations to local health authorities to 'intensify their efforts' to reduce the incidence of VD and to upgrade their publicity arrangements. Reference to contact tracing was limited to stressing the value of gaining information from patients as to the likely source of their infection. The more advanced tracing procedures being implemented in the major urban centres of Scotland were neither mentioned nor endorsed.

This reactive approach of the DHS (reconstituted as the Scottish Home and Health Department in 1962) continued into the 1960s. The Department responded cautiously to the stress placed by the Standing Medical Advisory Committee for England and Wales in its 1962 report upon an efficient system of contract tracing as *the* vital control strategy for VD. It had particular reservations about the use of official circulars to expound matters of clinical care and treatment to the medical profession.[129] Given the low priority accorded to the VD services by the Regional Hospital Boards and their assurances that VD provisions were adequate, the SHHD was also reluctant to endorse the recommendation for increased staff resource for tracing in the *BMA Report on VD and Young People* issued in 1964.[130]

In the late 1960s, the Department came under renewed pressure to review Scottish contact-tracing policy. First, in 1965, a Scottish Medical Advisory Committee working party on 'The Incidence, Epidemiology and Control of Gonorrhoea in Scotland' urged the need for more intensive contact tracing by social workers, especially among younger age-groups. According to its report, contact tracing was not being pursued systematically in Scotland outwith Edinburgh and Glasgow, due to a lack of resources, poor liaison between medical social workers and the VD clinics, and the failure of Regional Hospital Boards to make full use of local authority health visitors.[131]

Secondly, in 1968, the Ministry of Health issued fresh regulations and guidelines. The National Health Service (Venereal Disease) Regulations 1968 were designed to facilitate contact tracing by extending statutory protection for the disclosure of information 'in the furtherance of the prevention of the spread of venereal disease'. Under previous regulations in England and Wales, confidentiality clauses had seriously constrained the development of tracing procedures. Meanwhile, the Ministry's memorandum on contact tracing of November 1968 highlighted the need for local health authorities and hospital boards to improve their tracing procedures and facilities as a means of 'breaking the chain of infection' and provided a set of detailed guidelines on interviewing patients, identifying and locating contacts, and monitoring success rates, along with an overview of the legal issues involved.[132] The subsequent debate surrounding the Private Member's Bill of Sir Myer Galpern, Labour MP for Glasgow Shettleston in March 1969, which sought to re-introduce VD controls 'similar to those formerly contained in Defence Regulation 33B', merely served to underline the lack of a similar Scottish directive.[133]

However, the SHHD remained resistant to following the example of the Ministry of Health. In the light of the more favourable VD figures for Scotland, assurances from the Hospital Boards as to the adequacy of existing clinical arrangements and resourcing, and continuing doubts as to the wisdom of publicizing and openly promoting procedures vulnerable to action for damages under Scots Law, its medical officers remained of the view that no new regulations should be issued in Scotland. Early in 1970, however, a guidance booklet on VD stressing the value of contact tracing *was* distributed to all doctors in Scotland.[134]

An additional constraint on SHHD policy was a concern not to interfere with the significant progress already being achieved in contact tracing in Edinburgh and Glasgow during the 1960s. In both cities, more systematic interrogation of infected patients was instituted and additional staff dedicated to contact tracing. The focus of 'social work' in the clinics shifted from the traditional preoccupation with defaulters to tracking down the 'hidden pool of infection within the community'.[135] Particular attention was paid to identifying the 'inmates' of the more notorious brothels and tracing prostitutes operating in the docks,[136] and tracers routinely visited 'bars, nightclubs and cafés'.[137] Each VD department gradually built up:

> a dossier of promiscuous people, usually women ... compiled from
> the descriptions of those who ... attended, together with their habits,

haunts, and family background; from reports of other health visitors of possible problem families in their districts; and from newspaper reports of women drunk and disorderly, in court for soliciting or prostitution ....[138]

As a result, by 1970, nearly 50 per cent of primary contacts named in Edinburgh male VD clinics were being traced and persuaded to attend for treatment and 44 per cent of all first-time female patients attended clinics in response to contact tracing, as compared with 16 per cent in 1951.[139] In Glasgow, efforts to upgrade tracing procedures, inspired by Dr C. B. S. Schofield, Regional Consultant on Venereology, and based upon his previous experience of contact tracing in the pioneering Tynecastle Scheme instituted in 1944, also achieved significant results, with the percentage of primary female contacts successfully traced and attending for examination and treatment more than doubling during the decade.[140] The changing efficiency of contact tracing could be inferred from the changing ratio of male to female patients with gonorrhoea attending 'special clinics' in Scotland: from 4.1:1 in 1961 to 1.8:1 in 1971.[141] However, there was growing concern among Scottish venereologists at the lack of headway in tracing homosexual contacts whose sexual relationships were perceived as predominantly casual and highly promiscuous.[142]

The report of the Gilloran Committee on Sexually Transmitted Diseases in Scotland, published in 1973, stressed the importance of contact tracing in controlling the spread of STDs, and in particular, in securing medical treatment for the 'promiscuous females' and 'passive homosexuals' who allegedly constituted the major 'reservoirs of infection'. It noted the lack of uniformity within Scotland in contact-tracing facilities and procedures, and recommended as a matter of urgency that adequate provisions and standardized procedures should be available at all special clinics and that appropriate recruitment and in-service training be introduced, along with a proper career structure for contact tracers.[143]

In the event, the Gilloran Report did not initiate any substantive new departures in Scottish contact tracing for STDs. As we have seen, in the mid-1970s, the SHHD was preoccupied with the reorganization of the health services and was reluctant to endorse recommendations involving additional resources in a period of severe financial restraint.[144] An additional constraint was the lack of consensus within the medical and social work professions as to the desirable mix of medical and counselling skills required for effective contact tracing. As a result, the progress review of STD facilities by the SHHD in 1978 revealed wide variations in the provision of contact tracing. In some areas, such as Greater Glasgow and Lothian Health Boards, provisions were well developed, although duties might vary from tracing *per se*, to broader social interviewing and psycho-sexual counselling. Elsewhere, however, as in Tayside and Inverness, reliance continued to be placed largely upon the efforts of patients to persuade their own contacts to attend for treatment.[145]

Despite clear evidence of an urgent need to upgrade tracing facilities in many areas of Scotland, the SHHD remained unpersuaded that increased funding for the establishment of new training and career structures could appropriately be urged upon the Health Boards in the prevailing financial climate. As a result, although the Department conducted a more focused review of Scottish contact-tracing facilities in 1984–5, and some form of practical training together with a handbook for contact tracers was gradually introduced, as it entered the era of AIDS and HIV, the provision of contact tracing for STDs in Scotland remained highly variable and significantly under-resourced.[146]

This enduring problem of resourcing reflected the broader struggle of venereology to maintain its professional identity and status as a specialty within the Scottish health services. However, the slow and often erratic development of contact tracing for VD/STDs in twentieth-century Scotland has also been a function of broader ideological conflict over issues of personal liberty and the inquisitorial role of the State in protecting public health. Contact tracing was introduced in interwar Britain as part of 'the new hygiene of the Dispensary' with its focus on the surveillance of social relationships. Moreover, as we have seen, in Scotland, the development of contact surveillance was accompanied by a sustained campaign for more stringent local authority powers to combat the spread of VD, including compulsory notification and/or treatment. Yet, as with the campaign for VD controls, more coercive and comprehensive forms of tracing and regulating contacts met with increasing resistance from women's organizations and libertarian groups concerned at the authoritarian and discriminatory aspects of compulsory procedures.

Medico-legal issues relating to the confidentiality of information supplied by patients and contacts have clearly represented a powerful additional constraint upon public health authorities. Government archives reveal a lasting preoccupation of the health departments of State with the need to encourage a wider geographical and professional exchange of contact data while preserving the code of confidentiality upon which the success of the interwar voluntary VD services had largely been based.[147] In Scotland, the vulnerability of practitioners and contact tracers to charges of defamation under Scots Law represented an added dimension to these concerns, and clearly inhibited the degree to which the DHS and SHHD were prepared actively to recommend more aggressive contact tracing in their guidelines to the regional health authorities. As D. H. H. Robertson, Consultant Venereologist at Edinburgh Royal Infirmary, conceded in 1972:

> The process of contact tracing, based as it is on a single allegation, unsupported by any satisfactory evidence whatsoever, would cause a lawyer or solicitor to grow hot and cold with indignation. He could complain about unconstitutional approaches by officials and defamatory implications.[148]

Above all, in resisting the more interventionist demands of some clinicians and civic leaders, policy-makers were sensitive to the social psychology surrounding the process of contact tracing for a disease commonly stigmatized in the press and the community. From the earliest years of contact tracing in Scotland, experience suggested that in the process of identifying and locating sexual contacts and of persuading them to attend for often painful and protracted treatment and for tests of cure, coercion would prove counter-productive. Accordingly, in later twentieth-century Scotland, calls for the retention of wartime controls as a means of breaking the chain of venereal infection were resisted and a voluntary system of contact tracing and surveillance maintained, despite the rising incidence of gonorrhoea and other STDs after 1960.

Notes

1 See, e.g., *Edinburgh Public Health Department [EPHD] Annual Report (1949)*, 96; National Archives of Scotland [NAS], HH 58/66, Correspondence on VD Policy, 1944–62, Minute by L. C. Watson, 28 April 1949.

2 *Lancet*, Vol. II (1966), 1289; Vol. I (1967), 159, 221, 328–9, 384, 510; *Hansard [HC]* 662, cols 291–4, 3 July 1962; 679, cols 1920–36, 28 June 1963.

3 *Hansard [HC]*, 774, col. 511, 27 Nov. 1968; 780, cols 944–76, 21 March 1969.

4 *Ibid.*, col. 950; J. de Moerloose and H. Rahm, 'A Survey of VD Legislation in Europe', *Acta Dermato-Venereologica*, 44 (1964), 146–63. The only European countries lacking specific legislative

controls for the regulation of VD in the mid-1960s were the Netherlands and the United Kingdom.

5 *Hansard [HC]*, 679, cols 1925–35, 28 June 1963; 780, cols 966–75, 21 March 1969; NAS, HH 58/66/93, Memorandum on Control of Venereal Diseases: Compulsory Examination and Treatment, 20 June 1962.

6 *The Guardian*, 22 March 1969, 'Funds – Not Law Urged to Stem VD'; Greater Glasgow Health Board Archive [GGHBA], HH 55/T88, D. H. H. Robertson, 'Medico-Legal Problems Relating to Sexual Behaviour'; Communication from former consultant venereologist, 15 May 1995.

7 See, e.g., *EPHD Annual Report (1956)*, 155; *(1957)*, 153; A. King, '"These Dying Diseases": Venereology in Decline?', *Lancet*, Vol. I (1958), 656.

8 On the wider implications of the campaign in England, see B. Towers, 'Politics and Policy: Historical Perspectives on Screening', in V. Berridge and P. Strong (eds), *AIDS and Contemporary History* (Cambridge: Cambridge University Press, 1993), 55–73.

9 See, e.g., *Aberdeen Medical Officer of Health [MOH] Annual Report (1959)*, 5; *Glasgow MOH Annual Report (1958)*, 164; *EPHD Annual Report (1957)*, 153; *Health Bulletin*, 31, no. 2 (March 1973), 62.

10 R. C. L. Batchelor Papers, 'Changing Concepts and Changing Patterns in Venereology', Lecture to Tees-Side Division of BMA, 21 Oct. 1963.

11 R. C. L. Batchelor and M. Murrell, *Venereal Diseases Described for Nurses* (Edinburgh: E. & S. Livingstone, 1951), 196, 202–3.

12 Robert Lees, 'VD – Some Reflections of a Venereologist', *British Journal of Venereal Diseases [BJVD]*, 26 (1950), 160.

13 *Report of Committee on Homosexual Offences and Prostitution [Wolfenden Report], PP 1956–7 (Cmnd. 247) XIV*; NAS, HH 60/265, Wolfenden Committee, Correspondence and Papers; Debate on Report, *Hansard [HC]*, 596, cols 365–507, 26 Nov. 1958; Public Record Office [PRO], MH 55/2189, VD Publicity: Policy and Planning 1952–7, Minute, 24 Oct. 1957.

14 *Wolfenden Report*, 91.

15 *Ibid.*, 93–4.

16 *The Times*, 29 July 1960, 27 Aug. 1960.

17 NAS, HH 57/568, Treatment of Venereal Diseases in Prison: General Questions, Minutes by Dr I. D. Inch, 10 Jan. 1961, 18 April 1961.

18 *Ibid.*

19 *EPHD Annual Report (1961)*, 143; *(1964)*, 99; D. H. H. Robertson

and G. George, 'Medical and Legal Problems in the Treatment of Delinquent Girls in Scotland: II. Sexually Transmitted Disease in Girls in Custodial Institutions', *BJVD*, 46 (1970), 46–51.

20   D. H. H. Robertson, 'Medical and Legal Problems in the Treatment of Delinquent Girls in Scotland: 1. Girls in Custodial Institutions', *BJVD*, 45 (1969), 135.

21   J. M. Hunter and M. Neilson, 'Sexually Transmitted Diseases in Edinburgh: Patients under 18 years of Age', *Health Bulletin*, 38, no. 1 (1980), 24; *Edinburgh Health and Social Services Department [EHSSD] Annual Report (1968)*, 69. In contrast, no juvenile male patients were referred to the VD clinic from custodial institutions.

22   Medical Society for the Study of Venereal Diseases Scottish Branch [MSSVDSB], Correspondence and Papers relating to the Latey Committee on the Age of Majority.

23   *Ibid.*; Robertson, *op. cit.* (note 20), 135–6.

24   *Ibid.*, 132–5; *Report of the Committee on the Age of Majority, PP 1966–7 (Cmnd. 3342) 62*; Hunter and Neilson, *op. cit.* (note 21), 24.

25   Lothian Health Services Archives [LHSA], Uncatalogued, Correspondence on Treatment of Civilian Patients with Penicillin, 1944–5.

26   *EPHD Annual Report (1949)*, 94; *Glasgow MOH Annual Report (1948)*, 120; *Practitioner*, 171 (1953), 431; R. C. L. Batchelor and M. Murrell, *A Short Manual of Venereal Diseases and Treponematosis* (Edinburgh: Livingstone, 1961), 123.

27   *Dundee MOH Annual Report (1947)*, 129; *British Medical Journal [BMJ]*, (1947) Vol. II, 307; (1955), Vol. 1, 1430.

28   *Glasgow MOH Annual Report (1953)*, 120.

29   R. C. L. Batchelor, 'Recent Developments in Venereology', *Edinburgh Medical Journal [EMJ]*, 61 (1954), 370–2.

30   *EPHD Annual Report (1950)*, 150.

31   Northern Health Services Archives [NHSA], N-ERHB Admin. File 22/1, Film A20, Senior Administrative Medical Officer [SAMO] to Department of Health for Scotland [DHS], 11 Aug. 1959.

32   *EPHD Annual Report (1947)*, 89; *(1951)*, 97; *(1953)*, 104; Batchelor and Murrell, *op. cit.* (note 26), 134; NAS, HH 104/35/1, Continuation of Malarial Treatment for Neurosyphilis, Correspondence, 1959.

33   See, e.g., *EPHD Annual Report (1945)*, 35.

34   Batchelor and Murrell, *op. cit.* (note 26), 168; A. King, C. Nicol, and P. Rodin, *Venereal Diseases* (London: Bailliere Tindall, 4th edition 1980), 232–3. For early examples in Edinburgh of the dramatic success of penicillin in curing sulphonamide-resistant

patients, see LHSA, Uncatalogued, Correspondence on Treatment of Civilian Patients with Penicillin, 1944–5; R. C. L. Batchelor *et al.*, 'Penicillin in the Treatment of Venereal Disease: A Year's Experience in a Civilian Clinic', *EMJ*, LIII (1946), 31–6.

35 See, e.g., *EPHD Annual Report(1950)*, 153; *(1953)*, 105.

36 *EPHD Annual Report (1945)*, 36; Batchelor, *op. cit.* (note 29), 373.

37 See, e.g., *EPHD Annual Report (1950)*, 151.

38 *EPHD Annual Report (1955)*, 156.

39 Interview with former general practitioner involved in VD work in Aberdeen, 7 April 1997.

40 NAS, HH 58/66/59; HH 104/36/190, Review of the Organization of VD Services, 1978–9. In England and Wales, such payments were solely at the discretion of the clinic director (*Report of Joint Sub-Committee on Sexually Transmitted Diseases [Gilloran Committee]* (Edinburgh: HMSO, 1973), 6, 15).

41 NAS, HH 104/35, 'Laboratory Diagnosis of Venereal Diseases', Report of Working Party appointed by the Epidemiological Sub-Committee of the Scottish Standing Advisory Committee on Laboratory Services, 20 May 1966; HH 104/55, Second Interim Report, 2 June 1967; *Glasgow MOH Annual Report (1966)*, 315.

42 M. Schofield, *Promiscuity* (London: Victor Gollancz, 1976), 167.

43 *EHSSD Annual Report (1965)*, 190–1; *Glasgow MOH Annual Report (1963)*, 276–7; *(1971)*, 242; R. D. Stuart [Central Public Laboratory, Glasgow], 'The Diagnosis and Control of Gonorrhoea by Bacteriological Cultures', *Glasgow Medical Journal [GMJ]*, 27 (1946), 131–4; NAS, HH 104/35, 'Laboratory Diagnosis of Venereal Diseases', Report of Working Party.

44 *EPHD Annual Report (1950)*, 153; *(1951)*, 95; *(1956)*, 154; *(1961)*, 142–3; *Glasgow MOH Annual Report (1953)*, 117.

45 *EPHD Annual Report (1960)*, 143; *(1961)*, 143; *Glasgow MOH Annual Report (1960)*, 242.

46 *Glasgow MOH Annual Report (1958)*, 231; *(1963)*, 276–7.

47 *Ibid. (1963)*, 278–9.

48 NHSA, GRHB, B2/2/4, Aberdeen Special Hospitals, Group Medical Superintendent Reports (1960), 20; (1968), 28.

49 *EPHD Annual Report (1951)*, 96; Batchelor, *op. cit.* (note 29), 373–4; Batchelor and Murrell, *op. cit.* (note 26), 178–9; *Glasgow MOH Annual Report (1964)*, 248, 306.

50 *City of Edinburgh Health Department [CEHD] Annual Report (1972)*, 69.

51 *EPHD Annual Report (1952)*, 135–6.

52 *Ibid. (1957)*, 151; *(1958)*, 195; *(1959)*, 142; *Glasgow MOH Annual*

Report (1964), 253–4.

53 *Glasgow MOH Annual Report (1967)*, 229–30; *(1972)*, 222.

54 *Annual Report of DHS for 1960: Pt 1: Health and Welfare Services, PP 1960–61 (Cmnd. 1320) XVII*, 27; NAS, HH 58/66/59a, Observations of I. N. Sutherland, 10 Oct. 1960.

55 *EHSSD Annual Report (1967)*, 71. According to an article in the *Readers' Digest*, circulated to Scottish local health authorities in 1964, whereas in the mid-1940s, 100,000 units of penicillin had been sufficient to cure uncomplicated cases of gonorrhoea, by the early 1960s doses of one million units were commonplace and many doctors were administering doses of more than two million units (NAS, HH 58/66/71, 'Once More – VD', extract from *Readers' Digest*, Aug. 1961).

56 Schofield, *op. cit.* (note 42), 162–3; Edinburgh University Library, BBC Newscuttings, Box 1437, Venereal Disease.

57 See especially, C. B. S. Schofield, *Sexually Transmitted Diseases* (Edinburgh: Churchill Livingstone, 2nd edition, 1975). Penicillin was still described as the 'sheet anchor of treatment for gonorrhoea' in the Western Region in 1966 (*Glasgow MOH Annual Report (1966)*, 316).

58 See, e.g., *DHS, Annual Report for 1955, PP 1955–56 (Cmd. 9742) XXI*, 30.

59 *EHSSD Annual Report (1968)*, 70.

60 *DHS, Annual Report for 1949, PP 1950 (Cmd. 7921) XI*, 27; *Glasgow MOH Annual Report (1946)*, 79; *EPHD Annual Report (1946)*, 34; *(1947)*, 36; *(1949)*, 14; *Aberdeen MOH Annual Report (1946)*, 49; NAS, HH 58/108, Scottish Council for Health Education [SCHE] Minutes, 31 Dec. 1946, 16 April 1947, 28 Oct. 1947, 31 Dec. 1947. In 1947, the SCHE organized seven public meetings in the larger burghs on VD attracting a total audience of 6,350, and distributed 23,000 leaflets on VD and sex education.

61 For VD and social hygiene posters, films and leaflets that were distributed by the SCHE in the late 1940s and 1950s, see especially, National Library of Scotland, Miscellaneous Pamphlets, Central Council for Health Education, *Facts on Sex for Men; Yourself and Your Body; Women in War and Peace; What are the Venereal Diseases, The Approach to Womanhood; From Boyhood to Manhood; For Men on the Sea; For Men on the Road;* PRO, INF 6/639, Papers relating to *Subject Discussed;* INF 6/406, Papers relating to *The People at No. 19;* National Film Archive, *Subject Discussed*, shotlist and viewing copy.

62 NAS, HH 61/1099/26, 28, 47, Health Education in Schools 1960–66, Minutes and Papers.

63 See also, SCHE, *Teaching Health: A Working Guide* (1961), 25: 'girls should not behave in any way which might cause a normally-passioned boy to forget himself'.

64 Significantly, there was no female counterpart for the poster: '*VD–A Shadow on His Future*'.

65 NAS, HH 48/65/19, *DHS Circular 64/1960, Venereal Disease in Scotland: Increase in Incidence of Gonorrhoea.*

66 NAS, HH 58/112/11, Draft of Leaflet: 'A Personal Word', March 1962.

67 *EPHD Annual Report (1959)*, 15, 144.

68 *EPHD Annual Report (1962)*, 158. For similar findings in England in the mid-1960s, see M. Schofield, *The Sexual Behaviour of Young People* (London: Longmans, 1965), 115–18.

69 *EPHD Annual Report (1961)*, 16; *(1962)*, 158.

70 *Dundee MOH Annual Report (1965)*, 25; *(1966)*, 27–8; *Aberdeen MOH Annual Report (1966)*, 32; *(1967)*, 35.

71 *Health Education: Report of a Joint Committee* (London: HMSO, 1964), 9–10.

72 'Publicity Material on VD', *Health Bulletin*, XXVIII, no. 1 (1970), 6; G. D. Rees, 'The Menace of Venereal Disease and the need for Education', *Health Education Journal*, XXVIII, no. 4 (1969), 209–10. Strictly speaking, the display of VD posters was, until 1970, illegal under the 1889 Indecent Advertisements Act. However, no prosecutions had ever been brought against local health authorities and it was the concern of civic leaders for public decency that had been the primary constraint. See, debate on Indecent Advertisements (Amendment) Bill, *Hansard [HL]* 310, 11 May 1970, cols 469–83.

73 NAS, HH 61/1099, Health Education in Schools 1960–66.

74 NAS, HH 58/112/26, R. M. Gordon to Chief Medical Officer, 29 Nov. 1965.

75 J. Weeks, *Sex, Politics and Society: The Regulation of Sexuality since 1800* (London: Longman, 2nd edition 1981), 256.

76 *Dundee MOH Annual Report (1966)*, 27.

77 See, e.g., NAS, HH 58/66, Venereal Disease, Minutes by A. M. Stephen, 20 Sept. 1961, 2 Oct. 1961; HH 58/113, SCHE, Minutes of Educational Advisory Committee, 30 June 1959.

78 NAS, HH 104/35, Report of Working Party on The Incidence, Epidemiology and Control of Gonorrhoea in Scotland, Oct. 1965.

79 See especially, *Scottish Home and Health Department [SHHD]*, *Annual Report, for 1968, PP 1968–9 (Cmnd. 4012) 63*, 55; *for 1970, PP 1970–71 (Cmnd. 4667) 48*, 11.

80   *Health Bulletin,* XXVIII, no. 1, (1970), 6; B. P. W. Wells and C. B.
     S. Schofield, '"Target" Sites for Anti-VD Propaganda', *Health
     Bulletin, ibid.,* 75–7.
81   Significantly, it was the first time that the word 'sex' had appeared in
     VD posters.
82   *Health Bulletin,* XXVIII no. 1 (Jan. 1970), 6.
83   *Aberdeen MOH Annual Report (1969),* 8; *(1970),* 10, 12; *(1972),* 4;
     EHSSD Annual Report (1969), viii; *(1970),* x, 5; *(1972),* 51.
84   Scottish Education Department, *Health Education in Schools,
     Curriculum Paper 14* (Edinburgh: HMSO, 1974), 11–12. In the
     same year, the Scottish TUC passed a resolution to similar effect
     (*STUC Annual Report for 1974,* 303).
85   *EHSSD Annual Report (1970),* x, 60; *Glasgow MOH Annual Report
     (1971),* 173; *(1972),* 178.
86   NAS, HH 61/970/3, Scottish Health Education Unit, Current and
     Proposed Programmes, 1970–75; HH 61/1020/33, 37, SHEU,
     Minutes of Steering Committee, 22 July 1975, 12 Feb. 1976.
87   NAS, HH 104/36, Memorandum by D. H. H. Robertson, June
     1977, 6.
88   NAS, HH 61/1021/10, Memorandum by B. Schofield and F. M.
     Martin, 'Health Education in Schools, with Particular Reference to
     Sexually Transmitted Diseases', 31 March 1976; MSSVDSB
     Minutes, 7 April 1984, 5 Oct. 1985.
89   NHSA, GRHB A4/3 [8/9] Pt 1A, Health Education Files 1974–6.
90   C. B. S. Schofield, 'The Knowledge of Patients about Sexually
     Transmitted Diseases', in D. R. Billington, J. Bell *et al.* (eds),
     Research in Health Education (Edinburgh: SHEU, 1978), 26.
     According to a survey by the National Children's Bureau in 1977, 1
     in 4 Scottish children aged 16 were receiving no sex instruction
     compared with 1 in 30 in the South of England (*Glasgow Herald,* 9
     Jan. 1978). On the inadequacy of VD instruction in schools in
     England and Wales, see, Schofield, *op. cit.* (note 42), 17–18; I.
     Sutherland (ed.), *Health Education: Perspectives and Choices* (London:
     Allen and Unwin, 1979), 192–4.
91   NAS, HH 61/1021/18, H. Robertson [SED] to E. Redmond
     [SHHD], 2 July 1976; Scottish Education Department, *op. cit.* (note
     84).
92   NAS, HH 61/1019/1, SED to CMO, SHHD, 16 Oct. 1974.
93   NAS, HH 61/1019/26, R. M. Bell, 'Health Education in Schools', 4
     Dec. 1975.
94   NAS, HH 61/1019/44, A. F. Reid to I. M. Robertson, 7 May 1976.
95   NAS, HH 61/1019/42, E. Redmond to A. Mitchell, 5 May 1976;

Hansard [HL] 367, cols 134–270, 14 Jan. 1976.

96   *Free Church of Scotland, Annual Report to General Assembly (1971),*
     143; *(1976),* 138; *(1977),* 145; *Church of Scotland, Annual Report to
     General Assembly (1964),* 344; *(1973),* 424, 444; NAS, HH
     61/1019/9, Health Education in Schools. Policy and General
     Questions 1974–8. Thus, the Moral Welfare Committee of the
     Church of Scotland condemned the sex education film *Growing Up*
     for condoning extra-marital sex (*Glasgow Herald,* 21 May 1971).

97   *Free Church of Scotland, Annual Report to General Assembly (1980),*
     146–7.

98   See, e.g., *ESSD Annual Report (1972),* 72.

99   Schofield, 'The Knowledge of Patients', *op. cit.* (note 90), 26; NAS,
     HH 61/1020/6, SHEU Steering Committee Minutes, 24 July 1973.

100 *SHEU Annual Report for 1978–79,* 3.

101 C. B. S. Schofield, *Sexually Transmitted Diseases* (London: Churchill
     Livingstone, 3rd edition 1979), 43. See also, NHSA, N-ERHB
     Admin. Files, Film 29, File 22/1, Correspondence on VD, 18 Feb.
     1969.

102 L. Bland and F. Mort, 'Look Out for the "Good Time" Girl:
     Dangerous Sexualities as a Threat to National Health', in Open
     University (ed.), *Formations of Nation and People* (London:
     Routledge and Kegan Paul, 1984), 149.

103 *EPHD Annual Report (1962),* 157; *(1963),* 138. According to
     Robert Morton, President of the MSSVD, 'only a return to
     puritanism [would] stop the spread of disease' (*The People,* 11 Aug.
     1968).

104 See, e.g., Health Education Board for Scotland Library, *SHEU,
     Circular No. 1, 5 Jan. 1970.*

105 See, e.g., *EHSSD Annual Report (1968),* 66.

106 Weeks, *op. cit.* (note 75), 256.

107 *SHHD Annual Report for 1970, PP 1970–71 (Cmnd. 4667) 48,* 11.

108 *Dundee MOH Annual Report (1966),* 28.

109 R. Davenport-Hines, *Sex, Death and Punishment: Attitudes to Sex and
     Sexuality in Britain since the Renaissance* (London: William Collins,
     1990), 275–6.

110 A. Mcmillan and D. H. H. Robertson, 'Sexually-Transmitted
     Diseases in Homosexual Males in Edinburgh', *Health Bulletin,* 35
     (Sept. 1977), 270; Interview with former consultant venereologist, 2
     June 1998.

111 See, e.g., R. Lees, 'The Prevention of Venereal Disease', *The
     Practitioner,* 145 (1940), 119–23; *The Lancet,* 4 May 1940, 851.

112 *Report of Medical Advisory Committee for Scotland on Venereal*

Diseases, PP 1943–44 (Cmd. 6518) IV, 7–8.

113 NAS, HH 65/122/11, Notes of Conferences between Secretary of
     State for Scotland and Representatives of Scottish Protestant
     Churches and Roman Catholic Church in Scotland, 30 June and 17
     July 1944; National Library of Scotland, Papers of Executive
     Committee, East of Scotland Branch of National Vigilance
     Association, 7 Nov. 1941.

114 Contemporary Medical Archives Centre [CMAC], SA/PVD/5,
     NSPVD Scheme of Propaganda, 1939–40; Perth and Kinross
     District Archive, 395/1/7, Posters of NSPVD on 'Venereal Disease
     Prevention', 1943; NAS, HH 65/122/11, Minutes of Meeting,
     Secretary of State for Scotland and Roman Catholic Church in
     Scotland, 17 July 1944.

115 CCHE, *For Men on the Sea*, 14; *For Men on the Road*, 10; Perth and
     Kinross District Archive, 491/1/27, MOH to Town Clerk, Perth, 21
     Feb. 1950; NHSA, Aberdeen Public Health Committee Minutes, 7
     March 1949; Dundee City Archives, Dundee Public Health
     Committee Minutes, 10 Feb. 1949.

116 *Church of Scotland Report to the General Assembly: Annual Report of
     Committee on Church and Nation (1947)*, 316; *(1950)*, 349.

117 Interview with consultant venereologist, 9 April 1997.

118 NAS, HH 58/112/11, Papers of SCHE Medical Advisory
     Committee, March 1962; HH 104/55/12, *Ministry of Health,
     Circular, HM(68) 84, Nov. 1968, Control of Venereal Disease.*

119 NAS, HH 58/66, Minute I. N. Sutherland, 17 Oct. 1961.

120 See, e.g., *Glasgow Herald*, Editorial, 3 Feb. 1971, 'Policy on
     Morality'; NAS, HH 61/970/29, Scottish Home and Health
     Department, Family Planning and Health Education: Aide Memoire
     for Discussion, Nov. 1970.

121 NAS, HH 58/66/1–8, Minutes and Papers on Possible Circular on
     Contact Tracing, 1948.

122 NAS, HH 58/66, Minutes and Correspondence on Contact Tracing,
     1948–62.

123 British Medical Association [BMA] Archive, Venereologists Group
     Committee, 26 Feb. 1953, Memorandum by R. Lees.

124 *EPHD Annual Reports (1948–60)*; see especially *(1948)*, 95; *(1952)*,
     141; *(1953)*, 108; *(1958)*, 197; *(1960)*, 144.

125 See *Annual Reports of MOH for Glasgow (1948–60)*; Communication
     from former Regional Consultant on Venereology, 14 May 1993.
     For similar *ad hoc* arrangements in Aberdeen, see NHSA, N-ERHB
     Admin. Papers, Film A20, File 22/1, Note of Meeting, 19 May
     1959. Evidence suggests that much of the contact tracing work in

Aberdeen was routinely undertaken by a retired health visitor or one
of the technicians (Interview with retired GP and VD clinical
assistant, 9 April 1997).

126   *Ministry of Health, Circular 6/59, Prevention of Venereal Disease,* 27
       April 1959.

127   NAS, HH 58/66/11–30, Minutes and Correspondence on the
       Prevention of Venereal Disease.

128   See *ibid.*, items, 33–44; *DHS Circular 64/1960, Venereal Disease in
       Scotland: Increase in Incidence of Gonorrhoea,* 2 Sept. 1960.

129   NAS, HH 104/35/21a, Note by SHHD, May 1963.

130   NAS, HH 104/35/37, Minute by I. M. Macgregor, 14 July 1964.

131   NAS, HH 104/35/75, Report of Working Party, Oct. 1965. In
       Aberdeenshire, efforts by the Public Health Department to
       undertake tracing were seriously restricted for lack of information
       from the hospital authorities (NHSA, N-ERHB Admin. Papers,
       Film A20, File 22/1, MOH Aberdeen County Council to Assistant
       Senior Medical Officer, 24 Jan. 1969).

132   *National Health Service (Venereal Diseases) Regulations, 1968, S.I.
       1968 No. 1624. Ministry of Health, National Health Service: Control
       of Venereal Disease HM(68) 84, Nov. 1968.*

133   NAS, HH 104/55/55, Correspondence relating to Galpern's Bill;
       Control of Venereal Diseases Bill, PP 1968–69 (Bill 40) 1; *Hansard
       [HC],* 780, cols 944–76, 21 March 1969.

134   NAS, HH 104/35/49, 75, 79; NAS, HH 104/55/7, 92, Papers on
       Venereal Disease: Incidence and Control 1963–71.

135   *EPHD Annual Report (1962),* 144; *(1965),* 111; *EHSSD Annual
       Report (1967),* 77.

136   *Ibid. (1966),* 133.

137   LHSA, Pamphlet Box FS-GR, L. Scarth, 'Notes on VD Out-Patient
       Clinics' (1971).

138   C. B. S. Schofield, *Sexually Transmitted Diseases* (Edinburgh:
       Churchill Livingstone, 2nd edition 1975), 28.

139   *EHSSD Annual Report (1970),* 58; R. C. L. Batchelor and M.
       Murrell, *op. cit.* (note 11), 193. In contrast, only 3% of male
       patients attended the Royal Infirmary clinic in response to contact
       tracing.

140   *Glasgow MOH Annual Report (1964),* 252; *(1970),* 207. Prior to the
       appointment of a full-time Consultant Venereologist in Glasgow,
       there was little liaison between the male and female clinics over
       'follow-up' work. The two health visitors in the female clinics were
       often fully occupied assisting in medical examinations and
       treatment, and the only contact cards issued were to married male

patients for their wives. The doctors staffing the clinics largely ignored contact tracing and a 'calvinistic' attitude prevailed towards the welfare of possible sexual contacts (Communication from former consultant venereologist, 14 May 1995). On the Tynecastle Scheme, see especially, H. M. Johns, 'The Social Aspect of Venereal Diseases – 3: Contact Tracing', *BJVD*, XXI (1945), 17–21.

141 Gilloran Committee, *op. cit.* (note 40), 3.

142 See, e.g., *EHSSD Annual Report (1964)*, 99; *(1965)*, 110.

143 Gilloran Committee, *op. cit.* (note 40), 2, 6, 14–15.

144 The following account is based upon NAS, HH 104/36, Correspondence relating to Sexually Transmitted Diseases: Gilloran Report. Information on Services from Health Boards, 1975–80; Minutes and Papers of the MSSVDSB; C. B. S. Schofield and N. McNeil, 'Sexually Transmitted Diseases in Scotland 1972–75', *Health Bulletin,* 35, no. 1 (1977), 18–21.

145 For similar deficiencies in England and Wales, see *BMJ,* 24 April 1982, 1211. It should be stressed that in many areas, such as Dumfries and Galloway, or Argyll and Bute, it would have been economically unviable to attach contact tracers to every clinic. Many of the so-called 'peripheral clinics' had few cases of which only *c.*10% involved statutory VD that could legally be contact traced. Moreover, even in the absence of an officially designated contact tracer, a great deal of effective tracing was frequently carried out, often informally, by GPs and health visitors in liaison with clinicians in the urban centres. Similarly, in Forth Valley, a very successful tracing programme was initiated 'courtesy of one of the senior prostitutes in the area' who ensured that all the local prostitutes attended a special clinic (Communication from retired consultant venereologist, 15 May 1995). Scottish Returns for 1972–5 reveal that the contacts of 74% of patients with syphilis or gonorrhoea were 'sought' and that 66% of such contacts attended for treatment. As less than half the infections with primary or secondary syphilis were acquired in the locality of the VD treatment centres and over one-third acquired abroad, the proportion of syphilis contacts attending was consistently lower than for gonorrhoea. The regular consorts of patients with other STDs were also sought but no effort was made when the contact was merely a 'casual pick-up'. See Schofield and McNeil, *op. cit.* (note 144), 19; *Scottish Health Statistics (1977),* 34; *(1980),* 31.

146 See especially, MSSVDSB Papers, 'Sexually Transmitted Disease: Notes on Facilities in Scotland', 9 April 1984. The percentage of new cases of gonorrhoea in Scotland found by contact tracing

'Breaking the Chain of Infection'

actually fell from 36% in 1972 to 32% in 1980, as did the percentage of contacts sought who attended treatment centres – from 74% to 63% (*Scottish Health Statistics (1980)*, 31).

147 See, e.g., NAS, HH 104/25, VD Legislation: Correspondence with Citizenship Groups, Ministerial correspondence and Minutes on Statutory Provisions for Confidentiality of Treatment, 1948–66.

148 D. H. H. Robertson, 'Venereal Diseases', *Synapse: Journal of the Edinburgh Medical School*, 21, no. 3 (1972), 34.

13

Conclusion:
VD in the Age of AIDS

Sexually Transmitted Diseases in Scotland 1980–95

Incidence and Epidemiology
The pattern of Sexually Transmitted Diseases [STDs] in Scotland has changed dramatically since 1980 *(see Figures 13.1–13.3).*[1] A rise in total cases of 26 per cent between 1980 and 1985 was followed by a sharp fall between 1985 and 1990 of 28 per cent (a 36 per cent fall in male cases and 16 per cent fall in female cases), widely attributed to the fear of HIV and AIDS, the impact of health education campaigns, and the adoption, especially within the gay community, of 'safer' sexual practices.[2] Thereafter, the early 1990s witnessed a slight fall in overall numbers, with a continuing but slower decline in male cases being offset by a rise in female cases of some 8 per cent. As a result, the sex distribution of cases shifted significantly over the whole period, with the share of female cases rising from 36 per cent to 48 per cent. Age-specific data on new STD cases reveal that all age-groups shared in these trends, but that the share of the younger age-groups declined significantly, especially for male cases.[3]

Since 1980, syphilis has remained an uncommon STD in Scotland, accounting for less than 1 per cent of all new cases. The few cases that have been recorded have mainly been latent infections diagnosed on serological testing rather than recently acquired primary or secondary disease. *Treponima pallidum* has remained highly sensitive to penicillin and with the exception of small localized outbreaks, often the result of imported infections, appears to be under control. In the 1970s and 1980s, gay men were the group with highest rates of newly acquired infection, but over the past decade, even this has declined.[4]

The most striking feature of the Scottish STD figures for the period 1980–95 is the dramatic ten-fold fall in the prevalence of gonorrhoea. In 1980, gonorrhoea was diagnosed in 26 per cent of new male cases at treatment clinics and in 27 per cent of female cases. By 1995, these shares had fallen to 3.3 per cent and 1.4 per cent respectively. The initial fall in Scotland occurred mainly in gay men

315

with a lag of several years before heterosexuals perceived HIV as a problem and gonococcal rates among them began to decline sharply. In more recent years, although heterosexual transmission has continued to decrease, infections in gay men have remained steady or even increased slightly, indicating that the impact of the national HIV media campaigns on sexual practices may have been short-lived.

The incidence of non-specific genital infections also declined markedly in Scotland over the period, although part of the fall is accounted for by the separate recording of chlamydial infections after 1990. Other factors are thought to have been 'better patient awareness of STD, altered sexual practices in response to the threat of AIDS, and more efficient contact tracing'.[5] Although its rising incidence in the early 1980s was largely a function of improved diagnostic facilities, chlamydia caused increasing concern given that it was asymptomatic in many women, resulting in 'a pool of infection within the community'. However, the proportion of non-gonococcal urethritis caused by *chlamydia trachomatis* appears to have declined in recent years for reasons which are unclear.

The impressive decline in bacterial STDs in Scotland since 1985,

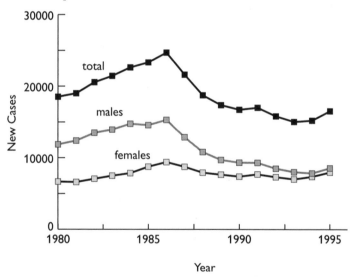

Figure 13.1
New Cases of Sexually Transmitted Diseases
at Scottish Treatment Clinics 1980–95
(*Source: Scottish Health Statistics*)

316

comparable to that associated with the introduction of penicillin, has been in marked contrast to the persistently high prevalence of viral infections such as genital herpes and warts.[6] The total number of reported cases of genital herpes has remained relatively constant but there has been a significant shift towards Type I infections, traditionally associated with oral cold sores, which may reflect more oral sex with its associated lower risk of acquiring HIV infection. Meanwhile, warts have in recent years become by far the commonest 'other STD' seen in genito-urinary medicine. Control is difficult since, as in the case of genital herpes, treatments and prophylactics are often ineffective and the long natural history of the disease means that many individuals remain infectious for a lengthy period.

Resourcing and Status of Venereology

Lack of resources and professional influence continued to plague Scottish venereology in the early 1980s. Despite repeated representations, the

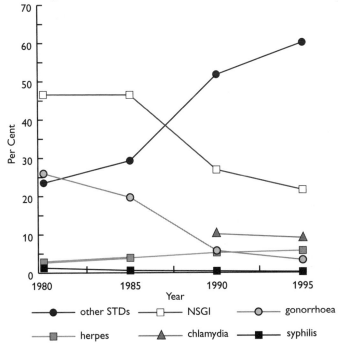

Figure 13.2
New Male Cases of STD at Scottish Clinics 1980–95:
By Disease %
(*Source: Scottish Health Statistics*)

317

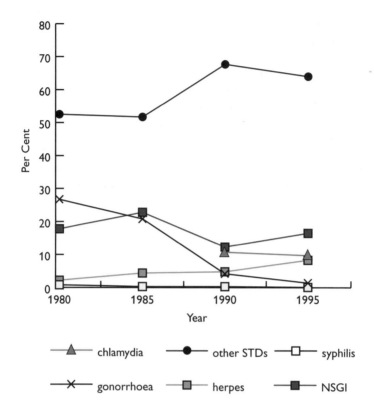

Figure 13.3
New Female Cases of STD at Scottish Clinics 1980–95: By Disease %
(Source: Scottish Health Statistics)

Area Health Boards continued to ignore many of the recommendations of the Gilloran Committee, and continued to appoint non-specialists to vacant posts and to accord the specialty low priority in their financial allocations.[7] In recognition of its widening scope and the change in emphasis away from the old statutory venereal diseases, and with the aim of removing some of the social stigma of attending a clinic, the specialty was renamed genito-urinary medicine (GUM).[8] However, as in England, it continued to be perceived as lacking in medical influence and prestige with poor facilities, a very variable calibre of staff, and training provisions that were marginalized within mainstream hospital teaching.[9]

As elsewhere in the United Kingdom, in Scotland, the onset of AIDS 'brought the area of STDs and genito-urinary medicine in from the cold', making it a 'primary career option' and promoting the role of the specialty in health policy formation.[10] The number of consultants and other clinical specialists in genito-urinary medicine rose by over 25 per cent between 1985 and 1990.[11] However, in many respects, the process was more protracted in Scotland because north of the border, AIDS initially emerged very much as a drug-related issue rather than of sexually transmitted disease. As a result, GUM departments had to compete for resources with infectious disease units and community drug-control programmes.[12]

Health Education

The threat of AIDS also had dramatic effects upon the scope and content of health education relating to STDs. Until the mid-1980s, STDs remained low on the agenda of health education authorities, priority being accorded to issues such as alcoholism, smoking, family planning, and dental health. Reference to STDs was markedly absent from the annual reports of the Scottish Health Education Group [SHEG] and the funding of sex education by the Area Health Boards remained inadequate.[13] Provision of sex education in schools remained 'poor and sporadic', with continuing resistance from many parents, civic leaders, education authorities, and religious institutions.[14] According to SHEG's evidence to the Social Services Committee on AIDS in 1987, there was still 'a widespread belief that there [was] no real infrastructure of health and social education in schools which carrie[d] a sex education programme to which AIDS [could] be added'.[15]

More generally, SHEG's efforts to promote more awareness of contraception among the young foundered on the political sensitivities of the Scottish Home and Health Department [SHHD]. The Scottish Office was reluctant to sanction STD material that might be interpreted as encouraging under-age sexual activity, and that might drag the Department into the highly contentious debate surrounding the provision of contraceptive advice to young girls, demanding that SHEG's approach should place 'more emphasis on abstinence and less on contraception'.[16] In the view of the SHHD, the promotion of contraceptive techniques in posters and telephone advice lines might actively encourage precocious and/or 'promiscuous patterns of sexual activity' and thus increase rather than inhibit the incidence of STDs, along with infertility and cervical cancer. SHHD officials privately bemoaned the fact that SHEG was not more disposed to promote abstinence as 'the ideal method for teenagers' and 'a strong ethical background' as 'the greatest protection of the cervix'.[17]

With the advent of HIV and AIDS, some of these constraints

were lifted. By 1990, SHEG had developed an entirely new range of multi-media materials relating to sexuality and health, in liaison with other statutory and voluntary organizations, including Scottish AIDs Monitor. It also launched a popular magazine, *The Issue*, dealing explicitly with all aspects of sexual relationships and disease, targeted at the 16–24 age-group, and circulated through retail outlets such as Virgin Records and as inserts in teenage magazines.[18] This was supplemented by a wide range of local initiatives involving roadshows, awareness training programmes, cinema commercials and outreach clinics for prostitutes, in which, for the first time, the use of condoms was officially endorsed as central to any prevention strategy for STDs.[19]

Yet, institutional, ideological, and cultural factors still inhibited preventive strategies towards STDs in Scotland. SHEG was marginalized within UK policy-making circles and hence much of the early health education material generated in response to AIDS gave low priority to the role of drug addiction in the cycle of transmission.[20] The area of sex education and sexual health remained politically contentious and a continuing rallying point for the 'moral majority', especially in Scotland.[21] Budgetary constraints and competing demands for time and resources within the educational curriculum perpetuated weaknesses in school provision for STD education, and evidence suggested that public understanding of diseases such as as genital warts and chlamydia remained poor.[22]

Although there was a partial shift in medical discourse surrounding venereal infection from diseased 'types' to particular sexual behaviours, arguably, medical aetiology and moral accountability remained conflated within the 'life-style'/'risk group' models of STDs advanced by epidemiologists in the late 1980s.[23] Health education material frequently straddled the 'thin definitional line between the epidemiologists' concept of risk and the lay interpretation in terms of blame and moral responsibility',[24] and some of the imagery in official posters continued to exploit traditional fears of the sexually active woman as a hidden reservoir of contamination and disease.[25] Above all, as with earlier VD propaganda campaigns, although AIDS-related health education initiatives raised awareness of STDs, there is little evidence that it effected any substantial and permanent change in patterns of sexual behaviour, especially amongst the heterosexual population. In a recent survey of sexual attitudes in Scotland, some 40 per cent of respondents in the 16–29 age-group 'admitted that they had done nothing to change their sexual lifestyle'.[26]

The Issue of Controls

The interplay and parallels between the medico-moral discourses surrounding VD and HIV and AIDS have perhaps been at their most evident in the continuing debate over the appropriate powers deployed by the State to protect public health against the spread of infection. In the British context, AIDS debate and policy-making has been heavily influenced by issues, rhetoric, and precedent drawn from the social history of VD.[27]

As with VD, moral panic surrounding HIV and AIDS led in the mid-1980s to a call, especially in the tabloid press, for a range of coercive measures including compulsory screening and notification, and the enforced isolation and treatment of infected persons.[28] As with VD, the campaign for AIDS-related public health legislation was informed by a moral epidemiology differentiating 'innocent' and 'guilty' victims and proscribing deviant behaviours perceived as immoral, if not criminal. Moreover, as before, much of the more coercive proposals increasingly focused on women as potential vectors of infection and especially on the role of female prostitutes as a 'bridging group' into the general population.[29] However, unlike earlier campaigns for compulsory controls, there is no evidence that public or professional opinion in Scotland was any more compulsionist than elsewhere in the UK.[30]

In the event, historical precedents relating to the attempted regulation of VD were successfully deployed to defend a voluntarist strategy towards AIDS. As Berridge has argued:

> The historical lesson was clear .... A voluntary and not a punitive approach had worked in the control of sexually transmitted disease. Confidentiality had helped control syphilis and gonorrhoea, not quarantine and stigmatisation. History and its 'lesson', in the UK at least, helped to establish a liberal consensual response to AIDS.[31]

It was an approach vigorously defended by Scottish clinicians and medical officials, before both the Expert Advisory Committee in 1985 and the Social Services Committee on AIDS in 1987. Although they were prepared to employ existing Scottish public health provisions for the compulsory detention of an AIDS patient posing a clear risk to the public health, and to support anonymous screening for epidemiological purposes, they were not in favour of AIDS becoming legally notifiable or its transmission being criminalized, other than in exceptional cases of so-called 'revenge sex'. Many of the arguments that were marshalled strongly echoed those advanced

321

earlier in the century: the danger of medical confidentiality being compromised, the need to protect civil liberties and to minimize stigma and discrimination, the medical and legal difficulties in establishing infectivity and the history of transmission, the absence of convincing evidence from legal controls overseas, and above all, the likelihood that compulsion would deter prospective patients from voluntary testing and treatment procedures. Echoes of former campaigns against regulated prostitution as a solution to the spread of STD also surfaced in the evidence of Scottish medical and police authorities.[32]

Attempts by the 'Moral Right', spearheaded by the Conservative Family Campaign, to introduce measures in the early 1990s for the compulsory screening and isolation of 'high-risk' groups met with a similar response from the Scottish press and medical establishment. An editorial in the *Scotsman* roundly condemned the Campaign's charter of responsibilities for HIV sufferers as 'foolish and wrong':

> It clearly sees the priority as protecting society from those with HIV, when experience points persuasively to the opposite conclusion: the dangers of isolating them. It seeks to exclude sufferers from activities in which there is not the slightest evidence that they risk infecting others. By isolating them on the margins of society, it could only deter individuals from ascertaining or admitting that they are infected, making the disease much harder to understand, contain and treat.[33]

Similarly, while many Scottish STD and public health consultants pressed in the early 1990s for more contact tracing for HIV to 'block the lines of transmission', and the Ministerial Task Force on HIV and AIDS in Scotland encouraged health authorities to undertake tracing with the voluntary consent of infected patients, the consensus view remained that, as formerly with VD, mandatory tracing was inappropriate, given the protracted gestation period of AIDS, its traumatic implications for contacts identified as sero-positive, and its possible deterrent effects.[34] As recently as 1997, renewed calls for the 'knowing' transmission of HIV to be a legal offence were prompted by a successful criminal prosecution by a British citizen in Cyprus,[35] but as with the social history of VD, the social history of AIDS would suggest that, even in a period of perceived epidemic emergency and moral panic, a voluntary, non-punitive response to sexually transmitted diseases is the likely outcome of social politics in Britain at the end of the twentieth century.

Reflections: VD and Scottish Society

The social history of VD in twentieth-century Scotland is as much a story of moral regulation as it is of public health. This study clearly reveals how the medical and legal discourses surrounding VD continued to be shaped by more general community concerns to regulate sexual behaviour and public morality. Moral panic engendered by 'the Hideous Scourge' provided a convenient peg upon which the local State could hang byelaws and procedures constraining patterns of social intercourse. Conversely, the desire of Scottish local authorities to maintain civic order and probity sustained an authoritarian tradition of public health administration in the handling of infectious diseases, including those that were sexually transmissible. In the Scottish cities, public order, public morality and public health remained inextricably linked both administratively and ideologically, and this was duly reflected within the operational philosophy of the VD services and the local health authorities that administered them.

Even in post-war Scotland, with the impact of new chemotherapies, public debate over VD continued to be shaped, and indeed triggered, as much by moral anxieties over the erosion of community and family values, as by the medical dimensions of the problem, and taxonomies of guilt and moral culpability have continued to circumscribe the social response to sexually transmissible diseases. In this context, the lasting role of the Churches in defining the moral climate of Scottish civil society and of local magistrates and church elders in sustaining 'the remarkable influence of puritanical religion' and 'an illiberal presbyterian theocracy' upon Scottish local government has been critical.[36] In addition, it might be argued that the moral surveillance traditionally exercised by the confessional and stool of penitence has in part been perpetuated by the 'disciplinary gaze and praxis of clinical medicine' within the VD/STD clinic.[37]

The relationship between the moral and medical dimensions of VD policy-making in Scotland appears at some variance with that prevailing elsewhere. For example, accounts of public health developments in the USA highlight a polarity between moral and biomedical approaches that was central to the debate over VD controls.[38] In many respects, Davenport-Hines' treatment of 'the dominant and conflicting mentalities' which have fashioned policies towards VD in twentieth-century England, focusing upon the ongoing conflict within the Social Hygiene Movement over prophylaxis, conveys a similar story.[39] In contrast, in Scotland, although the response of public health authorities to VD was often ambivalent, overt conflict between medical and moral viewpoints was strikingly absent. Instead, they were closely intertwined, with moral issues prescribing the boundaries within which debate took place and within which both social and medical strategies were formulated.[40]

This study would suggest that, in Scotland, as in many other countries,[41] this process of moral regulation, in which VD played such a central role, was heavily gendered. While medical arguments might be advanced for viewing women as 'reservoirs' of infection, it was also very much a social construction built upon long-standing cultural beliefs of 'woman as polluter'. Although the social epidemiology of VD shifted from the rhetoric of 'prostitution' to 'promiscuity' and 'high-risk behaviour' and the concept of a few core vectors was succeeded by that of a chain or network of infection, female sexuality and sexual behaviour long remained the focus of public concern over the incidence of VD and STDs and its implications for public health, especially in wartime. The processes by which medical, sociological and legal discourses surrounding VD in Victorian society criminalized and pathologized sexually active single women were clearly operative long after the First World War.

Gender discrimination also clearly characterized the formal and informal controls operating within Scottish social hygiene and public morality policy to regulate the sexual urges of the young. Shifts in the lifestyle of female adolescents, occasioned by changes in the labour market and family life, and by the onset of new forms of leisure and entertainment such as ice-cream parlours, dance-halls, and cinemas, with their appeal to illicit desires, were viewed as central to the spread of infection and the erosion of the sexual control so vital for social stability and racial health. New theories of sexual delinquency merely added a patina of scientific respectability to traditional fears identifying female sexual 'precocity' with pollution, and far into the second half of the twentieth century, medical and police authorities in Scotland continued to operate procedures that identified female juvenile offences with sexually transmitted disease. Within a comparative perspective, such procedures can be seen to be part of an international concern of urban authorities to regulate female adolescent sexuality in the interests of community health and morality.[42]

However, the Scottish experience also suggests that, within the process of medico-moral regulation, there was a class specificity to public order and public health controls and procedures relating to VD that could override or cut across considerations of gender. Thus, as we have seen, Scottish middle-class women's groups were highly instrumental in successive 'purity' campaigns to regulate working-class female behaviour in the interests of social hygiene. More generally, although 'propaganda' and health education materials often portrayed VD/STDs as a peril that affected all classes in society, and films often featured middle-class victims, it was predominantly patterns of working-class sexual behaviour that were enshrined within the social epidemiology that informed public health procedures. The association between deprivation and 'social disease' was perhaps appropriate, but given the continuing ignorance of the social distribution of VD, it was one that drew heavily on class assumptions about sexuality and compliance with treatment. The 'dark figure' of private patients will never be known, but it is clear that it has been the medical and social behaviour of the 'sexual proletariat' attending the clinics that has shaped the ideology of clinicians and administrators.

Yet, it would be wrong to constrict our interpretation of the dynamics of VD policy-making in twentieth-century Scotland within any narrow, deterministic social control theory. As Lucy Bland has observed, the formulation of social hygiene procedures 'clearly demonstrates the absence of a cohesive or unified state strategy', the State's view being 'fragmented in its expression at different levels of the State apparatus' and evolving as part of a symbiotic relationship with a range of pressure groups and ideologies.[43] In particular, the Scottish experience reveals the vital interplay between locally defined community interests and the broader concerns of central government (whether Whitehall or the National Executives of organizations such as the British Medical Association, British Social Hygiene Council, and National Council of Women) in the negotiation of policy options.

To some extent, these tensions reflected the strong tradition of civic authoritarianism in Scotland which was increasingly at odds with an English government intent on marginalizing the State from sexual politics. To some extent, they might also be construed as part of that broader historical process identified by political sociologists by which a quest for national identity has shaped sexual norms and 'respectabilities' in Western European societies.[44] At another level, they can be seen as the outcome of a dialogue between local middle-class political and professional interests and the State, in which the priorities of local and regional medical officials and pressure groups were overriden by the concerns of central government over the constitutional, medico-legal, and psephological implications of coercive health controls.

Mort has aptly remarked that the politics of sex 'point us towards the networks of professionalisms ... within civil society'.[45] As this study reveals, the debate surrounding the quest for social hygiene was primarily a debate conducted within middle-class, professional circles. While health and public order procedures relating to VD were often criticized for discriminating against the lower classes attending public clinics, and while working-class organizations passed sporadic resolutions on the issue, the debate rarely impinged upon working-class politics. For example, it figured only fleetingly in the proceedings of the Scottish Trades Union Congress and in local municipal elections. While at times, especially during the successive campaigns for compulsory notification and treatment, the rhetoric of class might be invoked, the content and outcome of the VD policy-making process was primarily shaped by horizontal contests for power and prestige between competing professional groups in Scottish society. The interplay within and between groups such as public health officials, private practitioners, venereologists, social workers, and civil servants in the local State was crucial, as was the negotiation between *their* imperatives and those of health advisers in regional and central government. This study therefore endorses recent models of social change and government growth advanced by historians of British medicine and society which focus on the rise and interaction of the professions.[46]

At the same time, it would be wrong to view the socio-sexual culture surrounding VD and STDs in twentieth-century Scotland as purely one imposed from above by a set of professional elites. Many labour organizations favoured more stringent measures regulating immorality and the wilful transmission of VD, and Mass Observation revealed significant working-class support for coercive measures in the interests of public health; a pattern of social response to be repeated in subsequent post-war moral panics surrounding STDs. It has also to be remembered that the enduring stigma and mythology surrounding the 'special' clinics and their treatment regimes was as much a function of working-class cultural taboos as of middle-class moralizing and propaganda.

Moreover, in focusing upon the social politics shaping VD provisions and their associated framework of formal and informal moral controls within the local community, there is a real danger of ignoring their arguably limited success in regulating the sexual behaviour of the mass of the population. For the story of VD administration in twentieth-century Scotland is as much a story of sexual 'wilfulness' as it is of control. The level of 'sexual recidivism' and reinfection was a constant lament of interwar venereologists and Medical Officers of Health. Similarly, a casual disregard for the risks of venereal infection by Scottish youth in practising its alleged 'cult of sexual sensuality' was a *leitmotiv* of post-war public health reports. Likewise, in recent years, despite the best efforts of a ministerial task force in Scotland to counter HIV and AIDS by inducing 'necessary behavioural change', evidence would suggest that patterns of sexual behaviour in the early years of the new millennium will remain remarkably resistant to change.

Although arguably the social, medical and cultural implications of HIV and AIDS are of a different order of magnitude, there are notable similarities between the social politics surrounding recent debate over sexually transmitted disease and the issues shaping earlier responses to VD. There is a similar concern in some political and medical circles that public health imperatives of breaking the chain of disease transmission have been unduly constrained by libertarian sentiment. Issues of resourcing, confidentiality and social discrimination have re-emerged along with the recognition that aggressive control strategies may deter patients from seeking treatment. Policy-makers have again had to address the problem of how to focus on high-risk groups without fostering prejudice and stigmatization. The debate has yet to be resolved, but the social history of VD in twentieth-century Scotland would suggest that its outcome will continue to be shaped as much by moral assumptions and social anxieties surrounding sexuality as by the medical dimensions of the issue.

Notes

1 The following analysis is based on *Scottish Health Statistics, 1980–95*; *Scottish Home and Health Department, Health in Scotland, Annual Reports by Chief Medical Officer, 1980–95*; J. D. C. Ross, 'The Changing Pattern of Sexually Transmitted Diseases in Scotland', *Answer* (Scottish Centre for Infection and Environmental Health, August 1995); C. Thompson, 'Genitourinary Medicine in Edinburgh: 1980–87', *Health Bulletin*, Vol. 47, no. 3 (May 1989), 120–32. It should be noted that official returns from treatment clinics almost certainly understate the incidence of STDs. A small but significant proportion of cases are not referred by general practitioners. In addition, these data do not include STDs such as hepatitis, treated at Infectious Diseases Units. For comparable data

Conclusion

for England, see Health Education Authority, *Health Update: Sexual Health* (London: HEA, 1997), 38–42.

2 Ross, *op. cit.* (note 1), 1; Thompson, *op. cit.* (note 1), 130–1.

3 Males under 24 accounted for 47.9% of new male cases at treatment clinics in 1980 as compared with 33.4% in 1995 (*Scottish Health Statistics*).

4 See, Ross, *op. cit.* (note 1), 2.

5 Thompson, *op. cit.* (note 1), 131.

6 However, the provision of Hepatitis B vaccine by STD clinics for 'high-risk' groups from the mid-1980s did lead to a dramatic reduction in its incidence among homosexuals (consultant venereologist Interview, July 1997; Medical Society for the Study of Venereal Diseases Scottish Branch [MSSVDSB], Minutes, 9 May 1987).

7 MSSVDSB, Minutes, 17 May and 17 Oct. 1980; 15 May and 2 Oct. 1981; 8 May 1982; 28 May and 8 Oct. 1983; 7 April 1984.

8 M. W. Adler, 'The Development of the Venereal Disease Services', in S. Farrow (ed.), *The Public Health Challenge* (London: Hutchinson, 1987), 109.

9 V. Berridge, *AIDS in the UK: The Making of Policy 1981–94* (Oxford: Oxford University Press, 1996), 25–6; V. Berridge and P. Strong, 'AIDS in the UK: Contemporary History and the Study of Policy', *Twentieth Century British History*, 2, no. 2 (1991), 156.

10 *Ibid.*, 156; Interview with consultant venereologist, 16 July 1997.

11 See, *Scottish Health Statistics*.

12 Interview with Consultant Venereologist, 16 July 1997; V. Berridge, 'AIDS, Drugs and History: The Scottish Dimension', George Bath Lecture, 7 May 1997, 16.

13 *Annual Reports of Scottish Health Education Group*; MSSVDSB, Minutes, 10 May 1986; NAS, HH 61/1227, Minutes of Community Medicine Specialist Group (Health Education).

14 *Ibid.*, 7 April 1984, 5 Oct. 1985.

15 *House of Commons Social Services Committee, Problems Associated with AIDS, Minutes of Evidence* (London: HMSO, 1987), 174, Memo. from S. Mitchell, Scottish Health Education Group [SHEG].

16 NAS, HH 61/1265, Sex Education and Family Planning 1984–5, Correspondence between Scottish Home and Health Department [SHHD] and SHEG.

17 *Ibid.*, HH 61/1265/76, Minutes of SHEG Family Planning Advisory Group, 22 Jan. 1985.

18 *Annual Reports of Scottish Health Education Board /Health Education Board for Scotland* [HEBS]. However, the traditional 'lavatorial'

328

Conclusion

aspect of VD propaganda was also preserved in the employment of a commercial company, *Convenience Advertising*, to target the toilets of higher educational establishments (*Annual Report of HEBS for 1992–3*, 6).

19 *Report of Ministerial Task Force, HIV and AIDS in Scotland: Prevention the Key* (Edinburgh: Scottish Office, Home and Health Department, 1992), 83–5.

20 *Social Services Committee on AIDS, op. cit.* (note 15), 173–4.

21 Berridge, *op. cit.* (note 9), 200, 258–9, 264–5.

22 Health Education Authority, *Health Update: Sexual Health* (London: 1994), 35–6; *ibid.* (London: 1997), 41; K. Milburn, *Peer Education: Young People and Sexual Health: A Critical Review*, HEBS Working Paper, no. 2 (Edinburgh: 1996), 12.

23 L. Bland and F. Mort, 'Look Out For the "Good Time" Girl: Dangerous Sexualities as a Threat to National Health', in *Formations of Nation and People* (London: Routledge and Kegan Paul, 1984), 147; G. M. Oppenheimer, 'In the Eye of the Storm: The Epidemiological Construction of AIDS', in E. Fee and D. M. Fox (eds), *AIDS: The Burdens of History* (Berkeley: University of California Press, 1988), 267–91.

24 Berridge, *op. cit.* (note 9), 31.

25 See especially, R. McGrath, 'Health, Education and Authority: Difference and Deviance', in V. Harwood, D. Oswell, K. Parkinson and A. Ward, *Pleasure Principles: Politics, Sexuality and Ethics* (London: Laurence and Wishart, 1993), 157–83.

26 *Scotland on Sunday*, 3 March 1996.

27 See, for example, V. Berridge and P. Strong, 'AIDS and the Relevance of History', *Social History of Medicine*, 4 (1991), 130–8; V. Berridge, 'AIDS, Drugs and History', *British Journal of Addiction*, 87 (1992), 364.

28 V. Berridge, 'AIDS, the Media and Health Policy', *Health Education Journal*, 50 (1991), 183.

29 V. Berridge, *op. cit.* (note 9), 97, 213.

30 Interview with consultant venereologist, July 1997.

31 V. Berridge, 'Where there's a Will ...', *Times Higher Educational Supplement*, 3 July 1992.

32 See especially, MSSVDSB Papers, Forth Valley Health Board, 'AIDS: Public Health Legislation', 1 April 1985; *Social Services Committee on AIDS, op. cit.* (note 15), Minutes of Evidence of Dr G. E. Bath, Dr R. Brettle, Dr I. S. Macdonald, and Chief Constable W. G. M. Sutherland, 180, 195–6, 221–2, 230–1.

33 *Scotsman*, 28 Aug. 1991.

34 *Report of Ministerial Task Force on HIV and AIDS, op. cit.* (note 19),
    48–9; *Focal Point,* BBC1, 15 Oct. 1992, 'Killing Without a Trace'.

35 *Scotsman,* 30 July 1997. The issue also arose in 1998 when a Home
    Office consultation document suggested that a review of the 1861
    Offences Against the Person Act might include proposals to penalize
    the intentional transmission of disease (*Guardian,* 9 Feb. 1998).

36 C. G. Brown, *The People in the Pews: Religion and Society in Scotland
    since 1780* (Dundee: Economic and Social History Society of
    Scotland, 1993), 44–5. There are strong parallels here with the
    influence of the churches in the Dutch VD debates. See A. Mooij,
    *Out of Otherness: Character and Narrators in the Dutch Venereal
    Disease Debates 1850–1940* (Amsterdam/Atlanta: Editions Rodopi,
    1998).

37 On these 'confessional' aspects of modern STD procedures, see
    especially, A. Pryce, 'Contamination, Penetration and Resistance:
    Male Clients in the VD Clinic', unpublished paper, British
    Sociological Association Conference, Edinburgh (1998).

38 A. M. Brandt, *No Magic Bullet: A Social History of Venereal Disease in
    the United States since 1880* (Oxford: Oxford University Press, 1985),
    46–7, 50–1, 113, 121; E. Fee, 'Sin Vs Science: Venereal Disease in
    Baltimore in the Twentieth Century', *Journal of the History of
    Medicine and Allied Sciences,* 43 (1988), 141, 161.

39 R. Davenport-Hines, *Sex, Death and Punishment: Attitudes to Sex and
    Sexuality in Britain since the Renaissance* (London: William Collins,
    1990), chs 6–7.

40 In this respect, Scotland more closely parallels the New Zealand
    experience. See, P. J. Fleming, 'Shadow over New Zealand: The
    Response to Venereal Disease in New Zealand 1910–45', Massey
    University, Ph.D. thesis (1989), 213–14.

41 For a fuller discussion of the comparative aspects of VD debate and
    ideology, see R. Davidson, 'Venereal Disease, Public Health and
    Social Control: The Scottish Experience in a Comparative
    Perspective', *Dynamis: Acta Hispanica ad Medicinae Scientarumque
    Historiam Illustrandam,* 17 (1997), 341–68.

42 See, e.g., C. Strange, *Toronto's Girl Problem: The Perils and Pleasures
    of the City: 1880–1930* (Toronto: Toronto University Press, 1995);
    R. M. Alexander, *The 'Girl Problem': Female Sexual Delinquency in
    New York, 1900–30* (Ithaca and London: Cornell University Press,
    1995); Mooij, *op. cit.* (note 36), ch. 3.

43 L. Bland, '"Cleansing the Portals of Life": The Venereal Disease
    Campaign in the early Twentieth Century', in M. Langan and B.
    Schwarz (eds), *Crises in the British State, 1880–1930* (London:

Hutchinson, 1985), 193–4. Foucault is similarly sceptical of the existence of a 'unitary sexual politics' (M. Foucault, *The History of Sexuality, Vol. 1: An Introduction* (London: Penguin, 1990 edition), 122).

44 See especially, G. L. Mosse, *Nationalism and Sexuality: Respectability and Abnormal Sexuality in Modern Europe* (New York: Howard Fertig, 1997 edition), ch. 1.

45 F. Mort, *Dangerous Sexualities: Medico-Moral Politics in England since 1830* (London: Routledge and Kegan Paul, 1987), 203.

46 See, e.g., H. Perkin, *The Rise of Professional Society: England since 1880* (London: Routledge, 1989); F. Honigsbaum, *The Division in British Medicine: A History of the Separation of General Practice from Hospital Care 1911–68* (London: Kogan Page, 1979).

Appendices

Appendix 1
Glasgow VD Treatment Provisions 1918–28

Institution	male i-p	male o-p	female i-p	female o-p	ch
Royal Infirmary	*	*			
Western I.	*	*	*	*	
Victoria I.	*	*	*	*	
Lock Hosp.			*	*	*
Belvidere Hosp. (1926-)	*				
Sick Children's Hosp. (1920-)					*
Eye I.	*	*	*	*	*
Bellahouston Dispensary	*	*	*	*	
Baird Street Clinic (1919-)			*	*	*
Black Street Cl. (1926-)		*			
Broomielaw Cl. (1919-)		*			
Maternity Hosp. (1928-)				*	

i-p = in-patients; o-p= out-patients; ch= children

333

Appendices

Appendix 2
Edinburgh VD Treatment Provisions 1919–28

Institution	male i-p	male o-p	female i-p	female o-p	ch
Royal Infirmary	*	*	*	*	*
R.I.E. Subsidiary Clinic (1923-)			*	*	*
Women's Hospital Bruntsfield			*m		*
Royal Maternity Hospital			*	*	*
Pilton Hospital (1923-)			*		*
Dispensaries:					
Grove Street				*	*
Windsor Street/Torphichen Street				*	*
Seamen's Dispensary Leith (1926-)		*			

m=married women

Appendix 3
Percentage Share of New Cases and Attendances in Edinburgh:
Out-Patients at Selected Dates

Year	RIE	WHB*	RMW	Leith
1920	85 [94]	11 [5]	4 [1]	–
1924	82 [94]	11 [5]	7 [1]	–
1928	66 [82]	14 [7]	14 [2]	6 [8]
1935	n/a	n/a [8]	n/a [3]	n/a [15]

[] attendances
* including subsidiary dispensaries.

Appendix 4
Percentage Share of In-Patients in Edinburgh:
Selected Dates

Year	RIE	WHB	RMH	Pilton
1920	65	20	15	–
1924	44	16	22	18
1928	39	23*	26	12
1935	40	24	22	14**

* including Elsie Inglis Hospital
** municipal hospitals

Sources and Select Bibliography

MANUSCRIPT SOURCES

Central Government Archives:

National Archives of Scotland
HH Series: Papers of:
Local Government Board for Scotland.
Scottish Board of Health.
Department of Health for Scotland.
Scottish Home and Health Department.
Scottish Council for Health Education.
Scottish Health Education Unit.
Scottish Health Education Group.
Private Legislation Procedure: Counsel Files.
Royal Sanitary Association of Scotland.
AD 15: High Court Precognitions.
ED 15: Scottish Education Department.
GD 333: Edinburgh Women Citizens' Association.
GD1/1076: Scottish Council of Women Citizens' Associations.

Public Record Office, Kew
MH Series: Papers of:
Ministry of Health, Public Health Administration and Services.
Ministry of Health, Joint Committees.
Medical Advisory Committee.
CAB 71: War Cabinet Papers: Lord President's Committee.
INF 6: Central Office of Information.
RG 23: Social Survey Reports and Papers.

Local Government Archives:

Dundee City Archives and Record Centre
Dundee Town Clerk, Correspondence and Papers.
Dundee Town Council, Minutes.

Edinburgh City Archives
Minutes and/or Papers of:
Convention of Scottish Royal Burghs.
Edinburgh Magistrates.
Edinburgh Public Health Department.
Edinburgh Town Council.
Lord Provost's Committee.
Public Health Committee.
Special Schemes Sub-Committee.
Town Clerk's Department.
VD Sub-Committee.

Glasgow City Archives
Minutes and/or Papers of:
Corporation of Glasgow.
Glasgow Corporation Provisional Order Proceedings.
Magistrates Committee.
Parliamentary Bills Committee.
Police Department.
Public Health Committee.
Special Committee on Farmed-Out Housing.
Special Sub-Committee on the Treatment of VD.
Sub-Committee on Clinical Services.
Sub-Committee on Infantile Mortality.
Glasgow Lock Hospital, Annual Reports.
Miscellaneous Prints.
Public Health Department Pamphlets and Newscuttings.
Scottish Co-operative Women's Guild, Annual Reports.

Perth and Kinross District Archive
Perth Public Health Department, Correspondence and Papers.
Perth Town Council, Minutes.

Medical Archives:

British Medical Association Archive
Minutes and Papers of:
Committee on the Increase of Venereal Diseases, 1960–62.
Committee on the Notification of VD, 1922–3.
Venereologists Group Committee.

Sources and Select Bibliography

Contemporary Medical Archives Centre
Minutes and/or Papers of:
BMA Venereologists Group.
Medical Women's Federation.
National Council for Combating Venereal Diseases/British Social Hygiene
  Council.
National Society for the Prevention of Venereal Disease.

Greater Glasgow Health Board Archive
Minutes and/or Papers of:
Chief Area Nursing Officer.
Medical Women's Federation: Scottish Western Association.
Scottish Regional Hospital Boards, Chairmen's Meetings.

Lothian Health Services Archives
Minutes, Papers or Annual Reports of:
Bruntsfield Hospital and Elsie Inglis Memorial Maternity Hospital.
Edinburgh Royal Maternity and Simpson Memorial Hospital.
Royal Edinburgh Asylum/Hospital.
Royal Infirmary of Edinburgh, Board of Managers.
Royal Infirmary of Edinburgh, Medical Managers' Committee.
Royal Infirmary of Edinburgh, Venereal Diseases Department.
Scottish Asylums.

Northern Health Services Archives
Minutes, Papers or Annual Reports of:
Aberdeen Burgh Insurance Committee.
Aberdeen General Hospitals Board of Management.
Aberdeen Public Health Committee.
Aberdeen Royal Infirmary, Admin. Misc. Files.
Aberdeen Royal Infirmary, Medical Committee.
Aberdeen Town Council.
Education Authority for County of Aberdeen.
Foresterhill and Associated Hospitals, Board of Management.
Grampian Health Board.
North-Eastern Regional Hospital Board.
Northern Regional Hospital Board.
Scottish Association of Insurance Committees.

Other Medical Archives and Manuscripts
BMA Scottish Office: Scottish Committee Minutes.
Health Education Board for Scotland Library:

339

Circulars, Posters and Annual Reports of Scottish Health Education Unit
and Scottish Health Education Group.
Medical Society for the Study of Venereal Diseases, Scottish Branch,
Minutes and Papers.
Royal College of Physicians of Edinburgh, Council Minutes.
Royal College of Surgeons of Edinburgh, Council Minutes.
Royal College of Physicians and Surgeons of Glasgow, Minutes of Faculty.
Royal Infirmary of Edinburgh, VD Registers.
Papers of Dr R. C. L. Batchelor.
Papers of Dr David Lees.
Papers of Dr Robert Lees.

Other Archives:

Edinburgh Central Library
Edinburgh Magdalene Asylum, Minutes.

Edinburgh University Library, Special Collections
Minutes of Faculty of Medicine, University of Edinburgh.
BBC Newscuttings Collection.

Falkirk District Museums History Research Centre
Falkirk Women Citizens' Association, Minutes.

Fawcett Library
Minutes, Papers and Journals of:
Association for Moral and Social Hygiene.
National Council of Women.
National Union of Societies for Equal Citizenship.
National Vigilance Association.

Fife Council Archives
Fife and Kinross Venereal Diseases Joint Committee, Minutes.

Mass Observation Archive, University of Sussex
File reports and letters of Scottish respondents.

National Film and Television Archive
Shotlists and Viewing Copies of VD Propaganda Films.

National Library of Scotland
British Social Hygiene Council, Pamphlet Collection.

National Vigilance Association for Scotland, Eastern Division, Minutes.
Scottish Trades Union Congress, William Gallacher Memorial Library
STUC General Council Minutes.

University of Reading Library
Nancy Astor Papers.

PRINTED SOURCES

Official Publications:

Bills, Acts, Regulations and Circulars

Public General Acts

2 Edw. 7, ch. 11, Immoral Traffic (Scotland) Act 1902.
1 & 2 Geo. 5, ch. 51, Burgh Police (Scotland) Amendment Act, 1911.
2 & 3 Geo. 5, ch. 20, Criminal Law Amendment Act, 1912.
3 & 4 Geo. 5, ch. 38, Mental Deficiency and Lunacy (Scotland) Act, 1913.
Local Government Board for Scotland, Venereal Diseases: Circulars Issued by
    the Local Government Board for Scotland on 31st October 1916.
    Edinburgh: HMSO, 1916.
7 & 8 Geo. 5, ch. 21, Venereal Disease Act, 1917.
Criminal Law Amendment Bill (Bill 25), 1917.
Defence of the Realm Act, Regulation 40D, 1918.
Scottish Board of Health, Instructions to Patients Suffering from Syphilis.
    Edinburgh: HMSO, 1919.
Scottish Board of Health, Instructions to Patients Suffering from Gonorrhoea.
    Edinburgh: HMSO, 1920.
13 & 14 Geo. 5, ch. 40, Merchant Shipping Acts (Amendment) Act, 1923.
Medical Practitioners' Communications Privilege Bill (Bill 206), 1927.
Edinburgh Corporation (Venereal Diseases) Bill, 1928.
Defence of the Realm Act, Regulation 33B, 1942.
Department of Health for Scotland, Memorandum on Venereal Disease,
    Memorandum 74/1961.
Control of Venereal Diseases Bill, PP 1968–69 (40) I.

Local and Private Acts

1 Edw. 7, ch. clxiii, Glasgow Corporation (Police) Provisional Order Act,
    1901.
6 Edw. 7, ch. clxiii, Edinburgh Corporation Act, 1906.
3 & 4 Geo. 5, ch. lxxiv, Edinburgh Corporation Act, 1913.

4 & 5 Geo. 5, ch. clxxviii, Glasgow Corporation Act, 1914.

Reports and Minutes of Evidence

Annual

Reports of Local Government Board for Scotland.
Reports of Scottish Board of Health.
Reports of Department of Health for Scotland.
Reports of Scottish Home and Health Department: Health Services in Scotland.
Reports of General Board of Commissioners in Lunacy for Scotland.
Reports of General Board of Control for Scotland.
Reports of the Ministry of Health on the State of Public Health.
Reports of the Department of Health and Social Security on the State of Public Health.
Reports of the Scottish Council for Health Education.
Reports of the Scottish Health Education Unit.
Reports of the Scottish Health Education Group.
Reports of the Health Education Board for Scotland.

Occasional

Inter-Departmental Committee on Physical Deterioration, Report and Minutes of Evidence, PP 1904 (Cd. 2175) XXXII; 1904 (Cd. 2210) XXXII.
Royal Commission on the Poor Laws and Relief of Distress, Oral and Written Evidence from Scottish Witnesses, PP 1909 (Cd. 4499) XXXVII; 1910 (Cd. 4978) XLVI.
Report and Minutes of Evidence on the Practice of Medicine and Surgery by Unqualified Persons, PP 1910 (Cd. 5047 and 5422) XLIII.
Local Government Board for Scotland, Report by Thomas F. Dewar on the Incidence of Ophthalmia Neonatorum in Scotland. Edinburgh: HMSO, 1912.
Royal Commission on Divorce and Matrimonial Causes, Report and Minutes of Evidence, PP 1912–13 (Cd. 6478) XVIII; PP 1912–13 (Cd. 6481) XX.
Local Government Board, Report on Venereal Diseases by Dr R. W. Johnstone, PP 1913 (Cd. 7029) XXXII.
Royal Commission on Venereal Diseases, Reports and Minutes of Evidence, PP 1914 (Cd 7475) XLIX; PP 1916 (Cd. 8189) XVI; PP 1916 (Cd. 8190) XVI.
Departmental Committee on Reformatory and Industrial Schools in Scotland, Report and Minutes of Evidence, PP 1914–16 (Cd. 7886) XXXIV.
Departmental Committee on Sickness Benefit Claims under the National

Insurance Act, Reports and Minutes of Evidence, PP 1914–16 (Cd. 7689) XXX; PP 1914–16 (Cd. 7690) XXXI.

Joint Select Committee on the Criminal Law Amendment Bill and Sexual Offences Bill, Minutes of Evidence, PP 1918 (142) III; PP 1920 (222) VI.

Medical Research Committee, Special Report No. 14: The Wassermann Test. London: HMSO, 1918.

Report on the Administration of National Health Insurance in Scotland, PP 1920 (Cmd. 827) XXII.

Scottish Board of Health, Interim Report of Consultative Council on Medical and Allied Services: A Scheme of Medical Service for Scotland, PP 1920 (Cmd. 1039) XVII pt I.

Medical Research Council, Special Report No. 66: Report of Salvarsan Committee. Toxic Effects Following the Employment of Arsenobenzol Treatment. London: HMSO, 1922.

Medical Research Council, Special Report No. 78: The Serum Diagnosis of Syphilis: The Wassermann and Sigma Reactions Compared. London: HMSO, 1923.

Ministry of Health, Report of the Committee of Inquiry on Venereal Disease. London: HMSO, 1923.

Medical Research Council, Special Report No. 82: Cruikshank, J. N., Maternal Syphilis as a Cause of Death of the Foetus and of the New-Born Child. London: HMSO, 1924.

Departmental Committee on Sexual Offences against Children and Young Persons in Scotland, Report, PP 1926 (Cmd. 2592) XV.

Scottish Board of Health, Hospital Services (Scotland) Committee. Report on the Hospital Services of Scotland. Edinburgh: HMSO, 1926.

Royal Commission on National Health Insurance, Minutes of Evidence. London: HMSO, 1926.

Report of the Committee on Scottish Health Services, PP 1935–6 (Cmd. 5204) XI.

Ministry of Health, Report on Anti-Venereal Measures in Certain Scandinavian Countries and Holland. London: HMSO, 1938.

Report of Scottish Medical Advisory Committee on Venereal Diseases, PP 1943–4 (Cmd. 6518) IV.

History of the Second World War: United Kingdom Medical Series: Medicine and Pathology. Edited Cope, Z. London: HMSO, 1952.

History of the Second World War: United Kingdom Medical Series: The Civilian Health and Medical Services: Vol. 1: The Ministry of Health Medical Services. Edited Macnalty, A. S. London: HMSO, 1953.

History of the Second World War: United Kingdom Medical Series: The Civilian Health and Medical Services: Vol. 2: The Colonies, The Medical Services of the Ministry of Pensions, Public Health in Scotland, Public

Health in Northern Ireland. London: HMSO, 1956.
Report of Committee on Homosexual Offences and Prostitution, PP 1956–7 (Cmnd. 247) XIV.
Report on Medical Staffing Structure in Scottish Hospitals. Edinburgh: HMSO, 1964.
Health Education: Report of a Joint Committee. London: HMSO, 1964.
Report of the Committee on the Age of Majority, PP 1966–67 (Cmnd. 3342), 62.
Report of Joint Sub-Committee on Sexually Transmitted Diseases. Edinburgh: HMSO, 1973.
Scottish Education Department, Health Education in Schools, Curriculum Paper 14. Edinburgh: HMSO, 1974.
House of Commons Social Services Committee, Problems Associated with AIDS, Minutes of Evidence. London: HMSO, 1987.
Report of Ministerial Task Force, HIV and AIDS in Scotland: Prevention the Key. Edinburgh: Scottish Office, Home and Health Department, 1992.
Health Education Authority, Health Update: Sexual Health. London: HEA, 1994 &1997.

Other Government Publications:

Hansard.

Local Government Reports:

Medical Officer of Health for Aberdeen, Annual Reports.
Medical Officer of Health for Dundee, Annual Reports.
Edinburgh Public Health Department, Annual Reports.
Edinburgh Health and Social Services Department, Annual Reports.
City of Edinburgh Health Department, Annual Reports.
Medical Officer of Health for Glasgow, Annual Reports.

Medical Journals*:

British Journal of Venereal Diseases.
British Medical Journal.
Edinburgh Medical Journal.
Genitourinary Medicine.
Glasgow Medical Journal.
Health Bulletin.
Health Education Journal.
Journal of State Medicine.
Journal of the Royal Institute of Public Health and Hygiene.

Journal of the Royal Sanitary Institute.
Lancet.
Medical Officer.
Medico-Legal and Criminological Review.
Practitioner.
Public Health.
Scottish Health Statistics.
Transactions of the Incorporated Sanitary Association of Scotland.

Purity and Social Hygiene Journals*, Proceedings and Enquiries:

Reports and Evidence of National Birth-Rate Commission. London: National
    Council of Public Morals, Chapman and Hall, 1916; 1920.
Birth-Rate Commission, Prevention of Venereal Disease. London: Williams
    and Norgate, 1921.
Proceedings of the Imperial Social Hygiene Congress. London: NCCVD,
    1924; BSHC, 1927.
Association for Moral and Social Hygiene, *An Inquiry into Ten Towns in
    England and Wales into Subjects Connected with Public Morality.* London:
    AMSH, 1916.
Health and Empire [Journal of the NCCVD/BSHC].
The Shield: A Review of Moral and Social Hygiene [Journal of the AMSH].

 * References to articles and reports appearing in these journals are given in
    the notes. With a few exceptions these are not included in the bibliography.

Other Printed Reports and Proceedings:

BMA Report on Venereal Disease and Young People. London: BMA, 1964.
Church of Scotland, Proceedings of General Assembly.
Church of Scotland, Reports of Committee on Church and Nation.
Church of Scotland, Reports of Committee on Temperance and Morals.
*Congregational Union of Scotland, Report of Temperance and Social Questions
    Committee.*
Edinburgh Council of Social Service, Annual Reports.
Edinburgh Magdalene Asylum, Annual Reports.
Edinburgh Rescue Centre, Annual Reports.
Free Church of Scotland, Reports to General Assembly.
Scottish Trades Union Congress, Annual Reports.
United Free Church of Scotland, Proceedings and Debates of General Assembly.
United Free Church of Scotland, Reports of Committee on Social Problems.
*United Free Church of Scotland, Reports of Committee on Temperance and
    Public Morals.*

Sources and Select Bibliography

Newpapers and Periodicals:

Aberdeen Press and Journal.
Edinburgh Evening News.
Edinburgh Review.
Forward.
Glasgow Evening News.
Glasgow Herald.
Scotsman.

BOOKS AND ARTICLES

Adler, M. W., 'The Terrible Peril: A Historical Perspective on the Venereal Diseases', *British Medical Journal*, 19 July 1980, 206–9.

Adler, M. W., 'The Development of the VD Services', in Farrow, S. (ed.), *The Public Health Challenge.* London: Hutchinson, 1987, 101–12.

Alexander, R. M., *The 'Girl Problem': Female Sexual Delinquency in New York, 1900–30.* Ithaca: Cornell University Press, 1995.

Armstrong, D., *Political Anatomy of the Body: Medical Knowledge in Britain in the Twentieth Century.* Cambridge: Cambridge University Press, 1983.

Batchelor, R. C. L. and Murrell, M., *Venereal Diseases Described for Nurses.* Edinburgh: Livingstone, 1951.

Batchelor, R. C. L. and Murrell, M., *A Short Manual of Venereal Diseases and Treponematosis.* Edinburgh: Livingstone, 1961.

Beardley, E. H., 'Allied against Sin: American and British Responses to Venereal Disease in World War I', *Medical History*, 20 (1976), 189–202.

Bernstein, F., 'Envisioning Health in Revolutionary Russia: The Politics of Gender in Sexual-Enlightenment Posters of the 1920s', *Russian Review*, 57 (1998), 191–217.

Berridge, V., *AIDS in the UK: The Making of Policy, 1981–1994.* Oxford: Oxford University Press, 1996.

Berridge, V. and Strong, P., 'AIDS and the Relevance of History', *Social History of Medicine*, 4 (1991), 129–38.

Berridge, V. and Strong, P., 'AIDS in the UK: Contemporary History and the Study of Policy', *Twentieth Century British History*, 2 (1991), 150–74.

Berridge, V. and Strong, P. (eds), *AIDS and Contemporary History.* Cambridge: Cambridge University Press, 1993.

Beveridge, A., 'Madness in Victorian Edinburgh: A Study of the Patients Admitted to the Royal Edinburgh Asylum under Thomas Clouston, 1873–1908', *History of Psychiatry*, VI (1995), 133–56.

Blaikie, A., *Illegitimacy, Sex and Society: Northeast Scotland, 1750–1900.* Oxford: Clarendon Press, 1993.

346

Blaikie, A., "'The Map of Vice in Scotland": Victorian Vocabularies of Causation', in Forrai, J., (ed.), *Civilization, Sexuality and Social Life*. Budapest: Semmel University of Medicine Institute, 1996, 117–32.

Bland, L., "'Guardians of the Race" or "Vampires upon the Nation's Health"?: Female Sexuality and its Regulation in Early Twentieth-Century Britain', in Whitelegg, E. *et al.* (eds), *The Changing Experience of Women*. Oxford: Martin Robertson, 1982, 375–88.

Bland, L., 'In the Name of Protection: The Policing of Women in the First World War', in Brophy, J. and Smart, C. (eds), *Women-In-Law: Explorations in Law, Family and Sexuality*. London: Routledge and Kegan Paul, 1985, 23–49.

Bland, L., "'Cleansing the Portals of Life": The Venereal Disease Campaign in the early Twentieth Century', in Langan, M. and Schwarz, B. (eds), *Crises in the British State, 1880–1930*. London: Hutchinson, 1985, 192–208.

Bland, L., 'Marriage Laid Bare: Middle-Class Women and Marital Sex 1880–1914', in Lewis, J. (ed.), *Labour and Love: Women's Experience of Home and Family 1850–1940*. Oxford: Basil Blackwell, 1986.

Bland, L., *Banishing the Beast: English Feminism and Sexual Morality 1885–1914*. London: Penguin, 1995.

Bland, L. and Mort, F., 'Look Out for the "Good Time" Girl: Dangerous Sexualities as a Threat to National Health', in *Formations of Nation and People*. London: Routledge and Kegan Paul, 1984, 131–51.

Boyd, H. A., *Leith Hospital: 1848–1988*. Edinburgh: Scottish Academic Press, 1990.

Boyd, K. M., *Scottish Church Attitudes to Sex, Marriage and the Family 1850–1914*. Edinburgh: John Donald, 1980.

Brand, J. L., *Doctors and the State: The British Medical Profession and Government Action in Public Health, 1870–1912*. Baltimore: Johns Hopkins, 1965.

Brandt, A. M., *No Magic Bullet: A Social History of Venereal Disease in the United States since 1880*. Oxford: Oxford University Press, 1985.

Brandt, A. M., 'Sexually Transmitted Diseases', in Bynum, W. and Porter, R. (eds), *Companion Encyclopaedia of the History of Medicine, Vol. I*. London/New York: Routledge, 1993, 562–84.

Bristow, E., *Vice and Vigilance: Purity Movements in Britain since 1700*. Dublin: Gill and Macmillan, 1977.

Brown, C. G., *The People in the Pews: Religion and Society in Scotland since 1870*. Dundee: Economic and Social History Society of Scotland, 1993.

Bryder, L., *Below the Magic Mountain: A Social History of Tuberculosis in Twentieth-Century Britain*. Oxford: Oxford University Press, 1988.

Buckley, S., 'The Failure to Resolve the Problem of Venereal Disease among the Troops in Britain during World War I', in Bond, B. and Roy, I. (eds), *War and Society: A Yearbook of Military History*, Volume 2. London: Croom Helm, 1977, 65–85.

Bynum, W. F., 'Treating the Wages of Sin: Venereal Disease and Specialism in Eighteenth-Century Britain', in Bynum, W. F. and Porter, R. (eds), *Medical Fringe and Medical Orthodoxy, 1750–1850*. London: Croom Helm, 1987.

Cage, R. A., 'Sexually Transmitted Diseases and the Economic Historian: Lessons from the Glasgow Experience', *University of Queensland, Department of Economics, Discussion Paper 92* (1992).

Carson, K. and Idzikowska, H., 'The Social Production of Scottish Policing 1795–1900', in Hay, D. and Snyder, F. (eds), *Policing and Prosecution in Britain 1750–1850*. Oxford: Oxford University Press, 1989, 267–97.

Cassel, J., *The Secret Plague: Venereal Disease in Canada, 1838–1939*. Toronto: University of Toronto Press, 1987.

Cathcart, C. W., 'Four and a Half Years' Work in the Lock Wards of the Edinburgh Royal Infirmary', in Gibson, G. A. *et al.* (eds), *Edinburgh Hospital Reports*, Vol. 5. Edinburgh: Y. J. Pentland, 1898.

Chalmers, A. K., *The Health of Glasgow 1818–1925: An Outline*. Glasgow: Glasgow Corporation, 1930.

Chamberlin, J. E. and Gilman, S. L. (eds), *Degeneration: The Dark Side of Progress*. New York: Columbia University Press, 1985.

Checkland, O., *Philanthropy in Victorian Scotland: Social Welfare and the Voluntary Principle*. Edinburgh: John Donald, 1980.

Cookson, R. P., *A Doctor's Life*. Lewes: The Book Guild, 1991.

Corbin, A., *Women for Hire: Prostitution and Sexuality in France after 1850*. London/Cambridge, Mass.: Harvard University Press, 1990.

Costello, J., *Love, Sex and War: Changing Values 1939–45*. London: Collins, 1985.

Cree, V. E., *From Public Street to Private Life: The Changing Task of Social Work*. Aldershot: Avebury, 1995.

Cullen, G. M., 'Concerning Sibbens and the Scottish Yaws', *Caledonian Medical Journal*, 8 (1909–11), 336–57.

Davenport-Hines, R., *Sex, Death and Punishment: Attitudes to Sex and Sexuality in Britain since the Renaissance*. London: William Collins, 1990.

Davidson, R., 'Measuring "The Social Evil": The Incidence of Venereal Disease in Interwar Scotland', *Medical History*, 37 (1993), 167–86.

Davidson, R., '"A Scourge to be Firmly Gripped": The Campaign for VD Controls in Interwar Scotland', *Social History of Medicine*, 6 (1993), 213–35.

Davidson, R., 'Venereal Disease, Sexual Morality and Public Health in

Sources and Select Bibliography

Interwar Scotland', *Journal of the History of Sexuality*, 5 (1994), 267–94.

Davidson, R., '"Searching for Mary, Glasgow": Contact Tracing for Sexually Transmitted Diseases in Twentieth Century Scotland', *Social History of Medicine*, 9 (1996), 195–214.

Davidson, R., 'Venereal Disease, Public Health and Social Control: The Scottish Experience in a Comparative Perspective', *Dynamis: Acta Hispanica ad Medicinae Scientarumque Historiam Illustrandam*, 17 (1997), 341–68.

Davidson, R., 'VD Propaganda, Sexual Hygiene and the State in Interwar Scotland', in Taithe, B. and Thornton, T. (eds), *Propaganda: Political Rhetoric and Identity 1300–2000*. Stroud: Sutton Publishing, 1998, 183–99.

de Moerloose, J. and Rahm, H., 'A Survey of VD Legislation in Europe', *Acta Dermato-Venereologica*, 44 (1964), 146–63.

Dewar, T. F., 'On the Incidence of Venereal Disease in Scotland', *Edinburgh Medical Journal*, XXX (1923), 313–36.

Dittmar, F., 'The Prevalence of Venereal Diseases in Scotland', *Transactions of the Incorporated Sanitary Association of Scotland* (1919), 45–55.

Duncan, A., *Memorials of the Faculty of Physicians and Surgeons of Glasgow*. Glasgow: Maclehose, 1896.

Dyhouse, C., 'Working-Class Mothers and Infant Mortality in England, 1895–1914', *Journal of Social History*, 12 (1978), 248–67.

Eder, F. X., Hall, L. and Hekma, G., *Sexual Cultures in Europe: Themes in Sexuality*. Manchester: Manchester University Press, 1999.

Evans, D., 'Tackling the "Hideous Scourge": The Creation of the Venereal Disease Treatment Centres in Early Twentieth-Century Britain', *Social History of Medicine*, 5 (1992), 413–33.

Eyler, J. M., *Sir Arthur Newsholme and State Medicine: 1885–1935*. Cambridge: Cambridge University Press, 1997.

Fee, E., 'Sin vs. Science: Venereal Disease in Baltimore in the Twentieth Century', *Journal of the History of Medicine and Allied Sciences*, 43 (1988), 141–64.

Fee, E. and Fox, D. M. (eds), *AIDS: The Burdens of History*. Berkeley/London: University of California Press, 1988.

Ferguson, T., *The Dawn of Scottish Social Welfare: A Survey from Medieval Times to 1863*. London: Thomas Nelson, 1948.

Findlay, L., *Syphilis in Childhood*. London: Hodder and Stoughton, 1919.

Fleck, L., *Genesis and Development of a Scientific Fact*. Chicago and London: University of Chicago Press, 1979 edition.

Fleming, P. J., 'Fighting the "Red Plague": Observations on the Response to Venereal Disease in New Zealand 1910–45', *New Zealand Journal of History*, 22 (1988), 56–64.

Foucault, M., *The History of Sexuality, Vol. I: An Introduction.* London: Random House, 1979.

Foucault, M., *The Birth of the Clinic: An Archaeology of Medical Perception.* London: Routledge, 1993.

Gaffney, R., 'Poor Law Hospitals 1845–1914', in Checkland, O. and Lamb, M. (eds), *Health Care and Social History: The Glasgow Case.* Aberdeen: Aberdeen University Press, 1982.

Giarchi, C., *Between McAlpine and Polaris.* London: Routledge, 1984.

Gilchrist, E., *An Account of a Very Infectious Distemper Prevailing in Many Places.* Edinburgh: John Balfour, 1770.

Gilman, S. L., *Difference and Pathology: Stereotypes of Sexuality, Race and Madness.* Ithaca/London: Cornell University Press, 1985.

Gilman, S. L., *Health and Illness: Images of Difference.* London: Reaktion Books, 1995.

Grant, M., *Propaganda and the Role of the State in Interwar Britain.* Oxford: Clarendon Press, 1994.

Hall, L. A., '"Somehow Very Distasteful": Doctors, Men and Sexual Problems Between the Wars', *Journal of Contemporary History,* 20 (1985), 553–75.

Hall, L. A., *Hidden Anxieties: Male Sexuality, 1900–1950.* London: Polity Press, 1991.

Hall, L., '"The Cinderella of Medicine": Sexually-Transmitted Diseases in Britain in the Nineteenth and Twentieth Centuries', *Genitourinary Medicine,* 69 (1993), 314–19.

Hall, L. A., '"War always brings it on": War, STDs, the Military, and the Civil Population in Britain 1850–1950', in Cooter, R., Harrison, M., and Sturdy, S. (eds), *Medicine and the Management of Modern Warfare.* Amsterdam/Atlanta: Rodopi Press, 2000.

Harrison, L. W., *Modern Diagnosis and Treatment of Syphilis, Chancroid and Gonorrhoea.* London: Constable, 1924.

Harrison, L. W., 'Those were the days! or Random Notes on then and now in VD', *Bulletin of the Institute of Technicians in Venereology,* I, *c.*1950s. Wellcome Institute Library Reprint Series.

Harrison, M., 'The British Army and the Problem of Venereal Disease in France and Egypt during the First World War', *Medical History,* 39 (1995), 133–58.

Haste, C., *Rules of Desire: Sex in Britain: World War I to the Present.* London: Chatto and Windus, 1992.

Henriques, F., *Prostitution and Society: A Survey, Vol. 3: Modern Sexuality.* London: MacGibbon and Kee, 1968.

Humphries, S., *A Secret World of Sex: Forbidden Fruit: The British Experience 1900–1950.* London: Sidgwick and Jackson, 1988.

Hunter, J., Bain, S. and Robertson, D. H. H., 'Sexually Transmitted Diseases in Edinburgh: A Changing Pattern 1961–76', *Health Bulletin*, 36, no. 5 (1978), 251–9.

Hunter, J. and Neilson, M., 'Sexually Transmitted Diseases in Edinburgh: Patients under 18 years of age', *Health Bulletin*, 38, no. 1 (1980), 23–8.

Hutchinson, J., *Syphilis*. London: Cassell, 1889.

Jenkins, P., *Intimate Enemies: Moral Panics in Contemporary Great Britain*. New York: Aldine de Gruyler, 1992.

Johnston, T., *Memories*. London: Collins, 1952.

Jones, G., *Social Hygiene in Twentieth Century Britain*. London: Croom Helm, 1986.

King, A., 'Venereology – A Backward Look', *British Journal of Venereal Diseases*, 48 (1972), 412–15.

Kuhn, A., *Cinema, Censorship and Sexuality 1909–25*. London: Routledge, 1988.

Kuhn, A., *The Power of the Image: Essays on Representation and Sexuality*. London: Routledge and Kegan Paul, 1985.

Lees, D., *Practical Methods in the Diagnosis and Treatment of VD*. Edinburgh: Livingstone, 1927.

Lees, R., 'Some Random Reflections of a Venereologist', *British Journal of Venereal Diseases*, 26 (1950), 157–63.

Lees, R., 'The "Lock Wards" of Edinburgh Royal Infirmary', *British Journal of Venereal Diseases*, 37 (1961), 187–9.

Leneman, L., 'Venereal Disease in Eighteenth-Century Scotland: Evidence from the Divorce Courts', *Proceedings of the Royal College of Physicians of Edinburgh*, 27 (1997), 242–5.

Levack, I. and Dudley, H., *Aberdeen Royal Infirmary: The People's Hospital of the North-East*. London: Bailliere Tindall, 1992.

Levine, P., 'Venereal Disease, Prostitution, and the Politics of Empire: The Case of British India', *Journal of the History of Sexuality*, 4 (1994), 579–602.

Levine, P., 'Rereading the 1890s: Venereal Disease as "Constitutional Crisis" in Britain and British India', *Journal of Asian Studies*, 55 (1996), 585–612.

Levitt, I., *Government and Social Conditions in Scotland 1845–1919*. Edinburgh: Scottish History Society, 1988.

Levitt, I., *Poverty and Welfare in Scotland 1890–1948*. Edinburgh: Edinburgh University Press, 1988.

Levitt, I., *The Scottish Office: Depression and Reconstruction 1919–59*. Edinburgh: Scottish History Society, 1992.

Lewis, M., *Thorns on the Rose: The History of Sexually Transmitted Diseases in Australia in International Perspective*. Canberra: AGPS, 1998.

Sources and Select Bibliography

Logan, W., *The Great Social Evil: Its Causes, Extent, Results and Remedies.* London: Hodder and Stoughton, 1871.

Lowndes, F. W., *Lock Hospitals and Lock Wards in General Hospitals.* London: J. and A. Churchill, 1882.

McGrath, R., 'Health, Education and Authority: Difference and Deviance', in Harwood, V., Oswell, D., Parkinson, K., and Ward, A. (eds), *Pleasure Principles: Politics, Sexuality and Ethics.* London: Laurence and Wishart, 1993, 158–83.

McKee, F., 'Ice-Cream and Immorality', in *Proceedings of the Oxford Symposium on Food and Cookery 1991: Public Eating.* London: Prospect Books, 1991.

McKlintock, A., *Imperial Leather: Race, Gender and Sexuality in the Colonial Conquest.* New York: Routledge, 1995.

McLachlan, G., *Improving the Common Weal: Aspects of Scottish Health Services 1900–1984.* Edinburgh: Edinburgh University Press, 1987.

MacLeod, R. M., 'Law, Medicine and Public Opinion: The Resistance to Compulsory Health Legislation, 1870–1907', *Public Law* (1967), 107–28, 185–211.

McMillan, A. and Robertson, D. H. H., 'Sexually-Transmitted Disease in Homosexual Males in Edinburgh', *Health Bulletin,* 35 (1977), 266–71.

McNeil, N. and Schofield, C. B. S., 'Sexually Transmitted Diseases in Scotland, 1968–71', *Health Bulletin,* no. 2 (1973), 61–6.

Mahood, L., 'The Domestication of "Fallen" Women: The Glasgow Magdalene Institution, 1860–1890', in McCrone, D., Kendrick, S., and Straw, P. (eds), *The Making of Scotland: Nation, Culture and Social Change.* Edinburgh: Edinburgh University Press, 1989, 143–60.

Mahood, L., *The Magdalenes: Prostitution in the Nineteenth Century.* London: Routledge, 1990.

Mahood. L., 'The Wages of Sin: Women, Work and Sexuality in the Nineteenth Century', in Gordon, E. and Breitenbach, E. (eds), *The World is Ill Divided: Women's Work in Scotland in the Nineteenth and Early Twentieth Centuries.* Edinburgh: Edinburgh University Press, 1990, 29–48.

Mahood, L., *Policing Gender, Class and Family: Britain 1850–1940.* London: UCL Press, 1995.

Mahood, L., and Littlewood, B., 'The "Vicious Girl" and the "Street-Corner" Boy: Sexuality and the Gendered Delinquent in the Scottish Child-Saving Movement, 1850–1940', *Journal of the History of Sexuality,* 4 (1994), 549–78.

Manderson, L., *Sickness and the State: Health and Illness in Colonial Malaya: 1870–1940.* Cambridge: Cambridge University Press, 1996.

Marwick, J. D., *Records of the Convention of Royal Burghs 1711–38.*

Sources and Select Bibliography

Edinburgh: Scottish Burgh Records Society, 1885.

Merians, L. E. (ed.), *The Secret Malady: Venereal Disease in Eighteenth-Century France and England*. Lexington: University Press of Kentucky, 1996.

Meyer, G. S., 'Criminal Punishment for the Transmission of Sexually Transmitted Diseases: Lessons from Syphilis', *Bulletin of the History of Medicine*, 65 (1991), 549–64.

Milburn, K., *Peer Education: Young People and Sexual Health: A Critical Review*. Edinburgh: HEBS, 1996.

Miller, A. G., 'Four and a Half Years' Experience in the Lock Wards of Edinburgh Royal Infirmary', *Edinburgh Medical Journal*, 28 (1882), 386–403.

Mooij, A., *Out of Otherness: Characters and Narrators in the Dutch Venereal Disease Debates, 1850–1990*. Amsterdam/Atlanta: Rodopi Press, 1998.

Mort, F., 'Purity, Feminism and the State: Sexuality and Moral Politics, 1880–1914', in Langan, M. and Schwarz, B. (eds), *Crises in the British State 1880–1930*. London: Hutchinson, 1985.

Mort, F., *Dangerous Sexualities: Medico-Moral Politics in England since 1830*. London: Routledge and Kegan Paul, 1987.

Morton, R. S., 'Some Aspects of the Early History of Syphilis in Scotland', *British Journal of Venereal Diseases*, 38 (1962), 175–80.

Morton, R. S., *Sexual Freedom and Venereal Disease*. London: Owen, 1971.

Morton, R. S., 'Control of Sexually Transmitted Diseases Today and Tomorrow', *Genitourinary Medicine*, 63 (1987), 202–9.

Mosse, G. L., *Nationalism and Sexuality: Respectability and Abnormal Sexuality in Modern Europe*. New York: Howard Fertig, 1997.

Murnane, M. and Daniels, K., 'Prostitutes as "Purveyors of Disease": Venereal Disease Legislation in Tasmania 1868–1945', *Hecate*, 5 (1979), 5–21.

Newman, D., 'The History and Prevention of Venereal Disease', *Glasgow Medical Journal*, 81 (1914), 88–100, 164–78.

Pierson, R. R., 'The Double Bind of the Double Standard: VD Control and the CWAC in World War II', *Canadian Historical Review*, 62 (1981), 31–58.

Porter, D. and Porter, R., 'The Enforcement of Health: The British Debate', in Fee, E. and Fox, D. M. (eds), *AIDS: The Burdens of History*. Berkeley/London: University of California Press, 1988, 97–115.

Porter, R. and Hall, L., *The Facts of Life: The Creation of Sexual Knowledge in Britain, 1650–1950*. New Haven/London: Yale University Press, 1995.

Quétel, C., *History of Syphilis*. Oxford: Polity Press, 1990.

Risse, G., *Hospital Life in Enlightenment Scotland*. Cambridge: Cambridge University Press, 1986.

Robertson, D. H. H., 'Medical and Legal Problems in the Treatment of Delinquent Girls in Scotland: I. Girls in Custodial Institutions', *British Journal of Venereal Diseases*, 45 (1969), 129–39.

Robertson, D. H. H., 'Venereal Diseases', *Synapse: Journal of the Edinburgh Medical School*, 21, no. 3 (1972), 23–40.

Robertson, D. H. H. and George, G., 'Medical and Legal Problems in the Treatment of Delinquent Girls in Scotland: II. Sexually Transmitted Disease in Girls in Custodial Institutions', *British Journal of Venereal Diseases*, 46 (1970), 46–53.

Rosebury, T., *Microbes and Morals: A Study of Venereal Disease*. London: Paladin, 1975.

Ross, J. D. C., 'The Changing Pattern of Sexually Transmitted Diseases in Scotland', *Answer*. Scottish Centre for Infection and Environmental Health, Aug. 1995, 1–3.

Sangster, J., 'Incarcerating "Bad Girls", The Regulation of Sexuality through the Female Refuges Act in Ontario 1920–45', *Journal of the History of Sexuality*, 7 (1996), 239–75.

Sauerteig, L. D. H., 'Sex, Medicine and Morality During the First World War', in Cooter, R., Harrison, M. and Sturdy, S. (eds), *War, Medicine and Modernity*. Stroud: Sutton Publishing, 1998.

Schofield, C. B. S., *Sexually Transmitted Diseases*. Edinburgh: Churchill Livingstone, second and third editions, 1975 and 1979.

Schofield, C. B. S., 'The Knowledge of Patients about Sexually Transmitted Diseases', in Billington, D. R. and Bell, J. *et al.* (eds), *Research in Health Education*. Edinburgh: SHEU, 1978.

Schofield, C. B. S. and McNeil, N., 'Venereal Disease in Scotland', *Health Bulletin*, 28, no. 4 (1970), 19–25.

Schofield, C. B. S. and McNeil, N., 'Sexually Transmitted Diseases in Scotland 1972–75', *Health Bulletin*, 35, no. 1 (1977), 10–21.

Schofield, M., *The Sexual Behaviour of Young People*. London: Longmans, 1965.

Schofield, M., *Promiscuity*. London: Victor Gollancz, 1976.

Simpson, J. Y., 'Notices of the Appearance of Syphilis in Scotland in the Last Years of the Fifteenth Century', *Edinburgh Medical Journal*, 6 (1861), 683–7.

Simpson, J. Y., *Antiquarian Notices of Syphilis in Scotland in the 15th and 16th Centuries*. Edinburgh: Edmonston and Douglas, 1862.

Soloway, R. A., 'Counting the Degenerates: The Statistics of Race Deterioration in Edwardian England', *Journal of Contemporary History*, 17 (1982), 137–63.

Soloway, R. A., *Birth Control and the Population Question in England 1877–1930*. Chapel Hill: UNC Press, 1982.

Sources and Select Bibliography

Soloway, R. A., *Demography and Degeneration: Eugenics and the Declining Birth-Rate in Twentieth-Century Britain*. Chapel Hill: UNC Press, 1990.

Spongberg, M., *Feminizing Venereal Disease: The Body of the Prostitute in Nineteenth-Century Medical Discourse*. Basingstoke: Macmillan Press, 1997.

Stoler, A. L., 'Making Empire Respectable: The Politics of Race and Sexual Morality in Twentieth-Century Colonial Cultures', *American Ethnologist*, 16 (1989), 634–60.

Strange, C., *Toronto's Girl Problem, The Perils and Pleasures of the City: 1880–1930*. Toronto: University of Toronto Press, 1995.

Sturdy, S. and Cooter, R., 'Science, Scientific Management, and the Transformation of Medicine in Britain c1870–1950', *History of Science*, XXXVI, 421–66.

Sturma, M., 'Public Health and Sexual Morality: Venereal Disease in World War II Australia', *Signs*, XIII (1988), 725–40.

Tait, H. P., *A Doctor and Two Policemen; The History of Edinburgh Health Department 1862–1974*. Edinburgh: Mackenzie and Storrie, 1974.

Tait, W., *Magdalenism: An Enquiry into the Extent, Causes, and Consequences of Prostitution in Edinburgh*. Edinburgh: P. Richard, 1840.

Thompson, C., 'Genitourinary Medicine in Edinburgh: 1980–1987', *Health Bulletin*, 47 (1989), 120–32.

Tomkins, S. M., 'Palmitate or Permanganate: The Venereal Disease Prophylaxis Debate in Britain, 1916–1926', *Medical History*, 37 (1993), 382–98.

Towers, B. A., 'Health Education Policy 1916–26: Venereal Disease and the Prophylaxis Dilemma', *Medical History*, 24 (1980), 70–87.

Towers, B., 'Politics and Policy: Historical Perspectives on Screening', in Berridge, V. and Strong, P. (eds), *AIDS and Contemporary History*. Cambridge: Cambridge University Press, 1993.

Turner, A. L., *Story of a Great Hospital: The Royal Infirmary of Edinburgh*. Edinburgh: Oliver and Boyd, 1937.

Valenstein, E. S., *Great and Desperate Cures: The Rise and Decline of Psychosurgery and Other Radical Treatments for Mental Illness*. New York: Basic Books, 1986.

Vaughan, M., *Curing Their Ills: Colonial Power and African Illness*. London: Polity Press, 1991.

Walkowitz, J., *Prostitution and Victorian Society: Women, Class and State*. Cambridge: Cambridge University Press, 1980.

Watson, D., *Gonorrhoea and its Complications in the Male and Female*. London: Henry Kimpton, 1914.

Weeks, J., *Sex, Politics and Society: The Regulation of Sexuality since 1800*. London/New York: Longman, 1989.

White, B., 'Training Medical Policemen: Forensic Medicine and Public Health in Nineteenth-Century Scotland', in Clark, M. and Crawford, C. (eds), *Legal Medicine in History.* Cambridge: Cambridge University Press, 1994, 145–63.

Wigfield, A. S., 'The Emergence of the Consultant Venereologist', *British Journal of Venereal Diseases,* 48 (1972), 549–52.

Willcox, R. R., 'Fifty Years since the Conception of an Organized Venereal Diseases Service in Great Britain: The Royal Commission of 1916', *British Journal of Venereal Diseases,* 43 (1967), 1–9.

Wilson, S., 'The Incidence of Gonococcal Ophthalmia, Syphilis and Gonorrhoea since the Inception of the Glasgow Schemes of Prevention and Treatment', *Medical Officer,* CXXI, no. 3 (1969), 27–30.

Wilson, T., *Engendering AIDS: Deconstructing Sex, Text and Epidemic.* London: Sage Publications, 1997.

Woodward, J., *To Do the Sick no Harm: A Study of the British Voluntary Hospital System to 1875.* London: Routledge and Kegan Paul, 1974.

Wyke, T. J., 'Hospital Facilities for, and Diagnosis and Treatment of, Venereal Disease in England, 1800–1870', *British Journal of Venereal Diseases,* 49 (1973), 78–85.

Unpublished Theses and Articles:

Austoker, J., 'Biological Education and Social Reform', MA thesis, University of London (1981).

Davis, G. L., 'The Cruel Madness of Love: Syphilis as a Psychiatric Disorder: Glasgow Royal Asylum 1900–30', M.Phil. thesis, University of Glasgow (1997).

Fleming, P. J., 'Shadow over New Zealand: The Response to Venereal Disease in New Zealand 1910–45', Ph.D. thesis, Massey University, (1989).

Innes, S., 'Feminism, Family and Ideas of Equality and Citizenship: Britain 1900–39', Ph.D. thesis, University of Edinburgh (1998).

Kehoe, J. M., 'Medicine, Sexuality and Imperialism: British Medical Discourses Surrounding Venereal Disease in New Zealand and Japan', Ph.D. thesis, Victoria University, New Zealand (1992).

Lees, R., 'The Treatment of General Paralysis of the Insane', M.D. thesis, University of Edinburgh (1938).

Mackenzie, E., 'Chronic Gonorrhoea in Women and its Treatment', M.D. thesis, University of Edinburgh (1927).

Percival, G. H., 'Some Aspects of the Development of Dermatology with Special Reference to the Contribution of the Edinburgh Medical School'. Unpublished manuscript, Edinburgh University Library,

Special Collections (1982).

Smart, C., 'The Historical Struggle Against Child Sexual Abuse', Centre for Research on Family, Kinship and Childhood, University of Leeds, Working Paper No. 4 (1998).

Thomson, E., 'Women in Medicine in Late Nineteenth and Early Twentieth-Century Edinburgh: A Case Study', Ph.D. thesis, University of Edinburgh (1998).

Tibbits, D. R., 'The Medical, Social and Political Response to Venereal Diseases in Victoria 1860–1980', Ph.D. thesis, Monash University (1994).

INDEX

359

Index

Index

children *51, 109*
untreated females *170*
Victoria Infirmary *18, 55, 83, 88*
Western Infirmary *19, 55, 57, 96*
Glasgow Corporation Bill (1914) *30*
Glasgow Corporation (Police) Provision Order Bill (1901) *30*
Glasgow Royal Infirmary *17–18, 34, 93*
accommodation problems *50*
Lectureship in Syphilis *95*
lock wards *18*
medical training *96*
treatment of gonorrhoea *23*
withdrawal from VD scheme *56*
gleet *83*
Glengore Act *7*
gonococcus *6*
vaccine *80*
gonorrhoea *6–7, 10*
abortive treatment *81, 121, 108*
age distribution *87*
and alcohol consumption *246*
asymptomatic *86, 170*
cure *80, 170–71, 188*
defaulter statistics *112*
diagnosis *79, 82, 237, 279*
diathermy *59, 80*
epididymitis *23, 278*
gender distribution *85, 239*
general practitioners *82, 91*
homosexual transmission *251, 315–16*
incidence *36, 119–20, 157, 164, 215, 263, 288–9, 298, 315–16*
interwar trends *157, 162, 170*
intractable ('gleet') *83*
irrigation *see* irrigation

local authority guidelines *36–7*
myths about *170*
ophthalmia neonatorum *see* ophthalmia neonatorum
post-war *238, 288–9, 298*
prevalence *159*
as punishment *18*
racial distribution *241–2*
seamen *see* seamen
sequelae *17*
sterility *7, 17, 150*
surgical treatment *18, 80*
treatment *4, 22–3, 83, 113, 278*
treatment centres *79–81*
and trichomonas infection *280*
trivialized *170*
untreated women *57*
urethritis *6, 23, 84*
women *164, 215*
working-classes *242*
young people *239*
good neighbour courts *221*
Grampian *266, 292*
Greenock *51*
Greenwood, Arthur *194*
Guy, John *107*
gynaecology departments *109*

H

Haddow, T.D. *297*
Harrison, L.W. *54, 62, 186, 193, 205–6, 210, 216, 219*
Harrison clinics *55, 56, 63*
health education *119, 185, 190, 205*
campaigns *35*
funding *319, 320*
moral prophylaxis *293–7*
post-war *5, 282–97*
schools *142–4*
sex education *142–3, 289–97*
since *1980 319–22*

367

222
Lothians *52, 62, 302*
Lowe, Peter *9*
LSD *247*
lues venerea *10*
lumbar puncture *54, 77, 113*
lunar caustic *84*
Lysol *84*

M
McDonald, Archbishop *220*
Macdonald, Murdoch *194*
Macgregor, A.S.M. *107, 215*
Macgregor, I.M. *260*
Mackenzie, Leslie *17, 19, 141, 192*
Macnicol, M.H. *116*
Magdalene Asylums *11, 20, 26, 115, 116*
magistracy *11, 24, 323*
    double standards *225*
    Glasgow *28, 30*
    moral reform *26*
Mahood, Linda *11, 20*
malarial therapy *79, 167–8, 277–8, 280*
marriage *246*
Mass Observation *213, 326*
masturbation *121*
Matron's Association *139*
Maude, John *210, 219*
Medical Guild *61*
medical negligence *84*
Medical Officers of Health *35, 81, 157*
    compulsion *206*
    controls *206, 207–8, 214*
    and general practitioners *189–90*
    moral agenda *107–10*
    organization of local schemes *49*
    policing *11*

powers *177–81, 185–6*
propaganda *135, 136, 139–42*
running clinics *94*
medical practitioners *see* general practitioners
medical societies *4*
Medical Society for the Study of Venereal Diseases *92, 93–4, 211, 227, 250, 265, 267, 275*
Medical Women's Federation (MWF) *190–91, 206*
men
    married *110*
    promiscuity *111–12*
    as recipients of disease *148–9, 225*
    sexuality *248*
mental deficiency *113, 275*
Mental Deficiency and Lunacy (Scotland) Act (1913) *27*
merchant seamen *see* seamen
mercury *8–9, 10, 19, 22, 23, 77, 79, 83, 122*
metronidazole *279*
microscopy *82*
midwives *96*
Midwives Act (1902) *24*
militarization of VD *7, 117, 207–14*
military camps
    contamination of forces *33, 205–14*
    prostitutes *32–3*
    women patrols *33*
military efficiency *32, 178, 207–14, 211, 225*
military health *3, 26, 31–3*
Milton *84*
Ministerial Task Force on HIV and AIDS *322*
Ministry of Health *195, 218, 221*
    compulsory treatment *210, 219*

Index

Index

post-war *282–97*
Public Health Committees *170*
risk to public morality *141–2*
seamen *66, 138, 295*
social hygiene agencies *5, 135,
136, 144–8*
social purity groups *136,
138–9, 141–3, 148*
prophylactic packets *37, 108, 111,
121, 183*
prophylaxis *295–6*
ante-natal *78*
medical *3, 81*
moral *293–7*
prostitutes *26–9*
16ᵗʰ century penalties *8*
accommodation for infected
191
amateur *27, 31–3, 114–18,
148, 207, 210, 248–9*
child prostitutes *29*
compulsory examination *26–7,
275*
compulsory treatment *26–7,
218, 274–5*
controls *184, 274*
dangerous sexuality *20*
detention *26–7, 275*
and epidemiology *245*
farmed-out houses *29–30*
military camps *32–3*
moral dangers *2*
moral rehabilitation *26–7*
problem girls *114*
as reservoir of infection *149,
208, 274–6*
scapegoating *190*
social politics *1, 11–12*
VD registers *243–5*
wartime *208–10*
Provisional Order Bill (1927) *191*
pubic lice *239*

Public Assistance Departments *118*
public health *23–4*
authorities *2, 324*
debate *2, 7*
measures *166–72*
and morality *4, 17–37*
policy, development *3*
Public Health Acts *36, 180*
Public Health Amendment Bills
(1907–9) *30*
Public Health Committees *32, 49,
215, 224*
Edinburgh *64, 116, 179, 250,
289*
ignorance of incidence of VD *50*
propaganda *170*
socio-sexual engineering *5*
Public Health Departments *107–8,
183*
Public Health Institute *120*
Public Health (Scotland) Act
(1897) *178, 184*
Public Health (Venereal Diseases)
Regulations (Scotland) (1916)
36–7, 52
public morality *see* morality
public opinion
controls *195, 219, 221, 222,
226*
DORA 33B *213*
free treatment *49*
policy *205, 211*
view of infected patients *171*
public order measures *5, 11, 23–4*
purging *10*
purity groups *see* social purity
groups
purity legislation, punitive *32*

Q

quack remedies *8–9, 10, 22–3, 34,
147, 171, 186, 189*

374